CHRONIC PAIN

Volume II

Chronic Pain

Volume II

edited by

Thomas W. Miller, Ph.D., A.B.P.P.

INTERNATIONAL UNIVERSITIES PRESS, INC.
Madison **Connecticut**

Library of Congress Cataloging in Publication Data

Chronic pain / edited by Thomas W. Miller.
p. cm.
Includes bibliographical references.
ISBN 0-8236-0850-6 (v. 1) —ISBN 0-8236-0851-4 (v. 2)
1. Intractable pain. I. Miller, Thomas W., 1943–
[DNLM: 1. Chronic Disease. 2. Pain. WL 704 C55691]
RB 127.C4753 1990
616′.0472—dc20
DNLM/DLC
for Library of Congress 90-4262
CIP

Manufactured in the United States of America

Table of Contents for Volume II

IV Perspectives on Chronic Pain

Table of Contents for Volume I

II Diagnostic Issues in Chronic Pain

Contributors

FRANK ANDRASIK, PH.D., Professor, Department of Psychology, University of West Florida, Pensacola, Florida

RICHARD T. BECK, PH.D., Associate Professor, Department of Rehabilitation Counseling, Mankato State University, Mankato, Minnesota

CYNTHIA D. BELAR, PH.D., Chief Psychologist and Clinical Director, Behavioral Medicine, Kaiser-Permanente Medical Program, Los Angeles, California

DANIEL BLAZER, M.D., Professor, Department of Psychiatry, Duke University Medical School, Durham, North Carolina

STEVEN F. BRENA, M.D., Professor and Director, Pain Control and Rehabilitation Institute of Georgia, and Clinical Professor, Rehabilitation Medicine, Emory University, Atlanta, Georgia

DOROTHY BROCKOPP, PH.D., Associate Professor, College of Nursing and Markey Cancer Center, University of Kentucky, Lexington, Kentucky

GENE BROCKOPP, PH.D., Associate Professor, Department of Anesthesiology, College of Medicine, University of Kentucky, Lexington, Kentucky

JOSEPH P. BUSH, PH.D., Professor, Department of Psychology, Virginia Commonwealth University, Richmond, Virginia

ERIC J. CASSEL, M.D., Professor, Department of Public Health, Cornell University Medical College, New York City

ERLING ENG, PH.D., Clinical Professor, Department of Psychiatry, VA and University of Kentucky Medical Centers, Lexington, Kentucky

RANDAL D. FRANCE, M.D., Psychiatrist, Private Practice, Salt Lake City, Utah

EDITH W. M. HERMAN, PH.D., Assistant Professor, Department of Medicine, McMaster University, Hamilton, Ontario, Canada

FRANK W. ISELE, PH.D., Psychologist, Private Practice, Glens Falls, New York

LOUIS L. JAY, R.PH., Consulting Pharmacist and Graduate, University of Buffalo, Buffalo, New York

KAY RANGA RAMA KRISHNAN, M.D., Department of Psychiatry, Duke University Medical School, Durham, North Carolina

WOLFGANG F. KUHN, M.D., Professor, Department of Psychiatry and Behavioral Sciences, University of Louisville, Louisville, Kentucky

ROBERT LAKOFF, M.D., F.R.C.P. (C), Associate Professor of Psychiatry, University of Alberta, Canada

PAUL LUSTIG, PH.D., Clinical Psychologist, Private Practice, Madison, Wisconsin

GUIDO MAGNI, M.D., Visiting Professor, Department of Psychiatry, University of Western Ontario, London, Ontario and Department of Psychiatry, Institute of Clinical Psychiatry, Padua, Italy

ROBERT D. MARCIANI, D.M.D., Professor, Department of Oral and Maxillofacial Surgery, University of Kentucky Medical Center, Lexington, Kentucky

H. MERSKEY, D.M., F.R.C.P., F.R.C. Psych., Professor, Department of Psychiatry, University of Western Ontario and Director of Education and Research, London Psychiatry Hospital, London, Ontario, Canada

THOMAS W. MILLER, PH.D., A.B.P.P., Professor and Chief, Psychology Service, VA and University of Kentucky Medical Centers, Lexington, Kentucky

NANCI I. MOORE, PH.D., Clinical Associate Professor and Chief, Psychology Service, Veterans Administration Medical Center and University of Louisville, Louisville, Kentucky

JAMES C. NORTON, PH.D., A.B.P.P., Associate Professor of Psychiatry and Neurology and Associate Program Administrator, Area Health Education Center Program, University of Kentucky, College of Medicine, Lexington, Kentucky

STEWART PAGE, PH.D., Professor, Department of Psychology, University of Windsor, Windsor, Ontario, Canada

MARGARET A. RANKIN, R.N., D.S.M., M.A., Professor, College of Nursing, University of Iowa, Iowa City, Iowa

VICKIE J. REID, M.A., Department of Psychology, Virginia Commonwealth University, Richmond, Virginia

RANJAN ROY, ADV. DIP. S.W., Professor, School of Social Work, the University of Manitoba, Manitoba, Canada

STEVEN SANDERS, PH.D., Executive Director, Pain Control and Rehabilitation Institute of Georgia and Clinical Associate Professor of Rehabilitation Medicine, Emory University, Atlanta, Georgia

DOUGLAS K. SNYDER, PH.D., Professor of Psychology, Department of Psychology, Texas A & M University, College Station, Texas

CRAIG WAGGONER, PH.D., Clinical Psychologist, Thomas Rehabilitation Hospital, Ashville, North Carolina

MARK B. WEISBERG, PH.D., Metropolitan Clinic, Brooklyn Centre, Minnesota

WILLARD WHITEHEAD, III, M.D., Department of Psychiatry and Behavioral Sciences, University of Louisville, Louisville, Kentucky

JOHN F. WILSON, PH.D., Associate Professor, Department of Behavioral Sciences, University of Kentucky, College of Medicine, Lexington, Kentucky

Preface

In writing this two-volume work, the goal has been to bring together a multidisciplinary perspective and to make available to all professionals in the health care delivery system an overview of theory, diagnostic, and treatment issues and a multiplicity of therapeutic perspectives in addressing the diagnostic entity of chronic pain. It is hoped that this unique contribution will provide both conceptual clarity and scholarly direction. This book presents an area of inquiry which has emerged quite recently and is designed to inform the reader, clinician, and scientist, to stimulate new hypotheses, and to generate innovations in both research and clinical intervention in this growing area of study.

This two-volume compendium of empirically based observations is intended for readers who include students, as well as professionals, interested in understanding and helping a broad spectrum of patients who experience chronic pain. The work has four sections. The first section, The Nature of Pain, deals with the nature of pain from both a medical and psychological perspective. Included in this discourse are issues related to the neurosis of pain, economic, ethical and psychosocial considerations, ethnic factors, and the impact of compensation and litigation.

In Section II, Diagnostic Issues in Chronic Pain, is a conjoint effort from both the medical and psychological communities and provides a broad spectrum of approaches to the assessment and diagnostic considerations in addressing the chronic pain patient.

Section III, The Multiple Strategies in the Treatment of Chronic Pain, includes chapters by some of the most well-respected multidisciplinary leaders from the United States, Canada, and Europe. It attempts to address a wide variety of clinical issues regarding the treatment of pain patients, including patient motivation, treatment compliance, and specialized individual and group techniques that represent a multifaceted approach to the management of chronic pain.

Section IV, Perspectives on Chronic Pain represents a unique effort to bring together multidisciplinary perspectives in understanding the diagnosis, treatment, and impact of chronic pain across the life span.

In an effort to understand the nature and consequences of chronic pain for the individual, the family, and the professional practitioner, it is the intention in both of these volumes to address the following specific objectives:

1. To clearly define and provide a framework for understanding the nature and impact of chronic pain.
2. To explicate the critical concepts and variables associated with understanding chronic pain.
3. To identify the essential areas of research interests that converge on our state-of-the-art understanding of diagnostic and therapeutic issues faced by the chronic pain patient.
4. To elaborate on the most effective strategies for intervention by professionals, recognizing the important contributions from the variety of disciplines that have committed themselves to understanding and effectively treating the chronic pain patient.

I am indeed indebted and grateful to the number of people, agencies, publishers, and scientific societies who have provided their support over the years in compiling the collection of clinical and research expertise contained in these two volumes. While there is considerable enthusiasm for the material herein presented, my most sincere intention is to provide a provocative and hypothesis-generating compendium of expert opinion that allows the reader, the practitioner, and the clinical researcher to entertain new hypotheses, experiment with innovation, and encourage productive exchanges that will benefit all of humankind in our quest to relieve a condition known as chronic pain.

Dedication

This compendium on chronic pain is dedicated to all of humankind who have experienced chronic pain and who have come to know, understand, and adapt to this condition. It is also dedicated to the patients who have been diagnosed and treated through chronic pain programs in the Veterans Administration Health Delivery System, and finally, to my wife Jean, son David, and daughter Jeanine.

Part III

MULTIPLE STRATEGIES IN THE TREATMENT OF CHRONIC PAIN

Editorial Introduction

Psychological techniques in the treatment of chronic pain become the focus of Drs. Merskey and Magni. Both of these physicians are affiliated with the Department of Psychiatry of the University of Western Ontario, London, Ontario, and Dr. Magni is also a clinical professor at the Institute of Clinical Psychiatry, the University of Padua, Padua, Italy. An overview of several psychological approaches to the treatment of chronic pain are explored, including group psychotherapy, cognitive therapy, biofeedback, and muscle relaxation. In addition, specific reference to analytic and psychodynamic treatment, family therapy, milieu therapy, hypnosis, and combined techniques are also explored.

Dr. Frank Isele addresses biofeedback and hypnosis as specific treatment modalities in the management of chronic pain, noting that hypnosis appears most useful in enhancing cognitive restructuring and behavioral modification in pain management. Dr. Isele discusses biofeedback as an adjunct therapy to the treatment of chronic pain. Case presentations which allow the reader a clearer understanding of this strategy help to exemplify the value of both biofeedback and hypnotic suggestion in the management of chronic pain syndrome.

The employment of stress management programs in the treatment of chronic pain patients is presented by Dr. Cynthia Belar of the Department of Psychiatry, Kaiser Permanente Medical Program. Stress management within the realm of chronic pain is viewed as unique to the individual and one which addresses three main areas: an educational component, an intervention component, and a process component that addresses the control of outputs of stress in the chronic pain patient. An overview of the model for conceptualizing stress management in chronic pain is explored, together with appropriate assessment and intervention techniques discussed.

Group therapy in the management of chronic pain is

addressed by Dr. Edith Herman. Explored more specifically is the role of group therapy for pain patients and the nature of chronic pain, as well as the rehabilitation problems that lend themselves well to group therapeutic approaches. Specifically presented for the practitioner are the results of an evaluation of patient benefits derived from the McMaster Pain Program and its impact on the treatment of chronic pain patients.

Dr. Robert Lakoff, associate professor of psychiatry at the University of Alberta, Alberta, Canada, discusses the role and function of psychotherapy in the management of chronic pain. Such psychological characteristics as dependency, passivity, masochism, denial, regression, hostility, guilt, anxiety, and depression are all explored within both the clinical content and case illustration of this chapter. Dr. Lakoff notes that treatment should always be undertaken with the idea that it is a compelling and complex psychological experience which allows for a more clearer understanding of the human condition we have come to know as chronic pain.

The use of both pharmocologic and nonpharmocologic approaches to chronic pain management are discussed by Dr. Thomas W. Miller and Louis L. Jay in the next chapter in this section. Specific emphasis is placed on the broad spectrum of chronic pain related disorders and the multiple approaches to be considered for each category of chronic pain.

Finally, Drs. Gene and Dorothy Brockopp address chronic pain from the perspective of the family in treatment. Utilizing Rolland's model of chronic illness applied to the pain patient, the authors address various phases of the illness within the family life cycle. The family is viewed as the patient and the behaviors of family members are seen as largely directed toward the maintenance of the family structure.

12

Psychological Techniques in the Treatment of Chronic Pain

H. Merskey, D.M., F.R.C.P., F.R.C.P.(C), F.R.C.Psych. and Guido Magni, M.D.

Introduction

Much of the earlier writing on the psychology of pain did not separate acute pain from chronic pain. Many authors defined populations with chronic pain by the duration of the complaint. The differences between acute and chronic pain were particularly emphasized by Sternbach (1968, 1974). Bonica (1953) had earlier recognized that chronic pain was that pain which persisted past the usual time for the particular disorder to heal. Watson (1983) defined chronic pain in this light: ". . . persisting past one month or past the usual time for the particular disorder to heal. It usually lacks evidence of autonomic hyperactivity" (p. 1365). In theory chronic pain could be merely of two or three days duration if it followed from a brief remitting illness. In practice it is usually of more than six months duration, and most studies have taken that as

This chapter is an updated version of an article by H. Merskey, originally published in *The Postgraduate Medical Journal,* December, 1984, 8(4), 38–41, entitled "Psychological Techniques in the Treatment of Chronic Pain."

a point of departure. However, most cases of chronic pain that are established after three months from onset, do not remit wholly within a further three months. The Subcommittee on Taxonomy of the International Association for the Study of Pain (IASP, 1986) has chosen three months as the dividing line for coding acute from chronic conditions.

A number of the psychological observations which apply to acute pain also apply to chronic pain. But not all of them matter as much. For example, anxiety and anticipation often make acute pain worse; this is particularly notable before surgery. However, these are not nearly so prominent in respect to chronic pain. Similarly, a sense of control of the situation often eases acute anxiety or pain. This can be inferred from the animal literature (Mowrer and Viek, 1948) and has sometimes been shown in adults (Bowers, 1968; Thompson, 1981), and in children (McGrath, 1983).

It has been generally considered since the work of Beecher (1955) that a placebo effect can be found in 35 percent of patients with postoperative pain and other acute conditions. It is rarely the experience of anyone treating chronic pain. Acute pain is accompanied by anxiety and signs of sympathetic hyperactivity. These include tachycardia, an increase in blood pressure and in the secretion of catecholamines, and a decrease in salivary secretion. However, patients with chronic pain are more frequently depressed and show symptoms which resemble depression, such as disturbances of sleep and appetite, reduced energy, difficulty in concentration, irritability, and similar mood changes. Many patients with chronic pain who are depressed have learned, or have taught themselves, subjective techniques of pain control. Frequently, these involve distraction or an alternative method of occupation. Sometimes they find a way to occupy themselves with a task in the presence of distracting stimuli which are deliberately provided; usually this is the radio. Morgenstern (1964) demonstrated that a combination of tasks and distracting stimuli, like flashing lights and variable repeated noises, helped to reduce pain. However, if patients do reach the doctor for treatment it can be assumed that even though their efforts in this direction may have had some success, they have not been enough to produce the relief which is needed.

Basic Concepts of Pain

In the evaluation of patients with pain it is important to define basic concepts. Most people interested in the field favor the view that pain has to be regarded as a subjective phenomenon, whatever its cause. The pain from which psychiatric patients suffer is usually not distinguishable subjectively from pain which has other causes, although in a few cases the characteristics of the descriptions of pain, or the associated features, may help to achieve distinctions between pain which is due to psychological factors and pain which is due to lesions. Thus, most psychiatric patients with pain describe their pain in terms similar to the terms of organic disease, but in a few instances discriminating techniques will separate some members of the groups (Leavitt and Garron, 1979).

For some years we have felt it best not to use the description *psychogenic pain.* First, the original notion of a psychogenic symptom of any sort was one in which a physical disorder caused the psychological state (Lewis, 1972). The term has suffered a reversal of usage since it now, sometimes, but not always, means a symptom with psychological causes. Second, if *psychogenic pain* is accepted as an entity this gives credence to the idea that it is not really the same to the patients as true or so-called "genuine" pain—which of course has to be organic (whoever heard doctors, even psychiatrists or psychologists, talk of "genuine" learned behavior?). Accordingly, it seems best not to regard "psychogenic" pain as totally distinct from "organic" pain. This is not to say that we may not recognize some differences. We must recognize patterns in causation whether organic or psychiatric or both. Thus it is advisable to see pain as a fundamentally unitary phenomenon, albeit with various causes.

Those who have a philosophical interest may agree that this amounts to a monistic attitude to the properties of the condition and a dualistic, Descartian attitude to its causes. The approach recommended requires one to talk of pain of psychological origin or pain of organic origin or pain which has both causes. That is a little cumbersome, but it retains the unitary attitude to pain without giving up the clinical need for discrimination.

Psychiatric Considerations

A few cases of acute anxiety or hysteria present with pain. Cardiac neuroses such as effort syndrome, or precordial pain mimicking angina or resembling coronary disease, can be due to sudden stress or emotional conflict. The majority of pain problems in psychiatric practice represent pain of at least several months duration, and this is what will be discussed in this section.

If psychiatric considerations are important in patients with chronic pain, it becomes relevant to know what diagnoses should be considered. Five can be mentioned: First, it is very rare to find pain due to schizophrenia as a consequence of significant delusions or hallucinations. However, a significant minority of schizophrenic patients have headache or other somatic complaints. The somatic complaints often have a minor organic basis (e.g., from trauma). The headache seems to be associated with the illness but has not been well analyzed as to whether it is related to thought processes or muscle tension, or susceptible to any other explanation. In any case, these complaints are not often the source or a focus of major concern to the patient. Second, there is a well-recognized group of patients who are in the minority in all, or almost all, published studies and who have a classical endogenous depression. These cases may have pain on a delusional basis (e.g., jabbing pains from punishment being inflicted on them) or, much more often, because associated anxiety produces muscle tension. The majority of patients with endogenous depression, however, do not have notable pain symptoms. Everyone loves to comment on the few patients with pain and classical endogenous depression, and even more to diagnose them, because they represent one relatively small group where treatment is often very effective and the results are very gratifying.

Third, some have suggested recently, on the basis of clinical anamnestic data, that chronic pain without obvious depression or organic lesions could nevertheless represent two related psychological disorders (Terenius, 1980; Magni, Andreoli, & DeLeo, 1986). Depression usually presents itself with symptoms which reflect different psychological spheres: affective change, cognitive alternations, somatic symptoms, and behavioral manifestations. In some cases one of these aspects may dominate the clinical picture, covering or obscuring the others either wholly or partially. In such a case we could have a spectrum of possible forms or patterns of the illness, and among them those marked most by somatic disturbances would include chronic pain. Such a pattern without much evidence of depression presents diagnostic difficulty and has sometimes been defined as a depressive equivalent or a masked depression. It does not make a lot of sense semantically to call something depression, however, when it has neither the mood which is normally associated with depression nor the usual collection of typical depressive changes such as retardation, impaired concentration, guilt, and so forth. Indeed, until lately, no published evidence seems to have existed for the idea that there was any depressive element in so-called masked depression. However, some evidence is now emerging with regard to the prevalence of depression in chronic pain patients, and particularly in those who do not have overt depression but who might have a positive family history for depression or depressive spectrum disorder (alcoholism and sociopathy) (Magni et al., 1987a). Further, Magni et al. (1987b) have shown that 3H imipramine binding sites are decreased in the platelets of chronic pain patients who are not overtly depressed.

These data seem to give some weight to the idea that chronic pain without obvious organic pathology could be the expression of a disorder which has the same underlying physiology as depressive illness. However, this hypothesis is only applicable to a subgroup of subjects who have chronic pain without organic disease. It is interesting, nevertheless, because this subgroup could constitute a special sample in which to investigate the possible connections between psychological and somatic changes in this disturbance.

Fourth, there is a somewhat larger group of patients who have reactive depressions and in whom pain, especially headache, is a common symptom. These patients, too, respond quite well to the usual treatments for depression. They often show some neurotic mechanisms such as anxiety to which the pain can be attributed. Fifth, there are patients who have essentially neurotic conditions such as anxiety, often with hysterical symptoms or personality abnormalities. These form the bulk of psychiatric patients who are seen in pain clinics or who have chronic pain which is a major problem. There are a number of ways of categorizing them besides the traditional ones which we have used. The term *learned pain* or *operant pain* is one such set of terms which partly overlaps with these notions. The classification system of the American Psychiatric Association in the third *Diagnostic and Statistical Manual* (DSM-III) covers some of these patients with the term *somatization disorder* which is a version of what others have called *Briquet's syndrome* (Guze, 1970) and delineates a number of these patients but not all of them. Conversion disorders and histrionic personality refer to others, but not exclusively to patients with pain. There is also an understandable overlap between endogenous and reactive depressions, and a further overlap between reactive depression and the neurotic disorders.

Insofar as a distinct psychiatric diagnosis can be made, the guidelines for treatment are clear. Schizophrenic patients normally require phenothiazines as well as some quite specific social management and attention to the parts played by their families. Those with endogenous depression respond well to antidepressants and those with reactive depression also gain benefit from medication. In both categories, and especially in those with reactive depression, psychological support or exploratory psychotherapy is useful, and environmental manipulation is often required. Some of the patients with so-called marked depression also respond to the same treatments. Anxiety states respond somewhat to antidepressants and also to both exploratory psychotherapy and behavioral techniques such as relaxation and deconditioning. Benzodiazepines should be avoided since they do not provide satisfactory long-term medication and this population is at obvious risk of drug dependence.

Where the predominant phenomena involve hysterical or related intractable personality syndromes, the prognosis is poor. In cases such as these, management by a multidisciplinary team may be more effective than by a single specialized practitioner. Multiple techniques and mastery of these particular techniques will determine treatment strategies employed in these situations. These patients represent a very specialized psychiatric problem and need not detain us here. Overall, the general methods of psychiatric management of patients who focus on their body are very important in the care of many chronic pain patients. This applies also to patients with cancer pain.

Pain as a Behavior

Some authors have attempted other approaches which emphasize the aspects of behavior and interpersonal relations as being the principal determinants of the course of the disease of chronic pain and the outcome of the treatment. In doing this the most radical approach describes the condition not as "chronic pain" but rather as "chronic pain behavior." The behavioral model of pain derives particularly from the clinical practice and work of Fordyce (1976) who has developed treatment that shows good short-term results even though it raises some problems.

According to Fordyce, the behavior can be generally described as being of two kinds: respondent and operant. Respondent behavior is that which is determined in a subject by a stimulus and is not significantly influenced by learning or by the surrounding environment. In more conventional medical terms we would think of it as pain which is related to lesions. Operant behavior is, instead, directly related to the individual's past learning and is usually strongly influenced by the current environment. For example, if a certain action is followed by pleasurable events it will be reinforced. In the case of chronic pain, operant pain responses are manifested by the expression of pain, some verbal and nonverbal communications, a request for treatment, and so on. These behavioral manifestations can become habits of the patients if they are reinforced with rewards from the environment. The more intense the reward, the greater the probability that the action which is being rewarded will be repeated.

Within this framework, pain has been conceptualized in terms of respondent pain; for example, when it is linked to a noxious external stimulus, or else due to operant or learning mechanisms. Many types of pain, of course, do not fit only one of the two descriptions but instead are a mixture of both, and the behavior associated with the pain is similarly due to a mixture of causes. The attention of the therapist should be based on the ways in which the patient stimulates the interest of the environment (his movements, protective reflexes, requests for help or requests for medication, etc.) and the circumstances that contribute to determine his behavior. This includes the assessment of both the positive direct reinforcers (such as the solicitude of the relatives or the feeling of well-being caused by the analgesic) and not indirect reinforcement (the possibility of avoiding problems or responsibilities because of pain). It also includes the failure to reinforce more adaptive behavior when the environment, for some reason, discourages self-sufficiency and manifestations of independence.

Secondary Emotional Changes

There is evidence (Woodforde and Merskey, 1972; Sternbach, 1974) that patients with significant lesions develop secondary emotional changes. This is hardly surprising. Some of these changes include irritability, frustration, subjective depression, and reduction of sexual interest (Pelz and Merskey, 1982). There is, of course, impairment of sporting and recreational activities as well as work, and a corresponding degree of dissatisfaction in many instances. The depression in about 10 percent of patients in pain clinics may reach the level of significant illness (Pilowsky, Chapman, and Bonica, 1977) but is much more often a pattern of symptoms as just indicated. Many of these secondary changes will respond to treatment of the primary condition or to organic procedures which produce pain relief. The latter include physiotherapy, exercise, transcutaneous electrical nerve stimulation (TENS), minor analgesics, and surgery. Psychotropic medication, especially phenothiazines and amitriptyline, has some organic basis for its effects, even when psychiatric illness is not to be found (Monks and Merskey, 1984).

THE MAIN PROBLEM

The commonest problem in pain clinics, and perhaps in the practice of most doctors, is the patient who has a lesion and also some evidence of emotional disturbance. The emotional disturbance may be independent and make the pain worse, whether the lesion is a major one or a minor one, and it may at times be the main factor in producing the pain. The most common situation in pain clinics is that personality disorders promote the complaint of pain and the emphasis upon it. Difficulties with the family, the possibility of compensation, complications from the use of drugs, and dependence on them all compound these problems. Frequently, there has been excessive somatic treatment and sometimes excessive psychiatric treatment.

In general, the first step is to convince the patient that the doctor truly believes that he has pain. Nothing works better in this context than a comprehensive evaluation of the patient's condition. It is essential for every practitioner who becomes involved with a patient with chronic pain to establish for the patient that he has taken the main complaint seriously. This means reviewing, and if necessary, recording in detail, the features of the pain, the extent to which it disturbs the patient's life, the things that have been done for it, and the measures that might or might not relieve him. If such an approach is adopted it then becomes very acceptable to the patient to have enquiries made into his psychological status, whether the pain has affected him, what emotional conditions may make the pain worse, and so forth. This pragmatic and sympathetic approach frequently enables the patient to express and discharge much feeling about the troubles which his pain has given him. It is essentially supportive but occasionally will serve to explore emotional difficulties.

Once the main lines of this approach have been established the next requirement is to work on any and every measure which is relatively harmless and which may produce some improvement. These measures may be physical but are important psychologically. It is obvious that physical measures of treatment like physiotherapy, exercise, nerve blocks, TENS, medication, all serve to encourage the patient in the belief that he may get better. There can be times when some of them serve in a disadvantageous fashion to help him believe that the responsibility for getting better is not in his hands. But there is no reason in principle why a variety of physical measures should not be employed, and have some placebo benefits, without committing either the patient or the doctor to the view that psychological issues must be neglected. In such a context of care and attention and support it may be more possible to look at different issues in the patient's life which need to be reviewed than in any other context. These issues include the obvious considerations as to whether family relationships are satisfactory, whether the patient has a difficult boss (if he or she is still employed), and whether the patient is engaging in enough activity or other steps to relieve the pain by distraction or concentration or any other psychological process. Against this background of general support and care, arrangements can then be made to review or introduce a number of other more specialized approaches.

More Specialized Methods

Table 12.1 shows a number of the approaches which have been adopted, with some sample references relating to their description or evaluation. Those interested in more detail of particular approaches can refer to the sources cited. Interestingly, there are few extensive discussions of supportive psychotherapy in pain, although it is the form which is perhaps most

TABLE 12.1

SPECIALIZED TECHNIQUES AVAILABLE FOR PSYCHOLOGICAL MANAGEMENT IN CHRONIC PAIN

Analytic Psychotherapy	Pilowsky, 1978
Psychodynamic Treatment	Pilowsky & Bassett, 1982; Bellissimo & Tunks, 1984
Supportive Psychotherapy	Apley & Hale, 1973; Beard et al., 1977
Family Therapy	Roy, 1982; Waring, 1982; Fordyce, 1976
Group Therapy	Pinsky et al., 1979; Baptiste & Herman, 1982
Milieu Therapy	Herman & Baptiste, 1981
Cognitive Therapy	Tan, 1982; Turner & Chapman, 1982; Turk et al., 1984
Operant Therapy	Fordyce, 1976; Turner & Chapman, 1982
Hypnosis	Barber & Adrian, 1983
Combined Techniques	Roy & Tunks, 1982

often recommended. Bellissimo and Tunks (1984), however, have provided an explicit statement.

The following represents general comments upon the various approaches. Analytic psychotherapy was originally fostered by authors like Hart (1947) and Engel (1951, 1959). On the whole, its success in the treatment of psychiatric patients with pain has been limited and it is little used in chronic pain patients in pain clinics. It has been reported recently that this kind of treatment could be useful, together with other forms of treatment such as physiotherapy, occupational therapy, behavior modification, when combined in a form of multimodal treatment (Lakoff, 1983). The author correctly points out that in some patients chronic pain can promote the development of capacities to adjust to the symptoms, whilst in other patients it is more likely to provoke an increase in neurotic tendencies with consequent ego distortions and restrictions of personality development and impairment of human relations and behavior. Chronic pain can therefore be considered in the latter case, as a chronic situation in which ego functioning is variously impaired. Psychotherapy can be of some help in these patients, particularly when the neurotic traits are seen to be reinforced or uncovered by the symptoms of chronic pain. The help may be limited but the psychotherapeutic work will consist in building a psychological interpretation of the patient's pain behavior on the basis of the data derived from a deep and extensive knowledge of his or her developmental history.

Modifications of analytic psychotherapy offer some promise for a subgroup. Brief dynamic psychotherapy which is developed from the foregoing is the most attractive form of treatment to be considered. Malan (1976) and his colleagues have shown that brief dynamic therapy (say up to nine sessions) can define particular problems in patients' lives and resolve them with the participation of the patient. There is no reason to think that in some instances pain may not similarly resolve when it represents a major psychological problem in an individual's life. However, these instances will be limited to a small group.

Supportive psychotherapy is advocated strongly by Pilowsky and Bassett (1982) who write "[it] aims to support and strengthen the patient's own coping mechanisms . . . with no attempts . . . to challenge defenses. The therapist is usually more active and positive with maximal reality testing and encouragement . . . in the management of pain patients supportive psychotherapy is often the patient's major therapy" (p. 107). We concur fully with this, although in an unpublished study (Hall, 1980) it was shown that supportive psychotherapy was valuable.

So-called informal psychotherapy is substantially similar to supportive psychotherapy. The former has been shown to be useful in some forms of chronic pain such as chronic pelvic pain and recurrent abdominal pain in children (Apley and Hale, 1973; Beard, Belsey, Liebman, and Wilkinson, 1977; Berger, Honig, and Lukeman, 1977). This last condition is a kind of suffering of the child which is not linked to organic disorders in the great majority of cases. The pain symptomology is frequently so intense that it requires repeated medical attention. The treatment of recurrent abdominal pain (RAP) is not based on pharmacological interventions, which have been demonstrated to be ineffective, but on the use of informal psychotherapy, carried out directly by the pediatrician. The first goal of this treatment, once possible organic causes have been excluded by the necessary clinical and diagnostic processes, is to make the parents aware of the emotional nature of the disturbance whilst having them keep in mind also that the pain is real and not simulated or imagined. The therapist attempts to identify the stressful situations in which the whole family often lives and clarifies the role of these situations in the pathogenesis of the pain. Some interventions may also be made in the attempt to modify these situations. The interview is centered not only on the pain but also on the relationships within the family and the environment. This is only feasible if the doctor has established a good relationship with the child and his whole family through various meetings during which they have the opportunity to express themselves freely. Follow-up studies of RAP clearly indicate that in cases which are not treated, the pain persists for a longer period of time and is more frequently accompanied by symptoms which appear not to have an organic basis or are clearly neurotic. These studies seem to demonstrate the effectiveness of informal psychotherapy.

Group psychotherapy is probably of use in patients who have already entered into programs within specialized clinics. There are few, if any, reports of group psychotherapy for patients who have that modality of treatment alone. The results described by Pinsky, Griffin and Agnew, (1979), Catchlove and Cohen (1982), and Pinsky (1983) show, however, that group approaches based on a dynamic model and combined with other types of treatment can produce excellent results comparable with those from other types of programs.

Cognitive therapy is logical and has been shown by Khatami and Rush (1982) to work for specific individuals in pain at specific points in their care. Its overall value remains subject to assessment. Extensive reviews of this have been provided by Tan (1982) and also by Turner and Chapman (1982). Detailed methods of treatment can be found in the book by Turk, Meichenbaum, and Genest (1984). Miller and Berman (1983) review cognitive therapy in general. Perhaps the essential feature of cognitive therapy is to make systematic what we all think of doing empirically, such as distancing oneself from pain and saying "It isn't really me that is suffering," or favoring distraction techniques which emphasize something different like pleasant experiences (thinking about some nice experience with may help to reduce the impact of current pain) and so forth.

The methods which are classed as cognitive therapy are very varied. Tan (1982) mentions the provisions of preparatory information, prepared childbirth techniques and "coping skills." The latter comprise strategies like imaginative inattention ("think of a pleasant day at the beach"), imaginative transformation of the pain ("those sensations are really contractions, not pain"), imaginative transformation of the context ("that hurts but it's like being the hero in a James Bond film"), diversion of attention (counting ceiling tiles, doing mental arithmetic), and somatization (focusing on the part in pain but analyzing the experience as if for a biology report). Some workers, especially Turk, Meichenbaum, and Genest (1984), have developed "stress, inoculation procedures" in which the individual is exposed to painful or noxious stimuli, usually in the laboratory, as part of a process of becoming accustomed to the painful situation and adapting to it with the various cognitive techniques recommended.

On the whole, it seems that cognitive therapy may have some benefit, but this is still speculative. There is reason to think that it may work best in pain of mild or moderate severity (Melzack, Weisz, and Sprague, 1963). It tends not to prove popular with patients when the pain is severe. It then produces, apparently, only very limited gains. However, since all the gains with cognitive therapy are achieved at the expense of little or no risk to the patient, they deserve always to be considered and sometimes at least to be sought out.

Other self-management techniques which can be used alone or in combination are biofeedback and relaxation. Biofeedback gives the patients some ways to control the abnormal physiological responses which can cause pain or contribute to its persistence, particularly muscle tension of which the patient is unaware. During the learning phase superficial electrodes are applied to the target muscles and visual or acoustic signals give a feedback of the changes of the EMG. This technique is frequently associated with relaxation. Biofeedback may also involve attempted lowering or increases of the temperature of digits but this is mostly used for migraine. The technique of biofeedback is frequently associated with relaxation and can have a direct effect on muscle tension or an indirect effect on anxiety. It can be useful in distracting the attention of the patient from pain in providing him with a sense of control over his body. Unfortunately, biofeedback has for the most part, not been shown to be more successful or effective than simple relaxation procedures Cox, Freundlich, and Meyer, 1975; Haynes, Griffin, and Mooney, 1975; Hutchings and Reinking, 1976). Alone or combined, biofeedback and relaxation have been applied to patients with such different types of chronic pain as headache, backache, myofacial pain, rheumatoid arthritis, phantom limb (Chesney and Shelton, 1976; Sherman, Gall, and Gormly, 1979; Keefe, Black, and Williams, 1981). The results have sometimes been encouraging. However, many investigators have not found a particular benefit for biofeedback compared with relaxation, and its status is thus somewhat unsatisfactory.

A recent review on the relationship between familial problems of chronic pain states that the actual role of family dynamics in causing pain of obscure etiology is problematic. A causal relationship is not easily identifiable (Roy, 1985). Even though various kinds of family therapies have been utilized in the treatment of chronic pain, the data so far available are mainly of an anecdotal type, and methodologically sound studies that test the validity of this therapeutic technique are almost completely lacking. Careful assessment of familial dynamics in chronic pain patients is always helpful, but on the basis of present knowledge, family therapy requires cooperation of all parties concerned.

Hypnosis is sometimes linked with cognitive therapy. In the writers' view, hypnosis is just one form of suggestion and has nothing to commend it over other modes of suggestion and relaxation. The reader who wants a skeptical view of hypnosis can refer to Merskey (1971). A discussion of its place in treatment today by clinicians who use it is available in the volume by Barber and Adrian (1983).

Like hypnosis, behavioral methods are often linked with

cognitive ones in discussion. They have preceded cognitive techniques in development. Their formal development is principally due to Fordyce (Fordyce, Fowler, Lehmann, and DeLateur, 1968; Fordyce, 1976), and since his first description they have become increasingly popular, particularly in North America. As described above, the kernel of this approach is provided by the notion that conditioning will reduce or abolish "pain behavior." In operant conditioning, as distinct from classical conditioning, behavior is increased if it is rewarded ("negative reinforcement") or otherwise discouraged. Chronic pain patients are held to show much pain behavior which distorts their lives and which they may use as a form of interpersonal manipulation. Following from this it is argued that pain is "learned" or "unlearned" and that a successful operant program would enable patients to unlearn the pain which has been manifest in their pain behavior. There are conceptual problems in this viewpoint, and they will be discussed shortly.

It has long been recognized that active rehabilitative measures and concentration upon positive endeavors is beneficial to patients with both psychological and physical disorders. Exercise has also been seen to be valuable—despite initial pain from it—in many musculoskeletal disorders. Travell, Rinzler, and Herman (1942) observed that disuse gave rise to muscle pain. It is therefore appropriate to expect that any approach which includes these features will have advantages for at least some chronic pain patients. The specific operant procedure requires that patients be reinforced positively by the responses of staff if they are active and uncomplaining, and that they receive the reverse treatment if they do little or talk about their pain.

Some good results have undoubtedly followed from operant programs (Greenhoot and Sternbach, 1974; Newman, Seres, and Yospe, 1978; Roberts and Reinhardt, 1980). In a fairly representative report, Cairns, Thomas, Mooney, and Pace (1976) describe the results when behavioral approaches were employed in the second phase of treatment of a severely disabled group of low back pain patients, the first phase covering regional blocks and other somatic techniques. A postal survey of 100 patients, averaging ten months from discharge, elicited replies from ninety, of whom 70 percent were improved and 75 percent were working. Typically, in this report as in others, it is hard to disentangle the pure effects of the operant approach from other things which were going on at the same time. Increased activity and a reduction in medications used for pain, however, are common results of behavioral programs. The latter effect is often obtained by offering the patient a "pain cocktail" through which the medication taken is reduced without the patient being able to see the size of a decrease or when it is made. These particular types of change seem to be reported more often from behaviorally orientated centers.

Fordyce (1982) has no difficulty in making a sound case that the behavior of patients in pain is influenced by environmental factors. Sternbach (1983) has noted, however, that there is no proof that operant programs work any more than other interventions because operant programs have never been studied in an adequate, controlled fashion. Linton (1982) has assessed the situation in the treatment of chronic pain other than headache, not only in regard to studies of operant conditioning but also with respect to relaxation in cognitive and multimodal behavioral approaches. He says: "in general the quality of the studies were poor . . . few data were found which conclusively demonstrate that any of the approaches are effective or they are the treatment of choice" (p. 321). He adds, however, that the data do imply that behavioral approaches may help patients lead more normal and productive lives and agrees that the literature suggests that:

> (1) the operant methods lead to increased activity levels and decreased pain and drug intake; (2) the relaxation approach results in decreased electromyogram levels and some pain reduction; (3) the cognitive techniques are speculative at this time; and (4) the multimodal method regularly produced a variety of improvements but the diversity of the treatments makes general statements about utility impossible [p. 327].

The neglect of the experience of the patient is one aspect of the behavioral approach which remains unacceptable to the present writers. There need be no objection to recognizing that it is unhelpful for patients and their relatives to persist in ruminating about pain and avoiding any constructive activities. But it is also difficult to suppose that when pain is promoted by movement it will be abolished as a result of operant relearning, rather than because, after substantial exercise, the muscular status and respondent input of the individual will be changed. Likewise, even if unwanted behavior is diminished, it seems very unlikely that the experience of pain will go away unless some other change has been effected, either in the individual's physical status or in his thought processes. The patient is likely to comment that he still has his pain but he is not permitted to mention it. Special efforts are needed to get around this particular conflict of attitude between patient and practitioner. In any case, such methods would not resolve the conceptual dilemma. Any approach which insists on speaking only of "pain behaviors" whilst skirting around the nature of the subjective experience is likely to leave a significant group of doctors and patients dissatisfied with its comprehensive quality. The usual response to this is that the patient's descriptions of his experience are part of his behavior and should be taken into consideration by the clinician. Nevertheless, in practice the pure behaviorist approach seems to make a virtue of discounting the subjective experience, and is thus deficient.

One last important problem which deserves brief discussion has to do with the recurrence of pain symptoms in a percentage of patients who have been treated successfully in the past, either with one treatment or with a combination of different treatments. Unfortunately, precise data on this topic are not available and the estimate of how many patients are found in this condition is made particularly difficult by the fact that many patients who develop a recurrence may move to another center or therapist different from the one who provided the previous treatment. In the absence of precise figures it is possible, however, to state that approximately 20 to 30 percent of subjects develop a recurrence after successful treatment. The importance of this problem is obvious, and in future we should pay more attention to it and to know the dimensions of the phenomenon better. We wish to have more information about the characteristics of patients who relapse with particular treatments. Only such improved information will allow us to face the problem adequately.

Conclusions

The theme of this chapter has been to emphasize that there is an important field for psychiatric and psychological contributions in the management of chronic pain. Some of the limitations of these approaches have also been expressed. We believe that the best approach is founded upon a clear concept of pain. We have criticized attempts to discount the subjective experience. At the same time behavioral methods have a role to play in comprehensive management. As is often the case, an eclectic and comprehensive position should appeal to all those who agree that no single current theory is adequate on its own. This can also be expected to be more practical and to offer the best chance of effective treatments.

References

American Psychiatric Association (1980), *Diagnostic and Statistical Manual of Mental Disorders.* Washington, DC. American Psychiatric Press.

Apley, J., & Hale, B. (1973), Children with RAP; How do the grow up? *Brit. Med. J.*, ii:3–6.

Baptiste, D., & Herman, E. (1982), Group therapy: A specific model. In: *Chronic Pain: Psychosocial Factors in Rehabilitation,* eds. R. Roy & E. Tunks. Baltimore/London: Williams & Wilkins, p. 166.

Barber, J., & Adrian, C. (1983), *Psychological Approaches to the Management of Pain.* New York: Brunner/Mazel.

Beard, R.W., Belsey, E.N., Liebman, J.C.M., & Wilkinson, J.C. (1977), Pelvic pain in women. *Amer. J. Obstet. Gyncol.,* 128:566–570.

Beecher, H.K. (1955), The powerful placebo. *J. Amer. Med. Assn.,* 159:1602–1606.

Bellissimo, A., & Tunks, E. (1984), *Chronic Pain. The Psychotherapeutic Spectrum.* New York: Praeger.

Berger, H.G., Honig, P.J., & Liebman, R. (1977), RAP: Gaining control of the symptom. *Amer. J. Dis. Child.,* 131:1340–1344.

Bonica, J.J. (1953), *The Management of Pain.* Philadelphia: Lea & Febiger.

Bowers, K.S. (1968), Pain, anxiety and perceived control. *J. Consult. Clin. Psychol.,* 32:596–599.

Cairns, D., Thomas, L., Mooney, V. & Pace, B. (1976), A comprehensive treatment approach to chronic low back pain. *Pain,* 2:301–308.

Catchlove, R., & Cohen, K. (1982), Effects of a directive return to work approach in the treatment of Workman's Compensation patients with chronic pain. *Pain.* 14:181–186.

Chesney, M.A., & Shelton, J.L. (1976), A comparison of muscle relaxation and electromyogram biofeedback treatments for muscle contraction headache. *Behav. Ther. Exper. Psychiat.,* 7:221–225.

Cox, P.J., Freundlich, A., & Meyer, R.G. (1975), Differential effectiveness of EMG feedback, verbal relaxation instructions and medication placebo with tension headache. *J. Consult. Clin. Psychol.,* 43:892–896.

Engel, G.L. (1951), Primary atypical facial neuralgia: An hysterical conversion symptom. *Psychosom. Med.,* 13:375–379.

———(1959), "Psychogenic" pain and the pain-prone patient. *Amer. J. Med.,* 26:899–910.

Fordyce, W.E. (1976), *Behavioral Methods for Chronic Pain and Illness.* St. Louis: C.V. Mosby.

———(1982), A behavioral perspective on chronic pain. *Brit. J. Clin. Psychol.,* 21:75–87.

———Fowler, R., Lehmann, J., & DeLateur, B. (1968), Some implications of learning in problems of chronic pain. *J. Chron. Dis.,* 21:179–181.

Greenhoot, J.H., & Sternbach, R.A. (1974), Conjoint treatment of chronic pain. In: *Advances in Neurology: Pain,* Vol. 4, ed. J.J. Bonica. New York: Raven Press.

Guze, S.B. (1970), The role of follow-up studies: Their contribution to diagnostic classification as applied to hysteria. *Sems. In Psychiat.,* 2:392–396.

Hall, R.C.W. (unpublished), A comparison of tricyclic antidepressants and analgesics in the management of chronic post-operative surgical pain, 1980.

Hart, H. (1947), Displacement, guilt and pain. *Psychoanal. Rev.,* 34:259–263.

Haynes, S., Griffin, P., & Mooney, V. (1975), EMG biofeedback and relaxation instructions in the treatment of muscle-contraction headache. *Behav. Ther.,* 6:672–677.

Herman, E., & Baptiste, S. (1981), Pain control: Mastery through group experience. *Pain,* 10:79–83.

Hutchings, D., & Reinking, R. (1976), Tension headaches: What form of therapy is more effective? *Biofeedback & Self-Reg.,* 5:275–281.

International Association for the Study of Pain (IASP) (1986), *Classification of Chronic Pain: Description of Chronic Pain Syndrome and Definitions of Pain Terms,* Monograph for the Sub-Committee on Taxonomy, ed. H. Merskey. Pain Supplement 3. Amsterdam: Elsevier Science Publishers.

Keefe, F.J., Block, A.R., Williams, R.B., & Surwit, R.S. (1981), Behavioral treatment of chronic pain: Clinical outcome and individual differences in pain relief. *Pain,* 11:221–231.

Khatami, M., & Rush, A.J. (1982), A one year follow-up of the multimodal treatment for chronic pain. *Pain,* 14:45–49.

Lakoff, R. (1983), Interpretative psychotherapy with chronic pain patients. *Can. J. Psychiat.,* 28:650–653.

Leavitt, F., & Garron, D.C. (1979), The detection of psychological disturbance in patients with low back pain. *J. Psychosom. Res.,* 23:149–156.

Lewis, A. (1972), "Psychogenic": A word and its mutations. *Psycol. Med.,* 2:209–214.

Linton, S.J. (1982), A critical review of behavioural treatments for chronic benign pain other than headache. *Brit. J. Clin. Psychol.,* 21:321–330.

Magni, G., Andreoli, C., & DeLeo, D. (1986), Psychological profile of women with chronic pelvic pain. *Arch. Gynecol.*, 237:165–168.

———Andreoli, F., & Andreoli, C. (1987a), Modifications of [3H] imipramine binding sites in platelets of chronic pain patients treated with mianserin. *Pain*, 30:311–320.

——— ——— ———(1987b), [3H] imipramine binding sites are decreased in platelets of chronic pain patients. *Acta Psychiat. Scand.*, 75:108–110.

———Saleni, A., & DeLeo, D. (1984), Chronic pelvic pain and depression. *Psychopath.*, 17:132–136.

Malan, D. (1976), *The Frontier of Brief Psychotherapy.* New York: Plenum Press.

McGrath, P.A. (1983), Modulation of acute pain and anxiety for paediatric oncology patients. *Amer. Pain Soc. Abstr.*, 106.

Melzack, R., Weisz, A.Z. & Sprague, L.T. (1963), Stratagems for controlling pain: Contributions of auditory stimulation and suggestion. *Exper. Neurol.*, 8:239–243.

Merskey, H. (1971), An appraisal of hypnosis. *Postgrad. Med. J.*, 47:572–577.

Miller, R.C., & Berman, J.S. (1983), The efficacy of cognitive behavior therapies: A quantitative review of the research evidence. *Psychol. Bull.*, 94:39–43.

Monks, R., & Merskey, H. (1984), Treatment with psychotropic drugs. In: *Textbook of Pain*, eds. P.D. Wall & R. Melzack. London: Churchill Livingstone.

Morgenstern, F.S. (1964), The effects of sensory input and concentration on post-amputation phantom limb pain. *J. Neurol., Neurosurg, Psychiat.*, 27:58–61.

Mowrer, O.H., & Viek, P. (1948), An experimental analogue of fear from a sense of helplessness. *J. Abnorm. Soc. Psychol.*, 43:193–197.

Newman, R.I., Seres, J.L., Yospe, L.P. & Garlington, B. (1978), Multi-disciplinary treatment of chronic pain: Long-term follow-up of low back pain patients. *Pain*, 4:283–291.

Pelz, M., & Merskey, H. (1982), A description of the psychological effects of chronic painful lesions. *Pain*, 14:293–297.

Pilowsky, I. (1978), Psychodynamic aspects of the pain experience. In: *The Psychology of Pain*, ed. R.A. Sternbach. New York: Raven Press.

———Bassett, D. (1982), Individual dynamic psychotherapy for chronic pain. In: *Chronic Pain: Psychosocial Factors in Rehabilitation*, eds. R. Roy & E. Tunks. Baltimore/London: Williams & Wilkins.

———Chapman, C.R., & Bonica, J.J. (1977), Pain, depression and illness behavior in a pain clinic population. *Pain*, 4:183–187.

Pinsky, J.J. (1983), Psychodynamic understanding and treatment of the chronic intractable benign pain syndrome: Treatment outcome. *Sem. Neurol.*, 3:346–354.

———Griffin, S.E., & Agnew, D.C. (1979), Aspects of long-term evaluation of pain unit treatment program for patients with chronic intractable benign pain syndrome: Treatment outcome. *Bull. LA Neurol. Soc.*, 44:53–59.

Roberts, A.H., & Reinhardt, L. (1980), The behavioral management of chronic pain: Long-term follow-up with comparison groups. *Pain*, 8:151–157.

Roy, R. (1982), Marital and family issues in patients with chronic pain. A review. *Psychother. & Psychosom.*, 37:1–8.

———(1985), Family treatment for chronic pain: State of the art. *Intemate J. Fam. Ther.*, 7:297–309.

———Tunks, E. (1982), *Chronic Pain: Psychosocial Factors in Rehabilitation.* Baltimore/London: Williams & Wilkins.

Sherman, R.A., Gall, N., & Gormly, J. (1979), Treatment of phantom limb pain with muscular relaxation training. *Pain*, 6:47–56.

Sternbach, R.A. (1968), *Pain: A Psychological Analysis.* New York: Academic Press.

———(1974), *Pain Patients. Traits and Treatment.* New York: Academic Press.

———(1983), Fundamentals of psychological methods in chronic pain. In: *Advances in Pain Research and Therapy,* Vol. 5, eds. J.J. Bonica, U. Lindblom, & A. Iggo. New York: Raven Press.

Tan, S-Y. (1982), Cognitive and cognitive behavioural methods for pain control: A selective review. *Pain,* 12:201–206.

Terenius, L.Y. (1980), Biochemical assessment of chronic pain. In: *Pain and Society,* eds. H.W. Kosterlitz & L.Y. Terenius. Basel: Verlag Chemie, pp. 355–364.

Thompson, S.C. (1981), Will it hurt less if I can control it? A complex answer to a simple question. *Psychol. Bull.,* 90:89–94.

Travell, J., Rinzler, S., & Herman, M. (1942), Pain and disability of the shoulder and arm: Treatment by intramuscular infiltration with procaine hydrochloride. *J. Amer. Med. Assn.,* 120:417–424.

Turk, D.C., Meichenbaum, D., & Genest, M. (1984), *Pain and Behavioral Medicine.* New York: Guilford Press.

Turner, J.A., & Chapman, C.R. (1982), Psychological intervention for chronic pain: A critical review. II. Operant conditioning, hypnosis and cognitive-behavioral therapy. *Pain,* 12:23.

Waring, E.M. (1982), Conjoint marital and family therapy. In: *Chronic Pain: Psychosocial Factors in Rehabilitation,* eds. R. Roy & E. Tunks. Baltimore/London: Williams & Wilkins.

Watson, C.P.N. (1983), Chronic pain. *Mod. Med. Can.,* 38:1365–1369.

Woodforde, J.M., & Merskey, H. (1972), Personality traits of patients with chronic pain. *J. Psychosom. Res.,* 16:167–172.

13

Biofeedback and Hypnosis: Multifaceted Approaches in the Management of Pain

Frank W. Isele, Ph. D.

"I have such bad pain, maybe I'm going to die!" I used to carry that around with me all the time.

—Anonymous pain patient

Although perplexing and troublesome, the successful control and management of chronic pain has been, and continues to be, one of the most interesting aspects of clinical practice. There has been a fair amount of evidence and observation which suggests that pain is not simply a function of physical sensation but that personality factors, level of anxiety, the cognitive view the person has of the situation in which the injury occurred, suggestion, one's expectations, and other psychological variables contribute to the overall experience of pain (Melzack, Weisz, and Sprague, 1963; Volgyesi, 1972, Crasilneck and Hall, 1973; Levit, 1973; Melzack, 1973).

A recent review of research on chronic pain management has suggested a complex, multidimensional view of pain as an experience, as well as having implications for the assessment and treatment of chronic pain. Biofeedback and hypnosis as treatment approaches need to address more than just the symptoms of chronic pain. Trifiletti (1984) reviewed the use of operant, biofeedback, and cognitive–behavioral approaches in dealing with chronic pain. Cognitive–behavioral procedures were particularly consistent with a multidimensional framework and improved studies were suggested, using a wider range of assessment measures, involving cognitive and psychological factors, affective responses, and social, behavioral, and physiological measures.

The interpersonal aspects of pain have been explored in a number of recent studies. Adler, Bongar, and Katz (1982) discussed the importance of family interaction factors involved in stress-induced gastrointestinal symptoms of two preadolescent boys. Baker (1984) presented the case of a male cancer patient with whom hypnosis and behavior modification in the context of a family system proved successful in managing pain. O'Brien and Weisbrot (1983) suggested family psychotherapy as an adjunct to biofeedback or hypnosis, recognizing family conflicts that contributed to the aggravation of a chronic pain syndrome. Smith and Balaban (1983) used a combination of hypnosis, behavior therapy, and psychodynamic psychotherapy in dealing with a forty-one-year-old, single, registered nurse with systemic lupus erythematosus.

Cognitive and behavioral factors in combination with biofeedback and hypnosis have also been studied. A multifaceted approach was used by Schwartz, (1984) in dealing with a fifty-four-year-old woman with chest pain who was a frequent emergency room visitor. Schwartz's approaches consisted of reeducation, stress management training, and biofeedback, and he discussed the importance of psychological, social, and iatrogenic factors in managing this patient's chronic pain. Elkins (1984) needed to address guilt-producing belief systems in combination with hypnosis in managing the pain of a thirty-eight-year-old female with chronic myofibrositis. A thirty-six-year-old woman with multiple chronic pain was treated by LaCroix and Gauthier (1984). They reduced her overuse of medical facilities by means of a program which included relaxation training, EMG biofeedback, cognitive restructuring, contingency management, and social skills training. Finally, an important direction was suggested in the biofeedback treatment of chronic pain patients presented by Cram and Freeman

(1985). They treated ninety-eight Swedish, chronic pain patients and used an electromyograph (EMG) scanning protocol as an outcome measure for EMG biofeedback treatment of chronic pain. They found that EMG-assisted relaxation training protocols conducted in one static posture had limited effectiveness in reducing EMG scan readings for chronic pain patients. They concluded that the marginal effectiveness was due to poor response generalization. Cram and Freeman suggested that more dynamic (active) approaches would be more effective in training EMG-assisted relaxation for managing chronic pain.

Hypnosis seems to be useful in enhancing cognitive restructuring or behavioral modification in pain management. A study by Howard, Reardon, and Tosi (1982) clearly illustrates how hypnosis and hypnotic imagery can enhance the restructuring of negative cognitive, emotional, physiological, and behavioral states. They used the procedure of rational stage directed hypnotherapy to modify not just the subjective perception of pain but associated cognitive, emotional, behavioral, and physiological factors as well. They worked with a thirty-year-old woman with an eighteen-year history of migraine headaches. She was seen approximately one hour per week for a period of 6.5 months. Howard, Reardon, and Tosi conclude that rational stage directed hypnotherapy places great emphasis on the direct restructuring of belief systems and the resultant affective, physiological, and behavioral events. The primary measure of outcome in this study was the client's self-reported frequency of migraine headaches over time. An additional dependent variable included the client's Minnesota Multiphasic Personality Inventory (MMPI) profile. Pre- and posttreatment MMPI profiles showed a reduction of T scores on scales 1, 2, and 3 from mid-80s prior to treatment to mid-60s after treatment, suggesting significant alteration in her cognitive views of, and emotional responses to, illness.

Outcome measures of chronic pain are varied throughout the studies. Most of the studies above have used more than just the patient's subjective report of pain intensity in assessing outcome and effectiveness. In one case, the frequency of use of medical facilities was a measure of effectiveness. In another,

EMG scanning readings, conforming to a scanning protocol were used. Another used pre- and post-MMPI profiles.

One of the more traditional measures of pain has been subjective ratings of discomfort, often obtained by suggesting a rating scale (e.g., one through ten) and asking the subject to place a level of pain or discomfort that is being experienced at a given number (e.g., ten being maximum). However, as approaches to treating pain have become more multifaceted, so have measures of outcome. In a study employing the MMPI, Sweet (1981) presented three case studies and suggested that the MMPI was sensitive to changes in the patient's affect, thinking, and perceptions that resulted from biofeedback and relaxation training sessions and cognitive–behavioral intervention. The MMPI has also been found to be a useful tool in evaluating progress of chronic pain patients in Howard, et al.'s (1982) study. Onorato and Tsushima (1983) examined the relationship between frontalis muscle tension, a set of pain-related behaviors, and the MMPI's ability to predict the outcome of EMG biofeedback training for the reduction of pain. Tension headache and posttraumatic pain subjects succeeded in reducing forehead EMG to significantly low levels. However, no significant relationship between EMG levels and pain behaviors was observed. They hypothesized that personality factors appeared to be significantly related to therapy outcome. Factor analysis of the MMPI scores supported the predictability of the MMPI.

In addition to measuring pain directly, associated states may also be measured. Pitzele (1985) hypothesized a circle of pain. There were three components to the circle, one was pain, the other stress, and the other aggravation of the chronic condition. Pitzele felt that stress led to aggravation of the chronic physical condition which led to an increase in pain. Measures of various stressors impinging on a chronic pain patient then might be useful predictors of pain levels. Keefe, Crisson, and Trainor (1987) presented an observational method for assessing pain, using the concept of pain as a behavior drawn from Fordyce's (1976) work. They categorized pain behaviors into five types: guarding, bracing, rubbing, grimacing, and shying. They then devised an observational format, trained observers, and conducted reliability studies for such a systematic observation procedure. This procedure was presented as useful in primarily inpatient settings and could be done by nurses trained in the observation system. Keefe et al. felt that one of the major advantages of such a system was that it would be reliable as well as simple and objective. They felt that it may be helpful in augmenting or even replacing anecdotal observations of patient's pain behavior. Although developed with chronic low back pain patients, they felt that the observation method could be extended to patients suffering from a variety of other forms of chronic pain.

On an outpatient basis, other less systematic forms of the effectiveness with which pain is managed would include level and type of activity. In particular the resumption of preinjury activities or some approximation thereof may be useful outcome measures. Such changes are reported, albeit anecdotally, in the clinical case studies presented later in this chapter.

The above review suggests that current approaches in managing pain have emphasized multidimensional strategies often used in combination with one another. It is the general theme of this chapter that a multifaceted approach, including a combination of methods utilizing hypnosis, biofeedback, cognitive coping strategies, behavior modification programs, and expectation are perhaps most effective in managing and controlling chronic pain. Again, personality factors, level of anxiety and depression, one's cognitive view of the situation, expectations, as well as the interpretation of events contribute to the overall experience of pain.

Biofeedback

Biofeedback is a training procedure in which physiological learning occurs. With the aid of electronic instrumentation, subjects are made aware of selected physiological events, such as brain-wave activity, surface skin temperature, and muscle tension in the form of EMG values. Physiological responses become associated with thoughts and strategies developed by the subjects. The key features of biofeedback are (1) continuous and accurate monitoring of the chosen physiological response; (2) immediate feedback to the subject of changes in that response; (3) motivation to alter the response (Melzack and Perry, 1976). When the desired response (e.g., alpha wave production, increase in temperature, or reduction of EMG) occurs in the patient, visual and/or auditory feedback occurs which is both reinforcing and informational. Theoretically, such training permits the subject to modify the targeted physiological response significantly. Such an ability seems to provide subjects with a sense of control and effectiveness unavailable with other methods (Melzack and Perry, 1975).

Electroencephalographic (EEG) biofeedback in the form of alpha training has been successful in modifying response to pain (Pelletier and Peper, 1977) and alpha training produced a significant decrease in both sensory and affective dimensions of pain in 58 percent of patients suffering from chronic pain (Melzack and Perry, 1975). Melzack and Perry (1975) concluded, however, that the observed pain relief was not due to EEG alpha per se but to associated experiences, such as distraction, suggestion, relaxation, and a sense of control over pain. Temperature feedback as a method of modifying pain has been largely limited in the literature to migraine headache but does have other applications which will be illustrated in a case discussion later in this chapter.

EMG Biofeedback

The EMG as a form of biofeedback has been the most commonly studied intervention, and is, perhaps, the most widely used, although some of the latest research has begun to focus on multiple modality feedback (Christidis, Ince, Zaretsky, and Pitchfort, 1986).

Electromyographic biofeedback has been used with lower back pain (Grabel, 1973; Kravitz, 1978). However, recent studies of lower back pain (Nigl, 1981; Biedermann and Monga, 1985) have suggested that EMG levels of paraspinal muscles are unreliable measures of outcome in pain reduction. Although tension levels may be decreased, subjective measures of pain and discomfort are not necessarily diminished. Nouwen

(1983) found that EMG biofeedback training reduced standing paraspinal EMG levels but did not reduce subjective pain. Bush, Ditto, and Feuerstein (1985) divided sixty-six chronic low back pain sufferers into three equal groups. One group received paraspinal EMG biofeedback, one group received placebo treatment, and a third group received no intervention. Subjects were administered the Beck Depression Inventory, the State Trait Anxiety Inventory, the McGill Pain Questionnaire, and measures of paraspinal EMG, and were assessed before and after treatment conditions. There was also a reassessment using the same outcome measures at three-month follow-up. All groups showed significant reductions in pain, anxiety, depression, and paraspinal EMG, following treatment and at follow-up. There were no differences between groups. The conclusion to this study indicated that paraspinal EMG biofeedback was not a specific treatment for chronic low back pain.

In another study by Large and Lamb (1983), EMG biofeedback reduced EMG measures and there was a significant correlation between subjective pain levels and surface EMG activity. The EMG condition was found to be significantly greater than a control condition in training muscle relaxation, but again failed to reduce subjective pain levels, despite the high correlation between subjective pain and EMG biofeedback. Relaxation training accomplished using frontalis EMG biofeedback was used by Spence (1984) to assist twenty-one chronic pain patients. Results failed to support the use of EMG relaxation training as a standard procedure for chronic pain patients, and in fact, no significant alteration in mean pain and medication measures was found. In a study by Pearce and Morley (1981), tension headache and migraine headache were treated using EMG biofeedback. Pain ratings were not clearly related to induced EMG levels.

Expectations

Further studies involving lower back pain patients and EMG training (Adams, Pearson, and Olson, 1982; Biedermann, 1983) found that the amount of pain reduction was not significantly correlated with the amount of muscle tension reduction but did find that expectation of personal mastery contributed to a lowered pain experience due to EMG biofeedback. When patients succeed in reducing muscle activity and reducing pain, they become convinced that they can execute the behavior necessary to reduce their discomfort, and this expectation of personal mastery significantly affects their perception of pain. Along these lines of expectation, another group of studies involved heart-rate biofeedback in an attempt to reduce cold pressor pain (Magnusson, Hedberg, and Tunved, 1981; Reeves and Shapiro, 1982; and Subotnik and Shapiro, 1984). Expectancy was found to be a major determinant of pain reports in both the Magnusson, Hedberg, and Tunved (1981) and Subotnik and Shapiro (1984) studies. Subotnik and Shapiro provided two levels of outcome expectancy, increased pain and decreased pain. The increased pain expectancy subjects were told that decreasing their heart rate during the ice water immersion would cause more pain. The decreased pain subjects were told that decreasing their heart rate would cause less pain. Decreased pain subjects consistently reported less pain on the final cold pressor test, whereas the increased pain subjects consistently reported more pain. In the study by Reeves and Shapiro (1982) subjects were specifically instructed that increased heart rate was associated with increased pain and decreased heart rate with decreased pain. The group that received consistent instructions showed appropriate heart rate changes during biofeedback training and parallel changes in heart rate and pain perception during the final cold pressor test. The group that received inconsistent instructions produced no relationship between heart rate and pain perception changes during the final cold pressor test. It appears from these studies that expectations and instructional set are able to significantly modify the subjects' perception of pain.

In a study by Flor, Haag, Turk, and Koehler (1983), they found that attitude toward pain and its evaluation play an important role in the efficacy of biofeedback. Subjects suffering from chronic rheumatic back pain were treated with EMG biofeedback, psuedotherapy, or a conventional medical treatment alone during a four-week inpatient period. At the end of the treatment phase and at the four-month follow-up, the subjects in the biofeedback group showed significant improvement in the duration, intensity, and quality of their back pain as well as their EMG levels, negative self-statements, and utilization of the health care system. The psuedotherapy group showed minimal but nonsignificant improvements, and the medically treated group remained unchanged.

Apparently cognitive factors such as expectations and instructional set seem to combine to provide a sense of personal mastery or control. Pain reduction then may be the result of alterations in the patient's view or interpretation of the pain. Such a hypothesis would be consistent with the findings that EMG training failed to produce significant reduction in subjective pain.

However, studies in other areas have found useful effects from EMG biofeedback. Such studies have included rheumatoid arthritis (Achterberg, McGraw, and Lawlis, 1981), phantom limb pain (Tsushima, 1982), and whip-lash victims (Bissett, Mitchell, and Major, 1985). In these studies reduction of EMG tension was associated with subjective reduction in pain. Electromyograph biofeedback has also been used to facilitate work in the management of myofascial pain syndrome (Stenn, Mothersill, and Brook, 1979). Relaxation, sensory awareness training, EMG biofeedback, and cognitive skill training were utilized in that study. Although EMG-trained subjects experienced less subjective pain, there was no difference in EMG between groups that received EMG readings compared to those who were monitored but not provided with feedback.

It is apparent that the results of research in the area of EMG biofeedback have been somewhat unclear. Many studies indicate that reduction of EMG levels does not necessarily reduce subjective pain. The studies that do show correlations between subjective pain reduction and reduction of EMG levels often seem to employ more than EMG biofeedback training to accomplish the pain reduction. That is to say, a combination of methods, using instructions, expectations, and general relaxation training, often seem to be most effective.

The following case discussions are intended to illustrate the effectiveness of multifaceted approaches to chronic pain management. Each approach is specifically designed to meet the needs of the individual patient. The patient's interpretation of pain, associated affect, personality characteristics, and expectations of what can be accomplished with treatment are all considerations of developing successful strategies for coping with the pain.

Case of Mrs. A.

Presenting Problem and Background. Mrs. A. developed a pain in the lower lumbar region, radiating into her right buttock, and down the right leg. Her first experience with the pain began on an automobile trip when she was riding with her husband. The pain persisted and worsened after that time. Initial diagnosis was tendonitis and anti-inflammatory drugs were used with unpleasant side effects. She was also treated with a heating pad and hot soaks with minimal change in her level of pain. She began to work with EMG biofeedback approximately one year following the onset of the lower back pain. Biofeedback had been recommended by various sources and she was eager to begin.

Mrs. A. was fifty-one years old, married, and the mother of three children. She had been having periodic marital difficulties for most of her married life. She had completed two years of college, and her personality could be characterized as having a strong need to be in control. Mrs. A. was an extremely active woman physically prior to developing her lower back pain. Although socially outgoing her interests were so varied as to be probably quite erratic. She was excessively demanding and quite dominant in interpersonal relationships. Some of these personality characteristics were notably contributory to her marital difficulties as well as to her pain experience. Her husband, age fifty-three, presented similar difficulties in interpersonal relationships in that he, too, was a fairly dominant, aggressive individual for whom it was important to be in control.

Intervention. Mrs. A. served as her own control. A baseline–treatment–follow-up paradigm was used. Pain was measured by having Mrs. A. gauge her subjective discomfort in units ranging from one through ten, where ten was most intense.

Mrs. A. began treatment working with EMG biofeedback, applied directly to the lower back (paraspinal) region. Figure 13.1 presents EMG data for Mrs. A. during five training and three booster sessions. Figure 13.2 illustrates mean ratings of subjective units of discomfort (SUDS) for Mrs. A. before and during EMG training, during booster training, and at the beginning of alpha training.

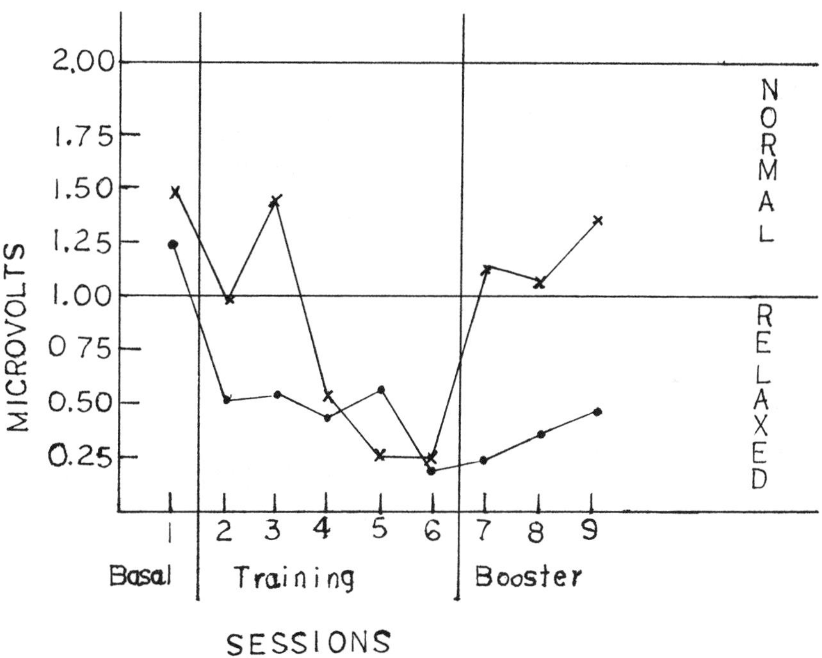

FIGURE 13.1. Initial (X) and final (o) microvolt values for Mrs. A.

Mrs. A. was seen for a total of five EMG training sessions, during which time her subjective units of discomfort were reduced and she also evidenced considerable control over muscle tension in the lower back area. Mrs. A. was seen for three follow-up sessions, during which time she reported increasing discomfort, although she continued to be able to reduce her muscle tension when she had the information provided by the EMG equipment. During the initial series of EMG training, it should be noted that she continued to use a transcutaneous electrical nerve stimulator (TENS) to also aid in pain reduction. During the period, Mrs. A. was reporting increased discomfort in the three follow-up sessions. This was a period of depression for her which she did resolve toward the end of the third follow-up session.

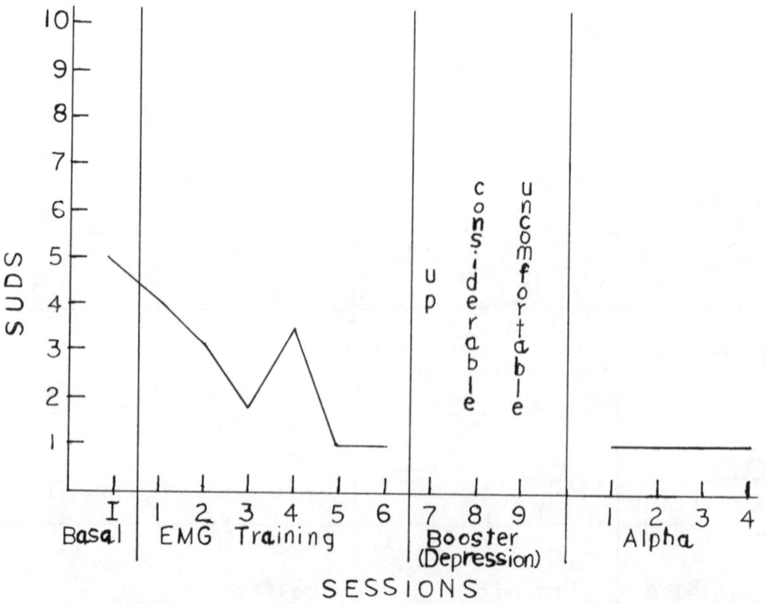

FIGURE 13.2. Mean ratings of subjective units of discomfort (SUDS) for Mrs. A. before and during EMG training, booster, and beginning of Alpha training.

Following the EMG biofeedback training and follow-up sessions, it was determined that Mrs. A. needed to continue with biofeedback work as she was not easily hypnotizable. She did, however, seem to have a negative feeling about EMG biofeedback. The utilization of EEG biofeedback was discussed, and Mrs. A. was quite receptive to these ideas. Alpha training began and continued for eleven training sessions and three follow-up sessions. Percent alpha was measured for 1000 second trials from the left temporal and left occipital lobes. Figure 13.3 presents the percent of alpha (defined as 8 to 12 hz and approximately 50 to 90 microvolts) and percent of TENS use for training and follow-up periods.

During the training sessions, it is notable that although Mrs. A. was able to maintain alpha frequency for gradually decreasing periods of time, she did, nonetheless, achieve reduction in the use of her TENS device and went for a period of approximately eight weeks where she didn't wear the TENS device at all.

Follow-up. Subsequent follow-up sessions revealed that Mrs. A. wore the TENS device approximately 50 percent of the time for a twelve-week period. In the last follow-up session, she reported that she felt satisfied that she was able to produce the alpha state on her own, without the use of the EEG biofeedback equipment. She also remained free of pain medication.

In addition, Mrs. A. began to work in conjoint psychotherapy, together with her husband, addressing issues having to do with their marriage relationship. One final note is that a little more than halfway through the period of alpha training sessions, Mrs. A. did develop a myofascial pain syndrome in the region of her left shoulder, but she was able to obtain reduction of that pain by using alpha. Informal follow-up occurred six months after the end of all treatment when Mrs. A. returned from vacation. No problem with pain and only minimal discomfort were reported. She indicated continued use of the number eight, her cue for alpha wave production. Mrs. A. was seen for a period of ten months.

Discussion. The number eight had great meaning for Mrs. A. in that it was the symbol or stimulus that she used to "zero in" on producing the alpha state for herself when she was not on training equipment. This effort by Mrs. A. suggests that for her the sense of being in control of her pain was necessary to its effective management and consistent with her overall view of the world as well.

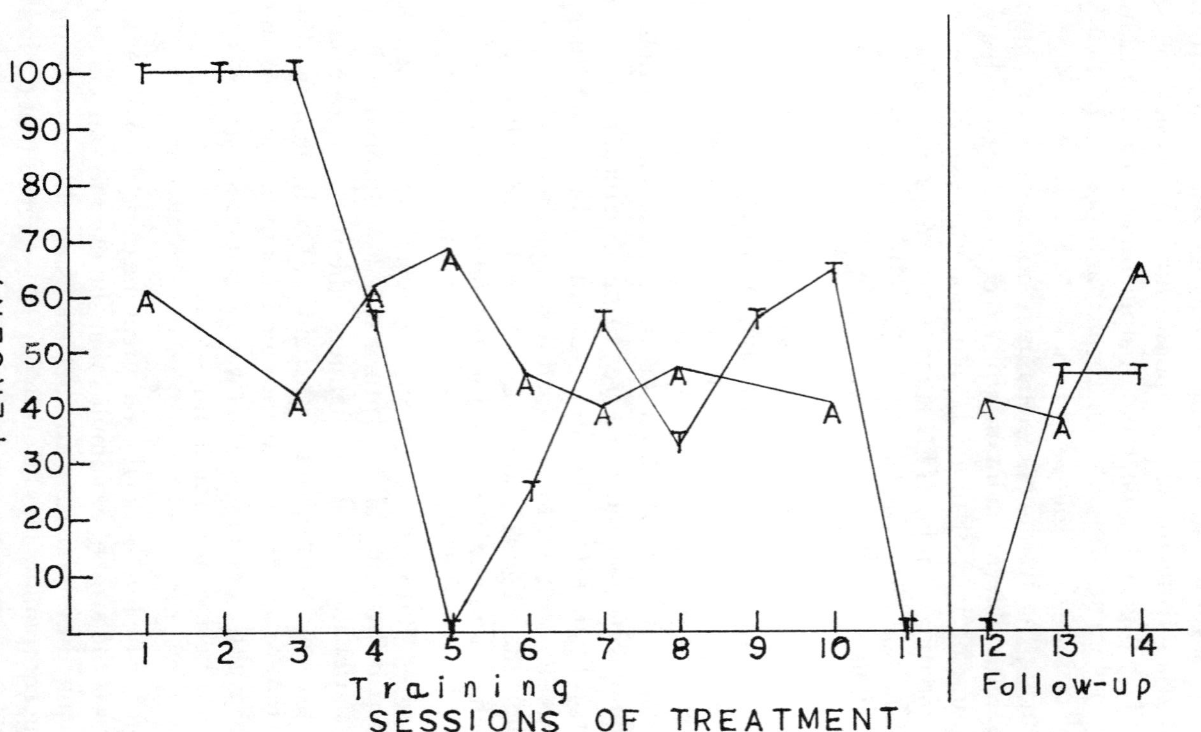

FIGURE 13.3. Percent alpha (A) and percent of TENS uses (T) for weeks of treatment and follow-up for Mrs. A.

Although there appears to be a strong positive correlation between reduction of EMG and subjective discomfort, initial EMG levels and pain perceptions increased during follow-up (see Figures 13.1 and 13.2). For this patient, alpha training was by her own report most effective in persistent reduction of chronic pain.

It is noteworthy to point out that Mrs. A.'s case reflects an integration of approaches, using not only two biofeedback modalities but also augmenting those methods with conjoint marital psychotherapy. It is noteworthy, too, that it appears even though her training session percentage of alpha production decreased slightly, the need for utilization of the TENS device also decreased as training continued. On the surface, these findings would appear to be contradictory; however, it seems that Mrs. A. had an increased sense of control over her pain by thinking of the number eight, which was the most consistent with her expressed personality needs to "be in charge." It may be that it was more the sense of control than the success at alpha training (as hypothesized above by Adams, et al., 1982; Biedermann, 1983) that might have produced the positive results for her to reduce her use of the TENS stimulator and medication.

Case of Mr. B.

Presenting Problem and Background; Mr. B. was fifty-nine years old and had a history of depression of about ten years duration. His personality could best be described as compulsive and overanxious, with periodic depressions during the previous ten years. He also had marital problems and a history of cardiac difficulties. Mr. B. sustained frostbite of both upper extremities, along with alcohol intoxication about six months prior to referral for biofeedback. He was found lying in a snowbank, not wearing any gloves, and on admission, his temperature was below 92 degrees fahrenheit. He was warmed up to 98 degrees. His hands were treated for frostbite, and upon discharge, all portions of the fingers appeared to be viable, but Mr. B. was complaining of constant pain with heat and cold intolerance. He was to continue physical therapy daily upon discharge. A series of appropriate nerve blocks followed, but these did not appear to have any effect on reducing the pain or sensitivity in his hands. He was referred for biofeedback six months after his injury, in order to improve skin blood flow by increasing surface skin temperature on the theory that such an effort would reduce the pain and sensitivity in his hands. Upon interview, Mr. B. was very apprehensive, as might have been evident from his extremely cold hands. He was also extremely aware of the coldness of his hands, insisting that they be touched in order to feel how cold they were. He indicated that he experienced pain in his hands which was seemingly correlated with a drop in temperature; the lower the ambient temperature, the more pain. He indicated his left hand was damaged more by the frostbite than the right hand, but gradually the hands were beginning to grow back nails on all fingertips. The pain was localized to the fingertips in both hands. There was also increased sensitivity, which was described as a cutting sensation, when he went to pick up any object that had edges on it. Mr. B. also indicated that he had problems with being irritable, and lately had become more quick tempered than he had been in a long time. He attributed this quick temper to the fact that his fingers had been frozen and that he had been more or less disabled for the few months after the occurrence.

Intervention. Mr. B. served as his own control. A baseline–treatment–follow-up paradigm was used. Pain was measured by having Mr. B. estimate his subjective discomfort in units ranging from one through ten, where ten was most intense.

Temperature biofeedback training was begun and continued for thirteen sessions. Thermistors were attached to the middle finger of each hand, and data were obtained by averaging the actual temperature in degrees Fahrenheit of both hands for initial and final readings in each training session. Figure 13.4 illustrates the initial and final temperature values for basal, training and booster sessions. Figure 13.5 presents mean ratings of subjective units of discomfort during treatment. These ratings were obtained by having Mr. B. estimate how uncomfortable his hands felt for each day during the training period. The ratings were then averaged to reflect a weekly SUD rating.

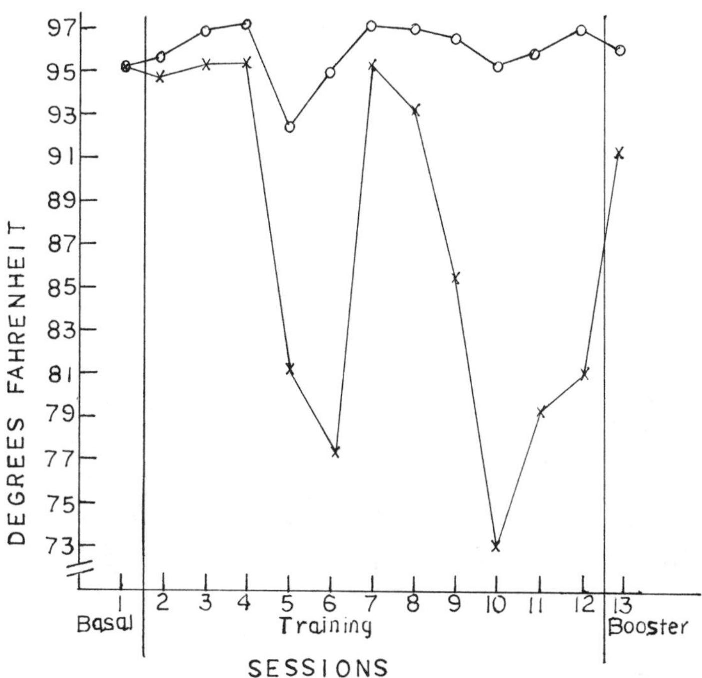

FIGURE 13.4. Initial (X) and final (o) temperature values for basal, training and booster sessions for Mr. B.

As can be seen in Figure 13.4, there was evidence that Mr. B. was able to obtain increased control over the amount he could raise his temperature during the session, to the point where in the tenth session, he was able to raise his hand temperature an average of 22 degrees Fahrenheit. In terms of his subjective ratings of discomfort (SUDS) during the training period, these ratings gradually diminished over time until they were rated at one SUD toward the end of the training period.

Discussion. Mr. B. improved dramatically over his thirteen sessions of temperature training. He had been accustomed to wearing gloves during most activities and also, almost regard-

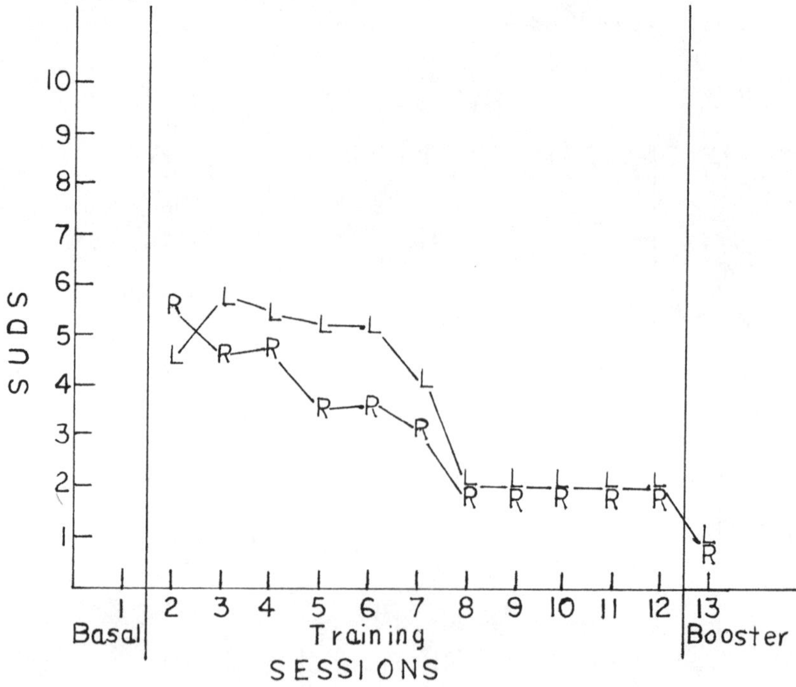

FIGURE 13.5. Mean ratings of subjective units of discomfort (SUDS) in each hand over treatment sessions for Mr. B.

less of ambient temperature. During follow-up, Mr. B. reported wearing gloves only in their appropriate ambient temperature conditions (e.g., winter). Figure 13.4 indicates marked variability in initial temperature values for each session. Some factors that contributed to this variability included environmental conditions, ambient temperature in the training room, and amount of time spent in discussion before training. Again, the increased sense of control is apparent. Such a sense of control was coincidental with an improvement in Mr. B.'s depressive symptomatology and a reduction in antidepressant medication use. Informal follow-up over a sixteen-month period after the final session indicated that the gains that Mr. B. had accomplished were well maintained. Mr. B's improvement in controlling his temperature might also be explained by the idea of increased personal mastery discussed by Biedermann (1983) and Adams et al. (1982). Such a hypothesis of increased expectation of personal mastery would be consistent with cognitive restructuring approaches to depression, and indeed, be consistent with the reduction in depressive symptomatology and the need for antidepressant medication.

Case of Mrs. C.

Presenting Problem and Background. Mrs. C. is thirty-five years old, married, an attorney. She sustained a whiplash-type injury in an automobile accident. She was riding as a passenger in the right rear seat of a vehicle that was stopped to make a left turn. The car was rear-ended by a second vehicle, caused to spin around, and then struck again by a third vehicle. She sustained a number of small cuts, one on her nose and one on her head. She was bruised in the head and taken by ambulance to the hospital following the accident. En route to the hospital, she became aware of difficulty in raising her head due to pain and weakness in her neck. X rays were negative for fracture and she was told that she had sustained a sprain of the neck and was provided with a cervical collar.

Gradually, her symptomatology stabilized and it was determined to basically involve the left neck and shoulder area. She described a radiating pain and numbness, going down the left arm and traveling into the little and ring fingers. She also described pain going up the back of her neck and she occasionally would get one-sided headaches. She was able to identify some "hot-spots" of pain in the left scapular area. On at least one occasion, she developed a severe pain in that area which lasted a matter of hours and caused great discomfort throughout the left upper extremities.

Mrs. C. was referred for treatment approximately eight months following her initial injury. She was treated during those eight months with a cervical collar, physical therapy, and medication. She was diagnosed medically as myofascial pain syndrome. Physical therapy was useful, although a great deal of spasm and tenderness throughout the left scapular area radiating up into the neck continued, even after the end of physical therapy. Range of motion, strength, and neurologic exam were essentially normal upon her referral for treatment. Upon initial referral, this patient was currently taking one-half a Norgesic Forte tablet, QID. She was also following a recommendation of exercise in the form of swimming.

In addition to the physical problems that Mrs. C. was experiencing, she also complained of fear and anxiety since the accident whenever she rode in an automobile.

As noted, Mrs. C. was an attorney by profession. She had no prior history of back injuries or difficulties with her left upper extremity. She was working as an attorney and continued to carry her workload upon referral and throughout treatment. She was able to report that during times of stress in her work, the pain tended to increase. She also associated increased pain with increased physical activity, such as working in her garden and exercising. She describes her preinjury life as "very active," including exercising, working in her garden, and so on. She had been married for approximately one year upon referral. She was an only child and her parents were deceased.

Intervention. Frontalis EMG biofeedback was begun following initial referral. Biofeedback training was combined with general relaxation training, using visual imagery for relaxation. Desensitization to riding in an automobile was also implemented as part of the overall intervention. Finally, cognitive approaches to stress management in terms of coping skill strategies were presented and employed having to do with Mrs. C.'s coping with pain as well as day-to-day stress in her work as an attorney. Electromyograph data in the form of microvolts, both frontalis EMG training, as well as multisite training involving the trapezius area are illustrated in Figure 13.6.

As can be seen from Figure 13.6, EMG measures decreased over treatment but then eventually plateaued, maintaining at a level slightly above normal tension state of the muscles. Figure 13.7 presents the Subjective Units of Discomfort (SUDS) which were Mrs. C.'s estimates of her level of discomfort during treatment. As can be seen from Figure 13.7, Mrs. C.'s SUDS declined gradually over treatment. It should also be noted that her level of activity and effectiveness in managing stress im-

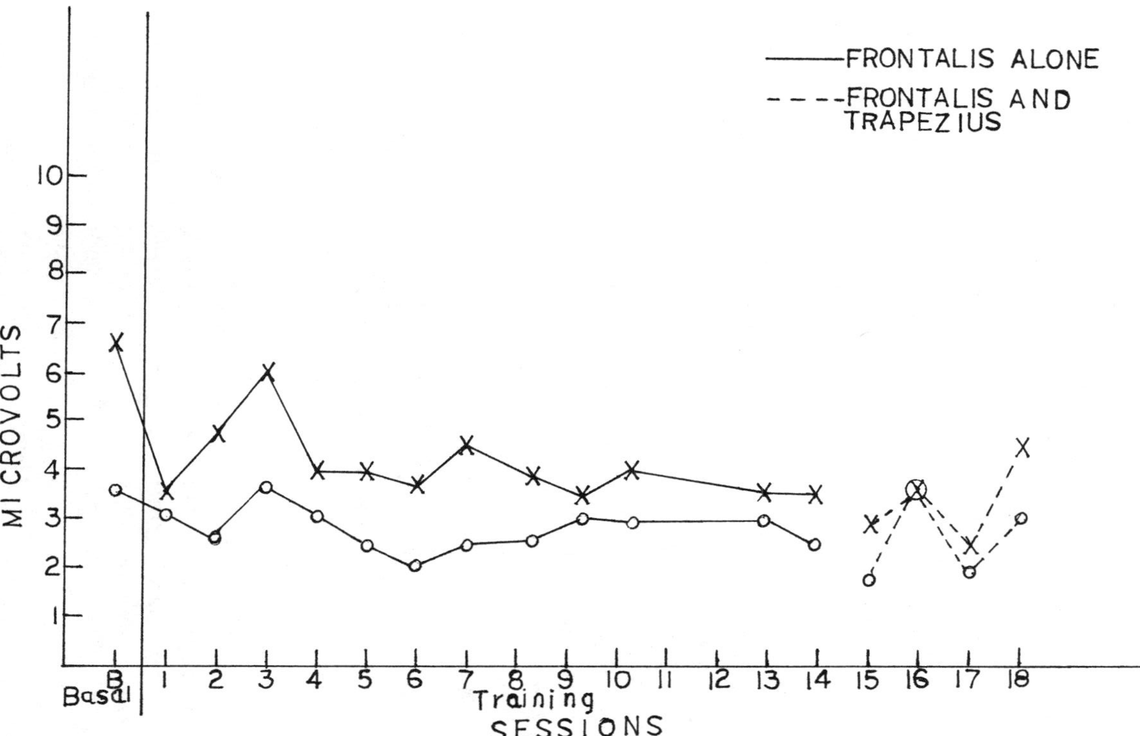

FIGURE 13.6. Initial (x) and final (o) EMG values for frontalis and combined frontalis and trapezius for Mrs. C.

proved over the course of treatment and her medication use diminished.

Discussion. Mrs. C.'s improvement occurred over a period of twenty-one sessions in seven months of treatment. During this time, a combination of approaches, including cognitive restructuring in the form of cognitive coping strategies for dealing with stress, relaxation, and biofeedback training were employed. It is interesting that Mrs. C.'s subjective perception of reduced pain was greater than the reduction of her EMG levels would suggest. Also, her use of medication as another measure of pain had decreased, suggesting considerable improvement in terms of her ability to manage the long-term myofascial pain.

As illustrated in the above cases, multifaceted approaches to pain management involve the identification of the patient's cognitive view and interpretation of his pain and then the development of procedures designed to address those views as well as alleviate the discomfort.

Biofeedback provides a specific tangible approach, probably more useful for patients whose personalities are interpersonally dominant, as in the cases of Mrs. A. and Mrs. C., or who are significantly depressed, and such helplessness can be challenged by the personal mastery offered by biofeedback, as with Mr. B. Such an association would be supported by the cognitive approaches taken to dealing with depression (Beck, 1976). However, not all patients have such personality characteristics nor interpretations of pain. Dumas (1980) found that subjects who scored high on hypnotic susceptibility tests did not gain significant control over EEG alpha but that subjects with moderate to low scores on hypnotic susceptibility tests did gain control of EEG alpha. Such a finding may suggest different approaches to pain "control," again dependent on cognitive and personality factors.

Hypnosis

The effects of suggestion on the perception of pain have been well known for centuries. Perhaps one of the oldest and

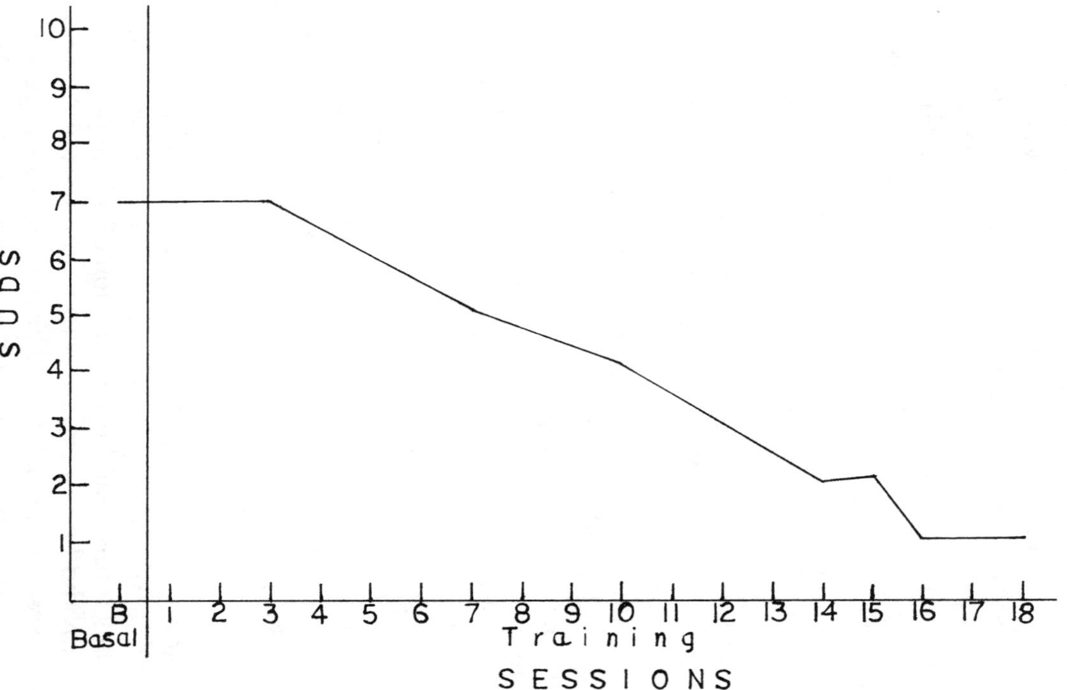

FIGURE 13.7. Mean ratings of subjective units of discomfort (SUDS) before and during EMG training for Mrs. C.

most persistent uses for hypnosis in clinical practice has been the management of pain (Crasilneck and Hall, 1973). Wickramasekera (1976) defines hypnosis as "a set of instructional-situational manipulations which have a high probability of success with an identifiable group of people [highly susceptible] under conditions of high motivation to participate" (p. 147). Hypnosis could also be viewed as a skill of an individual to focus attention, screen out extraneous stimulation, and alter perceptual events; for example, changing sensations. It should be noted that interpersonal variables are as much a part of instructional–situational manipulation as are many of the techniques and stimuli used in trance induction. As defined then, hypnosis and self-hypnosis are procedures that have been useful tools for chronic pain patients (Sacerdote, 1978) and also for those with terminal illness (Kleinsorge, 1967; Sacerdote, 1970; and Willard, 1974).

The uses of hypnosis as an assist to pain management in both adult and child cancer patients has been particularly successful. Harris (1985) reported the case of a forty-four-year-old female cancer patient and the use of hypnosis to reduce pain, eliminate nausea, and increase her appetite. A difference in the wording of the suggestion seemed significant. Instead of suggesting that she "bear" the pain, "control" of the pain was the focus of intervention. Davidson (1984) described a self-hypnosis technique for use with a thirty-two-year-old woman with terminal cancer. Araoz (1983) discussed how hypnotically facilitated, positive, mental imagery helps patients dissociate themselves from the cancer. Spiegel and Bloom (1983) studied fifty-four woman with metastatic carcinoma of the breast and compared self-hypnosis training, weekly group therapy, and a combination of both procedures in controlling the pain. They found that the combination of self-hypnosis and group therapy did best in measures of pain intensity. Margolis (1982) discusses another six cases where hypnotic imagery was used to reduce pain and discomfort in cancer patients. Alteration in perception and awareness were the primary suggestions used along with deep relaxation, ego strengthening, and imagery.

Work has also been done with children and adolescents

with cancer. Zeltzer and LeBaron (1983) reviewed interventions for pain that were the result of various medical procedures and chemotherapy used to treat cancer with children and adolescents. They found that hypnosis was more effective than supportive counseling, and that the techniques of hypnotic induction needed to be varied according to the age of the child. Kellerman, Zeltzer, Ellenberg, and Dash (1983) used hypnosis with sixteen adolescent cancer patients. They found significant reductions in anxiety, as well as a trend to greater self-esteem as a result of hypnotic interventions in managing the pain. Finally, Hilgard and LeBaron (1982) studied six nineteen-year-old cancer patients using hypnosis and found differences between self-reported pain and observed pain, but in general, effectiveness in the technique of hypnosis in reducing discomfort.

Hypnosis has also been used in dealing with other forms of pain and discomfort, most notably with severe burns (Dahinteroval, 1967; Schafer, 1975) and recurrent painful illnesses (Sachs, Feuerstein, and Vitale, 1977). Margolis (1985) presented case reports of three burn patients and four cancer patients, and discussed the use of hypnotic techniques as providing a significantly holistic approach to patients in relieving pain and strengthening the quality of their life. Dimond (1981) presented the case of the thirty-year-old female undergoing hemodialysis, and the effectiveness of hypnotically facilitated desensitization to deal with her ability to increase self-control and independence in accepting the procedure. Suggestions were made to help the patient incorporate the dialysis process into her personal needs for independence. It was also noted that a substantially increased blood flow during dialysis accompanied the psychological improvements. Williams (1983) reported the successful use of hypnosis to relieve pain in a sixty-three-year-old man injured in an industrial accident with chronic intractable shoulder pain for a duration of about thirteen years. Other uses of hypnosis have appeared with arthritis, ulcerative colitis, a variety of injuries, migraine headaches, phantom limb sensations, and damaged fascial nerves (Long, 1986). Finally, hypnosis has also been used in dealing with lower back pain following surgery (Lemmon, 1983), as well as chronic lower back pain (Medical Hypnoanalysis Society, 1984).

Studies of hypnotic susceptibility as a factor in one's response to pain reduction are mixed in their results. Spanos, McNeil, Gwynn, and Stam (1984) compared undergraduates high and low in hypnotic susceptibility, and found significantly lowered rated pain in high susceptibility subjects. The experimenters used three groups; one was given the suggestion to imagine their hand as numb and insensitive, another was asked to practice a distraction task, and a third received no special instructions. As already noted, the suggestion group that was also highly susceptible lowered rated pain. The low susceptibility distraction task group showed as much reduction in rated pain as high susceptibility subjects given the suggestion. Fricton and Roth (1985) found that an indirect hypnotic technique was significantly more effective than a direct hypnotic technique in reducing pain thresholds, regardless of hypnotic susceptibility. Hypnotic susceptibility was measured by the Stanford Hypnotic Susceptibility Scale. These findings suggested that low susceptibility subjects may still be able to achieve useful hypnotic reduction of pain, using hypnosis. Hypnosis has also been used with cognitive coping skills to deal effectively with temporal mandibular pain and dysfunction (Stam, McGrath and Brooke, 1984), as well as the pain associated with sickle cell disease (Thomas, 1984). A study by Toomey and Sanders (1983) used a group-based hypnotic approach to generating cognitive coping strategies with five chronic pain (head, facial, and back) patients. Results of self-rating depression scale, a self-esteem questionnaire, and global pain estimates suggested a reduction in subjective estimates of pain.

Hypnosis seems to be generally effective in reducing pain and discomfort. Often, however, suggestions are designed to modify not only perception and sensation but one's cognitive processes and beliefs as well. Significant alteration of pain, and skill in coping with it, is also possible even in low susceptibility subjects, depending on the focus of the suggestion (Fricton and Roth, 1985).

The following clinical cases are designed to illustrate multifaceted pain management approaches in detail.

Case of Mr. D.

Presenting Problem and Background. Mr. D. is twenty-six years old, single, and white, and he sustained an industrial accident. Injuries at the time consisted primarily of physical trauma following a fall at work. Mr. D. fell a vertical height of approximately four feet on his extended right lower extremity, receiving the full weight on his right foot. He then slumped to his right side, striking his right shoulder. Since that time, he had complained of marked pain in his right foot, paralysis of his right foot, and severe pain and limitation in his right shoulder. No clear diagnosis was made. Psychological trauma was also apparent in the incident as it happened early in the morning while he was working the 11 P.M. to 7 A.M. shift and he was admittedly quite frightened by the fact that there were few people around at the time of his accident.

Mr. D. was referred for psychological treatment approximately four months after his initial injury, after having been examined and found to have little in the way of any hard evidence of organic disease. There did appear to be definite pain, probably of a reflex sympathetic dystrophy or causalgia type. In short, symptoms seemed to be greatly exaggerated, although to Mr. D, they were very real. Medical follow-up continued after the initial referral.

Mr. D. had one year of college at the time of interview and was disabled from his job as a millworker on which he had been injured. He was the middle of three children and had strong interests in the area of art and craft work, even to the extent of having made his own furniture. He reported little difficulty in interpersonal relationships.

Intervention. Mr. D. served as his own control. A baseline–treatment–follow-up paradigm was used. Pain was measured by having him estimate his subjective discomfort in units ranging from one to ten, where ten was most intense.

Initial approaches to Mr. D.'s pain consisted of simple relaxation training efforts, involving controlled abdominal breathing, and the use of relaxing imagery. This approach was followed by hypnotic intervention and the hypnotic strategies were augmented with behavioral procedures such as shaping and monitoring. The overall thrust of the intervention consisted of shaping the use of Mr. D.'s right hand, arm, and foot in the form of simple exercises, consisting of right hand squeezes, right arm lifts, and seated as well as standing foot pressure. Prior to doing these exercises, Mr. D. was trained in self-hypnosis and used imagery of warmth and lightness as well as suggestions of increased self-control and feelings of success. Toward the middle of the course of treatment, Mr. D. experienced severe personal stress—his father was terminally ill. His father finally died, and this event caused a hiatus in treatment.

Data provided from Mr. D.'s behavior monitor are reflected in Figures 13.8 and 13.9.

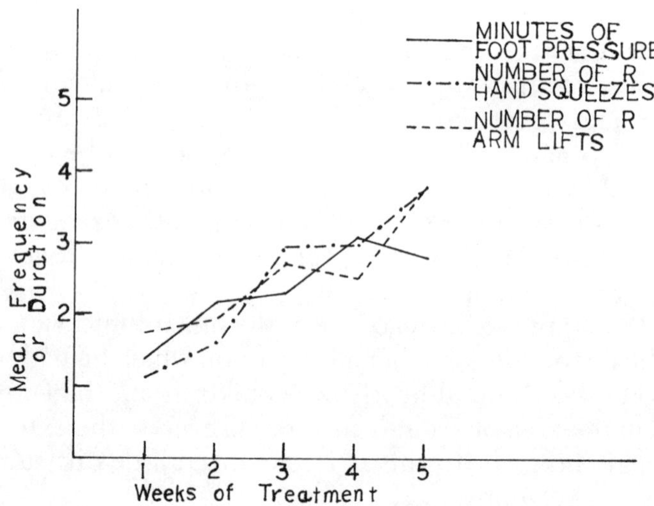

FIGURE 13.8. Weekly means for seated foot pressure, hand squeezes, and arm lifts for Mr. D.

Figure 13.8 illustrates the minutes of seated foot pressure on the right foot over a five-week period of treatment. As can be seen from the figure, the amount of time Mr. D. was able to put pressure on his foot in a seated position increased from a

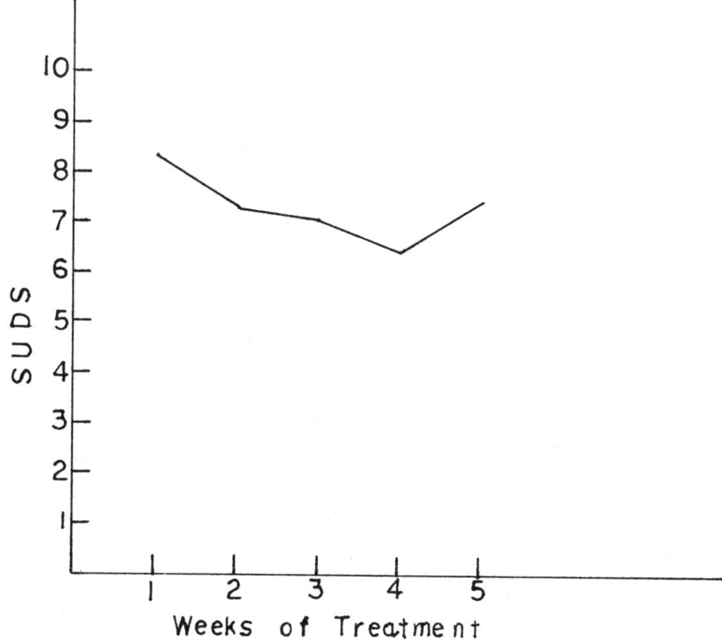

FIGURE 13.9. Weekly mean subjective units of discomfort (SUDS) for Mr. D.

mean of 1.43 minutes to a high of 3.07 minutes. Figure 13.8 also shows a steady increase in frequency of right hand squeezes (of a tension spring) and the number of right arm lifts. Hand squeezes start at a mean of 1.14 and tripled to a final mean of 3.7. Arm lifts began at 1.7 and have more than doubled to 3.7.

Figure 13.9 presents the subjective units of discomfort (SUDS) averaged for each week of treatment. As can be seen from Figure 13.9, Mr. D.'s SUDS declined only slightly over weeks in treatment.

Improvement began to occur during the five weeks of treatment, both in terms of objective measures of foot pressure, hand squeezes, and arm lifts as well as subjective ratings of discomfort. Mr. D. returned to treatment about two months after the fifth session. In that two months, his father had died and the first session that occurred upon his return consisted pretty much in helping him get his father's death into perspective. In terms of his shoulder, he was reporting that it felt better and was about 75 to 80 percent back to normal use. Six months previously, he had only had approximately 15 percent of use in his shoulder. He indicated that his arm would tire easily; however, with regard to his right hand, he was up to eight to nine squeezes of a tension spring per day, and he was able to keep approximately five minutes of seated foot pressure on his right foot.

Treatment was resumed the following week, continuing with hypnosis and suggestions to strengthen his muscles in his hand and shoulder and to numb his foot so he could put pressure on it. Also, his perceptions of his injury were reviewed, and suggestions made to reduce his initial fear that the residuals from the injury might be irreversible.

The following week Mr. D. started to lift weights with his arm and shoulder. Thus, monitors of hand squeezes on a tension spring and arm lifts were no longer appropriate as he had progressed beyond that point. Mr. D.'s foot, however, was still sensitive and heel pressure was painful. He continued to put seated foot pressure on his heel for over five minutes per day and used self-hypnosis to cope with the pain. Two weeks later his subjective discomfort levels had continued to drop and he was able to take five steps in the session without the aid of crutches or canes but under the anesthetic effects of hypnosis. Shoulder discomfort continued to drop.

Another hiatus in treatment occurred for an approximate period of two months, three weeks of which Mr. D. spent traveling. Upon return two months later, his right shoulder, arm, and hand were vastly improved. He reported some occasional aching but generally an almost complete return to normal functioning. He was walking with a cane and was able to put pressure on his right foot. Hypnosis was done to reinforce his hypnotic control of pain to reduce discomfort of his foot. A week later, he continued to walk fairly well but not very far. He had begun working on movement of his ankle, particularly heel and toe walking and rotation of the ankle. Upon his return, he also was discussing plans to get into college and take some business courses, demonstrating a goal-directed, future orientation. He talked of starting his own furniture business and was also planning to rebuild his mother's barn shortly.

A month later he was walking approximately one mile without significant discomfort and continued to do flexibility exercises for his foot. The shoulder was no longer a problem and he continued his future focus with plans to return to a local community college, asking about various courses he might take.

At another follow-up six weeks later, he reported continuing to walk now up to two miles per day. He complained of occasional aches from his foot but otherwise considerable improvement. He was no longer using a cane and had started his courses at a local community college.

The last follow-up session occurred two months later, at which time Mr. D. had completely improved, continuing to walk two miles daily and the use of his right arm, hand, and shoulder without discomfort. He continued his college courses and still had plans to go into his own furniture business.

The total course of treatment involved eighteen sessions over a period of eleven months, focusing initially on shaping behavior with hypnosis as an aid to alleviate pain. Later, self-hypnosis was used and the focus of hypnotic work shifted to suggestions involving cognitive–emotional changes as well as pain reduction.

Discussion. Mr. D. seemed to accomplish virtually complete return of function in his right arm, shoulder, and foot. It would seem that he was able to modify his perception of pain and also increase his sense of control over same, thereby alleviating the pain. In addition to the pain relief, however, Mr. D. also accomplished changes in his life, especially in terms of goals and direction. There may have been many factors responsible for such a change in addition to his injury. Certainly his father's untimely death contributed to his examination of where his life was going and in what direction.

For Mr. D., gradual, successful experiences with the use of his injured arm seemed initially inversely correlated with ratings of subjective discomfort (his perception of pain). Hypnosis in this case seemed to function to reduce pain, both directly while hypnotized and indirectly over time when Mr. D. began to achieve greater use of his arm, shoulder, and foot. Mr. D.'s personality was that of a fairly passive, unassuming individual who was also quite responsive to hypnosis. Although no standard measure of hypnotic susceptibility was obtained, Mr. D. was capable of entering moderate to deep hypnotic states. As mentioned already, self-hypnosis was also used by Mr. D., but he did seem to do better when provided with an external structure or source of hypnotizability. For example, Mr. D. worked best with the use of taped hypnotic sessions and would play these back for himself in an attempt to achieve a state of hypnotic pain reduction in between sessions.

Case of Mrs. E.

Presenting Problem and Background. Mrs. E. was thirty-five years old and she had sustained injury to muscles in her back and neck following an industrial accident. She was apparently bending down and pulling merchandise from a shelf in a stockroom when she felt muscles pull in her back and neck. Following her injury, she was treated medically, using hot packs, back massage, and whirlpool treatments, as well as exercise for her neck and left arm.

She indicated that following her injury, she would get headaches in the back of her neck and also aches and pains in the left trapezius muscle area of her back. To complicate matters, Mrs. E. was also in an automobile accident approximately three months after her injury. Mrs. E. was referred for psychological evaluation and treatment approximately nine months after her initial injury.

Mrs. E. was the mother of two children and had been married approximately four years when first seen. Her mother died when she was twelve years old and her father died when she was twenty-one years of age. She was the second from youngest in a family of ten children. She hadn't seen many of her family members since she had been married. Prior to marriage, she had been very close to her siblings. Her husband, at the time of her injury, was in the Service and frequently away from home for long periods of time. When asked what she had tried to do to alleviate her headaches and neck discomfort, she indicated that her husband would massage her neck and shoulders, and that massage would alleviate much of the discomfort. It was clear to some extent that she was probably more uncomfortable when her husband was not around and had less success in alleviating her discomfort during those times. To some extent, she was approaching pain relief in an interpersonally dependent position with some possible secondary gain in the form of increased attention from her husband.

Assessment. An MMPI performed on Mrs. E. was within normal limits. A mild depression, however, was noted, and was characterized by tendencies toward excessive self-blame, worry, and cynicism. She was also found to be somewhat predisposed to psychophysiologic illnesses and somatization. Complaints, headache and shoulder pains, and cramps were present as well.

Other personality characteristics included a tendency to be somewhat inhibited and to become uncomfortable when experiencing strong emotions. She had difficulty dealing with these emotions directly and was likely to somaticize tension. She tended to suffer from excessive guilt and responsibility and was also overanxious and difficult to get to know in social situations.

Initial functional analysis of Mrs. E.'s myofascial pain varied from five subjective units of discomfort (SUDS) to ten SUDS. This variation was on a scale ranging from one to ten where ten was the maximum intensity one could experience. Mrs. E.'s pains lasted from thirty minutes to twenty hours in duration. Her pain prevented her from carrying out routine household tasks when above six SUDS, and also prevented her from sleeping comfortably. Pain was intermittent in its duration and frequency. Mrs. E. attempted to deal with the pain by massages from her husband. No difference was observed in pain intensity or duration when her husband was at home or away.

Electromyograph biofeedback assessment of Mrs. E.'s pain was performed on three different sites: back of neck, right trapezius muscle, and left trapezius muscle. She was in a seated position during all EMG readings. Electromyograph readings from the back of neck averaged 7 microvolts (1 to 2 microvolts is the normal range of muscle tension for this particular EMG feedback monitor). Right trapezius area was 3.75 microvolts and left trapezius area was 6.5 microvolts. Subjective ratings of discomfort during testing were estimated by Mrs. E. at seven SUDS.

Intervention. Treatment initially consisted of hypnotically facilitated biofeedback. Principles and concepts of both biofeedback and hypnosis were explained. Mrs. E. was hypnotized at the beginning of the session immediately following EMG biofeedback readings on the left trapezius area. She was instructed under hypnosis to use imagery to facilitate relaxation and rest, and that this rest and relaxation would help her become better and better at relieving her muscle spasms. Initial and final EMG values and treatment session averages for SUDS are presented for treatment sessions in Figure 13.10. Figure 13.10 also shows EMG values for back of neck. In session 3, treatment began to focus on the back of the neck, as well as the left trapezius area, and both values are displayed, although not for every session.

As can be seen from Figure 13.10, Mrs. E.'s EMG values continued to increase during treatment. At session 16, the observation was made that her EMG values were increasing instead of declining. During this period of training, SUD levels declined slightly. In session 16, a "no treatment" strategy was employed as it was hypothesized that this patient was compounding existing tension and discomfort levels by "trying too hard" to be successful in her training.

Following a recess of six weeks, treatment was resumed. Evaluation of her daily routine revealed significant differences from the same routine at the beginning of treatment. A notable change in her family system also occurred at this time, when her husband came home during the recess from a tour of duty in Korea. He had been away for approximately three months—most of the time she had been in initial treatment. The differences in her daily routine included increased ability to

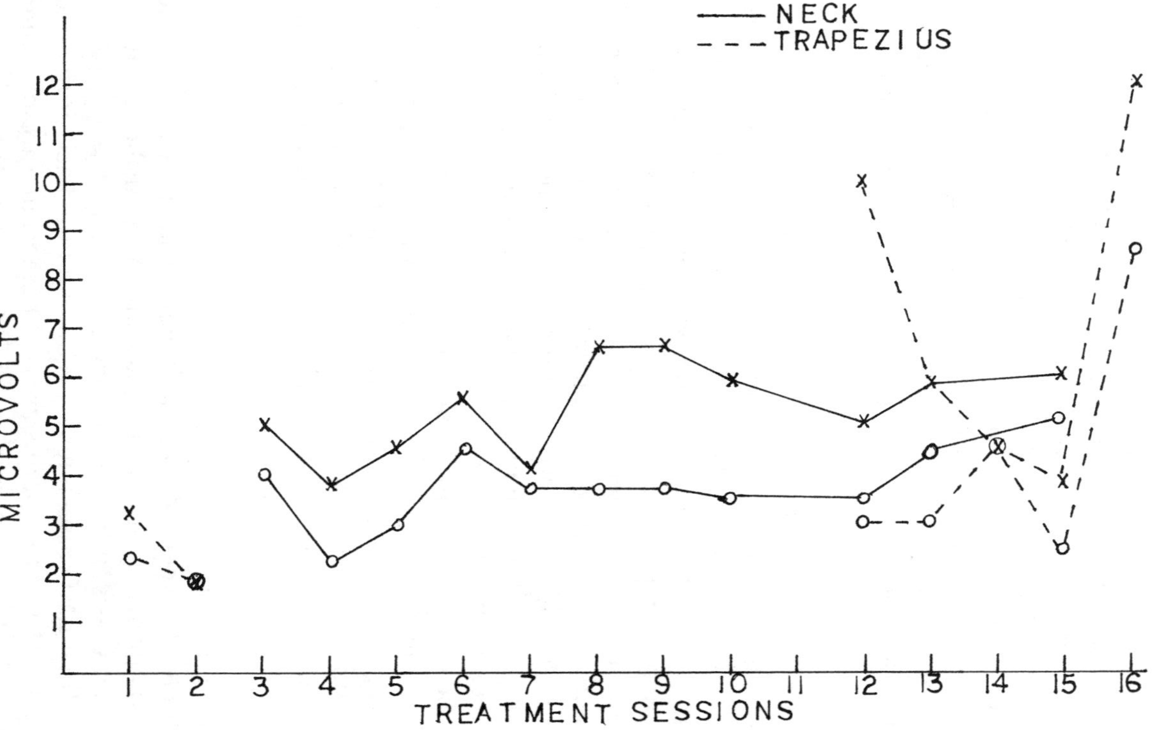

FIGURE 13.10. Initial (x) and final (o) EMG values for both neck and trapezius areas for Mrs. E.

grocery shop, clean house, and do laundry as well as increased socialization with friends.

The treatment focus shifted to changing her cognitive view of pain and introducing alternative methods of dealing with her emotions (e.g., assertive behavior) facilitated by hypnosis. Hypnotic imagery to let go of tension in neck and shoulders and for general relaxation was also employed. Electromyograph biofeedback monitoring was suspended. Following the first session of hypnotherapy, Mrs. E. began to iron clothes, an activity that since her injury she was unable to do. She stopped her antidepressant medication but continued her pain medication (Robaxin), and a minor tranquilizer (Xanax). She continued previous levels of housekeeping and socialization activities.

One month later, she began to show an increase in depressive symptomatology and pain. A hypnosis booster using "nourishing blood flow" imagery was employed with subsequent reduction of depressive symptoms and pain over the next two weeks. She also reported playing baseball and tennis with the kids and was beginning to taper off Robaxin and Xanax.

These suggestions were continued with "booster" sessions of hypnosis for thirteen more sessions, spaced at approximately two-week intervals.

Use of Robaxin and Xanax continued to decline. Hypnotic suggestions included increased activity and continued repair of damaged muscle tissue. Activities, both at home and in the community, continued to increase even to the point where Mrs. E. took charge of a church social activity. A muscle strengthening program was begun at a local rehabilitation facility to provide Mrs. E. with exercises to strengthen her flaccid back and neck muscles.

Issues between Mrs. E. and her husband were also addressed, primarily to clarify roles and responsibilities in the family and assist in problem solving.

A final EMG assessment was done on the back of the neck and left and right trapezius areas. These values are presented in Table 13.1 accompanied by the EMG values from the same sites prior to treatment.

TABLE 13.1

PRETREATMENT, POSTTREATMENT, AND DIFFERENCE MEASURES FOR BACK OF NECK, LEFT, AND RIGHT TRAPEZIUS AREAS FOR MRS. E.

Area	Pretreatment	Posttreatment	Difference
Back of Neck	7.0 μV	3.75 μV	3.25 μV
Left Trapezius	6.5 μV	3.0 μV	3.5 μV
Right Trapezius	3.75 μV	2.0 μV	1.75 μV

As can be seen from Table 13.1, all EMG values had declined appreciably at the end of treatment. Mrs. E.'s church social was very enjoyable, and by her report went well. Her activity level continued to be within normal limits and she even played tennis with little discomfort. Some soreness after tennis only lasted for approximately fifteen to twenty minutes. Use of Robaxin continued to decline, with Mrs. E. taking one tablet only occasionally (every two to three days).

Discussion. Mrs. E. was seen for a total of thirty-nine visits over a fifteen-month period, including initial evaluation. During initial intervention with hypnotically facilitated biofeedback, she seemed to increase rather than decrease muscle tension and SUD values did not decline appreciably. Levels of medication use and activities also did not change. After a prescribed period of no treatment, the hypnotic strategy was changed to focus on changing Mrs. E.'s cognitive views of pain (what was happening to her when she hurt) with positive imagery and her methods of dealing with her emotions about the pain by suggesting increased confidence, activity, and success. Such a change was also coincidental with her husband's return home from a three-month absence due to duty in the Service. His return, however, was brief as he was only back six months when he left again for duty out West. She subsequently joined him, leaving the area about six months later.

Mrs. E. seemed to respond best to cognitive, emotion, and activity changes suggested through hypnosis and practiced with self-hypnosis. Focus on her pain and muscle tension served, seemingly, to increase rather than decrease levels of EMG as noted when EMG monitoring was terminated (see Figure 13.10). Control and mastery for Mrs. E. was useful not when the target was her pain and tension but when it was her cognitive view of the pain and her resultant emotions about it.

Final medical opinion on Mrs. E.'s improvement was that she remained with a small percentage of permanent disability of the upper left extremity related to her injury two years before. Some restrictions of gainful employment were anticipated but none that would result in a major disability. She was discharged on Robaxin, 500 mg., PRN. Final diagnosis was myofascial pain syndrome related to a lifting injury.

Summary

A multifaceted approach in managing pain employs biofeedback and/or hypnosis as tools which address not only the felt symptom of pain but the underlying complex of affective, cognitive, behavioral, and interpersonal variables as well. The fear, anxiety, and depression that are associated with chronic pain are the emotional factors that appear to be addressed in either biofeedback or hypnosis. The parallels between addressing pain as fear and pain as depression seem most helpful. Indeed, Seligman's (1974) conceptualization of depression as learned helplessness is most apt as a consideration in dealing with chronic pain.

Ultimately, focusing solely on symptom relief is not enough. As observed in some of the above cases, relief from symptoms is only accomplished by an overall strategy of intervention that is useful in coping with pain. Restructuring one's beliefs about the pain with the aid of biofeedback or hypnosis is probably one of the most effective strategies that can be attempted.

Biofeedback and hypnosis have also been shown to be useful in facilitating the effectiveness of other procedures such as behavior modification, using shaping and reinforcement principles, to promote a return to preinjury behavior, as illustrated in the case of Mrs. C. and Mr. D., and also interpersonal relationships, cognitions, and the reduction of medication use as in the case of Mrs. A. and Mrs. E.

Successful coping with, or recovery from, chronic pain needs to be assessed, similarly, from a variety of aspects, including, but not limited to, ratings of subjective discomfort, systematic observation of behavior, description of belief systems, and level and type of activity.

Finally, certain personality variables, most notably along dimensions of personal mastery and interpersonal control seem to be important considerations and determinants for successful management of chronic pain. Studies and case histories presented have demonstrated that control, a sense of mastery, is a major variable in helping someone successfully manage pain. If one thinks of the anxiety that we know accompanies uncertainty, then a patient's quest for control, certainty of effort, is quite expected.

Increased control, independence, and self-esteem seem to be major psychological changes that accompany pain relief regardless of which method is utilized. Of course, each approach needs to be tailored to the particular needs and/or personality of the individual patient.

REFERENCES

Achterberg, J., McGraw, P., & Lawlis, F. G. (1981), Rheumatoid arthritis: A study of relaxation and temperature biofeedback training as an adjunctive therapy. *Biofeed. & Self-Reg.*, V. 6/2:207–223.

Adams, J., Pearson, C. S., & Olson, N. (1982), Innovative cross-modal technique of pain intensity assessment with lower back pain patients given biofeedback training. *Amer. J. Clin. Biofeed.*, 5/1:25–30.

Adler, R., Bongar, B., & Katz, R. E. (1982), Psychogenic abdominal pain and parental pressure in childhood athletics. *Psychosom.* 23/11:1185–1186.

Araoz, D. L. (1983), Use of hypnotic techniques with oncology patients. *J. Psychosoc. Oncol.*, 1/4:47–54.

Baker, S. R. (1984), Amelioration of phantom-organ pain with hypnosis and behavior modification: Brief case report. *Psycholog. Rep.*, 55/3:847–850.

Beck, A. T. (1976), *Cognitive Therapy and the Emotional Disorders*. New York: International Universities Press.

Biedermann, J. H. (1983), Mechanism of biofeedback in the treatment of chronic back pain: An hypothesis. *Psycholog. Rep.*, 53/3, P. 2:1103–1108.

——Monga, N. T. (1985), Relaxation oriented EMG biofeedback with back pain patients: Evaluation of paraspinal muscle activity. *Clin. Biofeed. & Health*, 8/2:119–123.

Bissett, A., Mitchell, K. R., & Major, G. (1985), The cervico-brachial pain syndrome: Muscle activity and pain relief. *Behav. Change*, 2/2:129–135.

Bush, C., Ditto, B., & Feuerstein, M. (1985), A controlled evaluation of paraspinal EMG biofeedback in the treatment of chronic low back pain. *Health Psychol.*, 4/4:307–321.

Christidis, D., Ince, L. P., Zaretsky, H. H., & Pitchfort, L. J. (1986), A cross-modality approach for treatment of chronic pain: A preliminary report. *Psychosom. Med.*, 48/3–4:224–228.

Cram, J. R., & Freeman, C. W. (1985), Specificity in EMG biofeedback treatment of chronic pain patients. *Clin. Biofeed. & Health*, 8/2:101–108.

Crasilneck, H. B., & Hall, J. A. (1973), Clinical hypnosis in problems of pain. *Amer. J. Clin. Hypnosis*, 15/3:153–161.

Dahinteroval, J. (1967), Some experiences with the use of hypnosis in the treatment of burns. *Internat. J. Clin. & Experiment. Hypnosis*, 15/2:49–53.

Davidson, G. P. (1984), Hypnotic augmentation of terminal care chemonalgesia. *Austral. J. Clin. & Experiment. Hypnosis*, 12/2:133–134.

Dimond, R. E. (1981), Hypnotic treatment of a kidney dialysis patient. *Amer. J. Clin. Hypnosis*, 23/4:284–288.

Dumas, R. (1980), Cognitive control in hypnosis and biofeedback. *Internat. J. Clin. & Experiment. Hypnosis*, 28/1:53–62.

Elkins, G. R. (1984), Hypnosis in the treatment of myofibrositis and anxiety: A case report. *Amer. J. Clin. Hypnosis*, 27/1:26–30.

Flor, H., Haag, G., Turk, D. C., & Koehler, H. (1983), Efficacy of EMG biofeedback, pseudotherapy, and conventional medical treatment for chronic rheumatic back pain. *Pain*, 17/ 1:21–31.

Fordyce, W. E. (1976), *Behavioral Methods for Chronic Pain and Illness*. St. Louis, MI: C. V. Mosby.

Fricton, J. R., & Roth, P. (1985), The effects of direct and indirect hypnotic suggestions for analgesia in high and low susceptible subjects. *Amer. J. Clin. Hypnosis*, 27/4:226–231.

Grabel, J. A. (1973), Electromyographic study of low back muscle tension in subjects with and without chronic low back pain. *Diss. Abstr. Internat.*, 34/6-B:2929–2930E.

Harris, J. E. (1985), Hypnosis in the relief of pain in the cancer patient. *Med. Hypoanal.*, 6/1–2:64–65.

Hilgard, J. R., & LeBaron, S. (1982), Relief of anxiety and pain in children and adolescents with cancer: Quantitative measures and clinical observations. *Internat. J. Clin. & Experient. Hypnosis*, 30/4:417–442.

Howard, L, Reardon, J. P., & Tosi, D. (1982), Modifying migraine headache through rational stage directed hypnotherapy: A cognitive experiential perspective. *Internat. J. Clin. & Experiment. Hypnosis*, 30/3:257–269.

Keefe, F. J., Crisson, J. E., & Trainor, M. (1987), Observational methods for assessing pain: A practical guide. In: *Applications in Behavioral Medicine and Health Psychology: A Clinician's Source Book*, eds: D. C. McKee & J. A. Blumenthal. Sarasota, Florida: Professional Resource Exchange, pp. 67–94.

Kellerman, J., Zeltzer, L., Ellenberg, L., & Dash, J. (1983), Adolescents with cancer:

Hypnosis for the reduction of the acute pain and anxiety associated with medical procedures. *J. Adol. Health Care*, 4/2:85–90.

Kleinsorge, H. (1967), Hypnosis, long term treatment of severe bodily suffering. *Revue De Medecine Psychosomatique et de Psychologie Medicale*, 9/1:39–43.

Kravitz, E. A. (1978), EMG feedback and differential relaxation training to promote pain relief in chronic low back pain patients. *Diss. Abstr. Internat.*, 39/3-B:1485–1486E.

LaCroix, R., & Gauthier, J. (1984), A successful treatment program for reducing chronic pain behaviors. *Scand. J. Behav. Ther.*, 13/3:163–171.

Large, R. G., & Lamb, A. M. (1983), Electromyographic (EMG) feedback in chronic musculoskeletal pain: A controlled trial. *Pain*, 17/2:167–177.

Lemmon, K. W. (1983), Chronic lower back pain differentiation of the real and imagined. *Med. Hypnoanal.*, 4/1:17–30.

Levit, H. I. (1973), Depression, back pain and hypnosis. *Amer. J. Clin. Hypnosis*, 15/4:266–269.

Long, P. (1986), Medical mesmerism. *Psychology Today*, 20/1:28–29.

Magnusson, E., Hedberg, B., & Tunved, J. (1981), Heart rate control and aversive stimulation. *Biolog. Psychol.*, 12/ 2–3:211–222.

Margolis, C. G. (1982), Hypnotic imagery with cancer patients. *Amer. J. Clin. Hypnosis*, 25/2–3:128–134.

———(1985), Hypnotic interventions for pain management. *Internat. J. Psychosom.*, 32/3:12–19.

Medical Hypnoanalysis Society (1984), Commentary on "Society." Annual meeting. In: *Proceeding* Ann Arbor: MI: Medical Hypnoanalysis Society. 6/3:117–119.

Melzack, R. (1973), *The Puzzle of Pain*. New York: Basic Books.

———Perry, C. (1975), Self-regulation of pain: The use of alpha-feedback and hypnotic training for the control of chronic pain. *Experiment. Neurol.*, Vol. 46(3), pp. 452–469.

——— ———(1976), Self-regulation of pain: The use of alpha feedback and hypnotic training for the control of chronic pain. In: *Biofeedback, Behavior Therapy and Hypnosis*; ed. I. Wickramasekera, Chicago: Nelson-Hall.

———Weisz, A. F., & Sprague, L. P. (1963), Strategems for controlling pain: Contributions of auditory stimulation and suggestion. *Experiment. Neurol.*, 8:239–247.

Nigl, A. J. (1981), A comparison of binary and analog EMG feedback techniques in the treatment of low back pain. *Ameri. J. Clin. Biofeed.*, 4/1:25–31.

Nouwen, A. (1983), EMG biofeedback used to reduce standing levels of paraspinal muscle tension in chronic low back pain. *Pain*, 17/4:353–360.

O'Brien, C. P., & Weisbrot, M. M. (1983), Behavioral and psychological components of pain management. *Nat. Inst. on Drug Abuse: Res. Monogr. Series,* Monogr.: 45, pp. 36–45.

Onorato, V. A., & Tsushima, W. T. (1983), EMG, MMPI, and treatment outcome in the biofeedback therapy of tension headache and post-traumatic pain. *Amer. J. Clin. Biofeed.*, 6/2:71–81.

Pearce, S., & Morley, S. (1981), An experimental investigation of pain production in headache patients. *Brit. J. Clin. Psychol.*, 20/4:275–281.

Pelletier, K. R., & Peper, E. (1977), Developing a biofeedback model: Alpha EEG feedback as a means for pain control. *Internat. J. Clin. & Experiment. Hypnosis*, 25/4:361–371.

Pitzele, S. K. (1985), *We Are Not Alone—Learning to Live with Chronic Illness.* New York: Workman.

Reeves, J. L., & Shapiro, D. (1982), Heart rate biofeedback and cold pressor pain. *Psychophysiol.*, 19/4:393–403.

Sacerdote, P. (1970), Theory and practice of pain control in malignancy and other protracted or recurring painful illness. *Internat. J. Clin. & Experiment. Hypnosis*, 18/3:160–180.

———(1978), Teaching self-hypnosis to patients with chronic pain. *J. Hum. Stress*, 4/2:18–21.

Sachs, L. B., Feuerstein, M., & Vitale, J. H. (1977), Hypnotic self-regulation of chronic pain. *Amer. J. Clin. Hypnosis*, 20/2:106–113.

Schafer, D. W. (1975), Hypnosis use on a burn unit. *Internat. J. Clin. & Experiment. Hypnosis*, 23/1:1–14.

Schwartz, D. P. (1984), A chronic emergency room visitor with chest pain: Successful treatment by stress management training and biofeedback. *Pain*, 18/3:315–319.

Seligman, M. E. P. (1974), Depression and learned helplessness. In: *The Psychology of Depression: Contemporary Theory and Research*, eds. R. J. Friedman & M. M. Katz. Washington: Winston-Wiley.

Smith, S. J., & Balaban, A. B. (1983), A multidimensional approach to pain relief: Case report of a patient with systemic lupus erythematosus. *Internat. J. Clin. Experiment. Hypnosis*, 31/2:72–81.

Spanos, N. P., McNeil, C. Gwynn, M. I., & Stam, H. J. (1984), Effects of suggestion and distraction on reported pain in subjects high and low on hypnotic susceptibility. *J. Abnorm. Psychol.*, 93/3:277–284.

Spence, N. D. (1984), Relaxation training for chronic pain patients using EMG feedback: An analysis of process and outcome effects. *Austral. N. Ze. J. Psychiat.*, 18/3:263–272.

Spiegel, D., & Bloom, J. R. (1983), Group therapy and hypnosis reduce metastatic breast carcinoma pain. *Psychosom. Med.*, 45/4:333–339.

Stam, H. J., McGrath, P. A., & Brooke, R. I. (1984), The effects of a cognitive-behavioral treatment program on temporo-mandibular pain and dysfunction syndrome. *Psychosom. Med.*, 46/6:534–545.

Stenn, P. G., Mothersill, K. J., & Brooke, R. I. (1979), Biofeedback and a cognitive behavioral approach to treatment of myofascial pain dysfunction syndrome. *Behav. Ther.*, 10/1:29–36.

Subotnik, K. L., & Shapiro, D. (1984), Heart rate biofeedback and cold pressor pain: Effects of expectancy. *Biofeed. & Self-Reg.*, 9/1:55–75.

Sweet, J. J. (1981), The MMPI in evaluation of response to treatment of chronic pain. *Amer. J. Clin. Biofeed.*, 4/2:121–130.

Thomas, J. E. (1984), Management of pain in sickle cell disease using biofeedback therapy: A preliminary study. *Biofeed. & Self-Reg.*, 9/4:413–420.

Toomey, T. C., & Sanders, S. (1983), Group hypnotherapy as an active control strategy in chronic pain. *Amer. J. Clin. Hypnosis*, 26/1:20–25.

Trifiletti, R. J. (1984), The psychological effectiveness of pain management procedures in the context of behavioral medicine and medical psychology. *Genet. Psychol. Monogr.*, 109/2:251–278.

Tsushima, W. T. (1982), Treatment of phantom limb pain with EMG and temperature biofeedback: A case study. *Amer. J. Clin. Biofeed.*, 5/2:150–153.

Volgyesi, F. A. (1972), Pain and hypnosis: Multidimensional psychotherapy and general medical practice. *J. Amer. Inst. Hypnosis*, 13/6:255–259.

Wickramasekera, I. (1976), *Biofeedback, Behavior Therapy and Hypnosis.* Chicago, IL: Nelson-Hall.

Willard, R. D. (1974), Perpetual trance as a means of controlling pain in the treatment of terminal cancer with hypnosis. *J. Amer. Inst. Hypnosis,* 15/3:111,131.

Williams, J. A. (1983), Ericksonian hypnotherapy of intractable shoulder pain. *Amer. J. Clin. Hypnosis,* 26/1:26–29.

Zeltzer, L., & LeBaron, S. (1983), Behavioral intervention for children and adolescents with cancer. *Behav. Med. Update,* 5/2–3:17–22.

14

Stress Management and Chronic Pain

CYNTHIA D. BELAR, PH.D.

The goals of stress management programs for chronic pain patients are to correct maladaptive behavior and to transfer the skills learned during treatment to real life situations. The maladaptive behavior involved may be affective, cognitive, physiological, or overt action in nature. In this model of treatment, the patient is not the passive recipient of some medical intervention, but rather must actively assume responsibility for return to health, or maintenance of it. The reduction of pain may be a goal, but where not possible, acceptance of, and coping with, pain is emphasized. Return to maximal functioning in recreational, occupational, social, and family activities or relationships is central to program goals. Change within the clinic setting alone is insufficient.

Stress management programs, although individually tailored, have three themes in common. (1) There is an educational theme in which the patient comes to understand the relationships among cognitions, affect, behavior, physiology, and pain. (2) There are interventions designed to help the patient control stressors (i.e., *inputs* to stress) and variables thought to exacerbate pain. These stressors may involve either actual environmental events or perceptions of environmental and/or internal events. Pain itself is considered a stressor. (3)

The chronic pain patient learns specific techniques in order to control the *outputs* of stress (behavior patterns, physiological responses).

The particular methods chosen for implementation of a stress management program should depend upon an understanding of the individual patient involved, which in turn requires a detailed initial patient assessment. Standardized "package" programs run the risk of (1) applying inappropriate interventions in an individual case, and (2) missing the opportunity to utilize a more precise (and perhaps less expensive) intervention which would be more appropriate to the individual case.

Assessments can be accomplished by one who is professionally and clinically trained in psychological and behavioral measurement. In addition to thorough interviewing and behavioral assessment methods, clinical psychologists have found some psychological tests to be useful. For example, scores on the Minnesota Multiphasic Personality Inventory (MMPI) have been used to predict surgical outcome (Wiltse and Rocchio, 1975: Blumetti and Modesti, 1976). However, it is important to note that the MMPI was originally normed on psychiatric patients, and that most currently available computerized interpretation systems would not be appropriate. Psychologists using the MMPI with chronic pain patients need to be aware of the data base associated with this population (Bradley, Prokop, Margolis, and Gentry, 1978).

Model for Assessment of Chronic Pain Patients

There are a number of different theories of pain, a review of which is outside the scope of this chapter. Suffice it to say that "specificity models" of pain have not been particularly useful; that is, in the study of pain it has been repeatedly found that there is only a loose link between specific noxious stimuli and the perception of pain, a link which is mediated by central nervous system (CNS) activity. While this fact appears intellectually obvious from a review of experimental data, health professionals in the clinical arena often tend to think in terms of specificity theory when assessing individual patients. If a particular noxious stimulus is thought to be insufficient to produce a patient's pain response, another "specific" process is often inferred (e.g., psychopathology).

Statements reflecting use of a specificity model of pain include: (1) "Mr. G.'s remaining pain is due to failure to sever some of the pain pathways during surgery." (2) "This patient is probably malingering; there's not enough tissue damage to cause the amount of pain this patient reports." (3) "Underlying conflicts concerning dependency needs account for this patient's pain problem." In the first case, the patient is likely to undergo further surgical or ablative procedures. In the second case, he or she may be shunted toward the mental health or legal system for intervention, while being denied further access to medical–surgical personnel. And in the third case, a conflict resolution type of psychotherapy is likely to be recommended. However, given the complexity of the phenomenon of pain, it is no wonder that focal interventions based on specificity models have often been ineffective for chronic pain patients.

Clinically it is important to view pain as a complex phenomenon with cognitive, affective, physiological, and behavioral components. This author has found that a combination of work by Melzack (1973) and Fordyce (1976) yields a model which is most useful in the understanding, assessment, and treatment of chronic pain patients from a psychological perspective. The components of this model are presented in Table 14.1. However, it is noted that the components described do not reflect mutually exclusive, noninteractive categories. They are presented for conceptual, organizing purposes only.

TABLE 14.1

TARGET AREAS FOR ASSESSMENT OF CHRONIC PAIN PATIENTS

Sensory Component

Stimuli From Disease Process
Attention/Distraction

Affective Component

Anxiety
Depression
Feelings of Control

Cognitive Component

Expectations
Attributions of Source and Meaning of Pain
Health Beliefs

Sociocultural Components

Familial Models
Cultural Features

Positive Reinforcement

Money
Attention
Nurturance
Drugs (type and regimen pattern)
Activity Pattern

Negative Reinforcement

Interpersonal Conflicts
Job Stressors
Family Responsibilities
Intrapersonal Conflicts (sex, aggression, dependency)
Perceptions of Problem as Psychogenic or Malingering
Psychopathology
Compensatory Behaviors (body positioning, medication usage)

Rewards for Well Behavior

Employment Opportunities
Family Members' Behavior
Consequences of Sick Role and Inactivity

SENSORY COMPONENT

Melzack (1973) describes sensory, affective–motivational and cognitive–evaluative aspects of pain. The sensory component involves noxious stimulation that results from the disease process or injury. However, this sensory component of pain does not exist in isolation, but can be affected by psychological variables such as the affective and cognitive components. The effects of anticipation of an injection is a good example. With the expectation of pain, there is increased anxiety, which results in increased muscle tension, which results in more pain when injected. With respect to chronic pain, while surgery might relieve the pressure on a nerve, other problems often remain (e.g., fears of disability, decreased sexual activity, financial concerns) which cause tension, muscle spasms, pressure on nerves, and an increase in pain, which in turn produces more anxiety and tension.

Attention can also affect the sensory component. At nighttime many pain patients report an increase in sensations of pain. While other variables might also be important, it is possible that a lack of external stimuli to attract attention at this time could result in increased internal focusing, and thus more pain. In conducting an assessment the clinician needs to understand not only sensory factors involved in the patient's disease process, but also attentional factors, opportunities for distraction, and the interrelationships with affective and cognitive components.

Affective Component

The affective component involves the feelings that the patient has about his or her pain problem, or while experiencing pain. A number of studies have demonstrated the relationships among pain, anxiety, and depression. In general, both experimental and clinical subjects who experience more anxiety or depression report more pain (Sternbach, 1974). An assessment is not complete without thorough exploration of these areas.

Feelings of helplessness and lack of control are also associated with reports of increased pain. Prior to the more recent application of self-efficacy theories to pain, work by Davison and his colleagues in the area of psychophysiology had demonstrated the importance of perceived control in mediating arousal to aversive stimulation. One of the most interesting findings from this work was that *belief* in control over aversive stimulation was actually more important than *real* control in producing lower levels of autonomic nervous system arousal. (Geer, Davison, and Gatchel, 1970). This particular finding is fundamental to a number of intervention strategies utilized in stress management programs for chronic pain patients.

Cognitive Component

Already alluded to in the discussion of perceived control, the cognitive component of pain refers to the judgments of the individual about the pain experience. What are his expectations about pain? What is the meaning of the pain to the individual? One reason why the soldiers that Beecher (1959) described may have required fewer narcotic analgesics than their civilian counterparts has to do with the meaning of pain to these individuals. For the soldiers, the injury meant relief (with honor) from the stress of the front lines. For the civilian counterparts, injury represented a disruption in everyday life and a withdrawal from loved ones.

Patient attributions with respect to source or meaning of pain must be carefully explored in order to design meaningful intervention programs. As an example, the author remembers well the patient whose aunt had died from a brain tumor that had gone undiagnosed despite her many complaints of headache. The patient, himself diagnosed as suffering from tension headache, believed that he was following in his aunt's footsteps and was quite fearful of another misdiagnosis. Had therapy been designed to correct a maladaptive physiological response (e.g., electromyographic biofeedback for scalp muscle contraction) without attention to this important variable affecting his experience of pain, it would have been unlikely to succeed.

The well-known placebo effect, also a cognitive component of pain, involves expectations concerning the experience of pain. Recent research has demonstrated that this effect has neurophysiological underpinnings related to the endorphins in that it can be blocked by nalaxone (a morphine antagonist).

Rather than viewing the placebo as a nuisance, stress management programs for chronic pain attempt to capitalize upon its effects, and train patients to exert more voluntary control over this phenomenon.

Sociocultural Components

It has been well established that cultural factors play a significant role in the way an individual perceives and responds to pain. Thus the clinician must understand the cultural background of the individual patient, exploring specific ethnic features with which he or she is unfamiliar. Familial models are powerful conveyors of cultural values, and may be models for either chronic pain or disability themselves. Careful history taking is an important component of the assessment process.

Behavioral Components

Fordyce (1976) described the behavioral components related to chronic pain. A fundamental premise is that since pain is a subjective experience, knowledge of pain is completely dependent upon patient *behavior*, either verbal or nonverbal. These behaviors are influenced by the same factors that influence all behavior (i.e., learning principles), even if the initial cause of the pain is not learned. In fact, the chronicity of a pain problem insures that even more opportunities for learning will occur, thus over time psychological factors may become increasingly important as bodily systems and behavior become conditioned. For example, if a truck driver who has spent many weeks away from home suffers an injury and is no longer able to work, he engages in a new behavior pattern—staying home. This in turn produces changes in reactions from family members, which in turn may affect his behavior, and so forth.

In summary, Fordyce asserts that there are psychological–behavioral components in *all* chronic pain patients. Thus, concepts such as "psychogenic pain," often reflect oversimplistic, dualistic mind–body thinking and are to be avoided. Psychological–behavioral components of pain should be assessed and described for every chronic pain patient in order to design comprehensive care. Specific areas to be assessed include direct positive rewards for pain, the avoidance learning aspects of pain behavior, and rewards that the patient experiences for the absence of pain.

Positive Reinforcement for Pain Behavior

Pain behavior can be positively reinforced through monetary awards for illness. In order to be seen as a legitimate recipient of disability payments, the patient must behave in a manner consistent with the socially accepted definition of "illness." While money is a powerful reward against which treatment supporting well behavior must compete, disability payments are not necessarily a contraindication to treatment. However, this author does defer treatment if it is known that liability litigation is in process. While it is not proposed that monetary aid be discontinued for patients with chronic pain problems, it is asserted that the design of these compensation systems should be reevaluated. Health professionals who are seriously interested in treatment of chronic pain patients would do well to spend a part of their time interfacing with health policymakers in this regard.

Another direct reward which might exacerbate pain is medication. Many analgesics produce a sense of well-being. When medication is taken on a PRN basis, the experience of pain must increase before medication (and the resultant sense of well-being) is warranted. Thus a contingency is set up in which pain becomes directly reinforced by the taking of medication. Many treatment programs use a fixed interval of pain medication in an attempt to avoid this difficulty. Other investigators report that withdrawal of analgesics alone is sometimes sufficient to decrease pain (Sternbach, 1974). The pattern of pain report in these cases closely resembles the well-known extinction curve which suggests that the behavior was under the influence of a positive reinforcer. (Following withdrawal of a positive reinforcer, the behavior initially increases, then decreases to a level lower than prior to treatment.)

Pain can also be directly reinforced by the programming of rest. Activity to the point of maximum pain tolerance (common advice given by physicians) can result in the relief or pleasant aspects of rest becoming contingent upon the experience of pain. Thus activity patterns need to be assessed.

The special attention, sympathy, and nurturance that patients receive for pain are other potential reinforcers. This includes medical attention, which is usually contingent upon complaints of pain and which is needed as proof of illness to family and friends. Medical attention is also sometimes sought as a substitute when other kinds of personalized attention are lacking in an individual's life. Related to this is the hypothesis that early unmet dependency needs make one more susceptible to a chronic sick role in later life (i.e., certain reinforcers may be prepotent). Early work by Gentry, Shows, and Thomas (1974) did illustrate that chronic pain patients tended to be later-born, with many siblings. They began work at a young age (mean = 16 years), married early, and assumed family responsibilities while still quite young.

Negative Reinforcement For Pain Behavior

Pain can also be reinforced through serving a protective function; that is, experience of pain might actually increase because it results in the avoidance of an aversive situation. This avoidance learning is a very powerful form of learning which is often difficult to change (and which many believe is the mechanism underlying much of neurotic behavior). Areas of potential negative reinforcement of pain behavior which need to be assessed include interpersonal conflicts; job stressors; family responsibilities; and intrapersonal conflicts in the areas of aggression, sex, and dependency. The familiar saying, "Not tonight, dear, I have a headache," reflects how problems in the area of sex might be avoided through the experience of pain, and thus the frequency of painful episodes might increase. Family responsibilities or the need to assert oneself with one's boss might also be avoided through adoption of the sick role.

Pain behavior can also be increased by the need to avoid any suggestion of having "imaginary" or "psychogenic" pain, since these labels are socially unacceptable. Thus the clinician needs to understand what language the physician has used in discussing the patient's problem, and the perceptions of the patient which have been communicated by the health-care system and the patient's environment (family, friends, employer). Many of our patients have assumed that when their physician stated there was nothing more to offer medically or surgically, he meant that the problem was "all in my head."

It should also be recognized that chronic pain and the related sick role can serve as an organizing feature for an individual's thoughts or life, without which he or she might appear more seriously psychologically disturbed. However, on the surface these patients often appear quite normal. The assessment of this potential is crucial, as significant errors in treatment design can be made if the level of psychopathology is underestimated.

Interestingly, pain can also be exacerbated by the avoidance of pain itself. For example, medication use is reinforced by the avoidance of continued pain; thus, in addition to the positive reinforcement effects on pain noted above, patients become increasingly dependent upon pill taking as they attempt to avoid future pain. Finally, the compensatory body positions adopted by many patients in an attempt to avoid pain often produce other pain problems. Whereas a pain problem may begin with a low back injury, over time the pain "spreads"; several years later the patient may be complaining of neck and shoulder pain as well as chronic headache. Physicians are then often convinced that the problem must be "psychogenic"; more than one of our patients have been given such feedback. However, this pattern can be easily explained by the musculoskeletal consequences of years of compensatory body positioning, which in an attempt to avoid pain has created other pain problems.

The potential effects of avoidance learning on pain, like other aspects of pain, requires careful assessment. The health professional needs to understand *what* the patient might be avoiding through the experience of pain or related pain behavior, and *why*. Does this avoidance reflect a lack of skills in dealing with the situation, an unalterable aversive environment, or significant psychopathology? What part of the current problems might be due to the *consequences* of behaviors adopted as a means to avoid pain?

Lack of Rewards for Well Behavior

For many pain patients, there are insufficient rewards for well behavior (while pain behavior is being both positively and negatively reinforced). Employers often hesitate to reinstate chronic pain patients (on the advice of insurance companies), and families tend to overprotect the sick. Family members may actually prevent and punish self-care activities (e.g., "Don't do that! You know what will happen."). In addition, the consequences of being in the sick role with its concomitant inactivity are significant. The patient may lose occupational skills and social contacts. And inactivity per se has physiological consequences that diminish the probability of future successful performance of well behaviors.

In designing a stress management program for pain behavior, as with any other behavior change program, it is important to remember that the elimination of pain behavior will not insure that well behavior will replace it. In fact, the longer the history of the problem, the greater are the hazards in this area.

Developing a Stress Management Program

The experienced clinician, after thoroughly assessing the above pain problem components, makes decisions about what interventions to employ in a stress management program. Although specific algorithms for these choices are not yet available from the research literature, the clinician considers (1) the relative importance of the intervention target in the patient's overall chronic pain problem; (2) the effectiveness of the intervention; (3) the estimated probability of change in the intervention target given an understanding of its relationship with other patient features; (4) the cost and efficiency of the intervention; (5) the skill of the clinician in delivering the intervention. In all cases, it is the pain *patient* who is being treated, not chronic pain.

Concomitantly, referrals to other health professionals are made to insure adequate treatment of aspects not within the competence of the clinician. It should be emphasized here that chronic pain is not the province of any one discipline, but often requires a multidisciplinary approach for successful intervention. While the mental health professional may be competent to assess and treat psychological and behavioral components, other disciplines are required to provide information in the assessment process (e.g., disease process information, assessment of strength), or to participate in the treatment process (body mechanics training, analgesic prescription, vocational training).

As indicated previously, stress management programs involve (1) education; (2) use of techniques to control stressors and variables which exacerbate pain; and (3) learning of skills to deal with the behavioral and physiological outputs of pain and stress. The interventions commonly used for the various components of pain problems are presented in Table 14.2. However, as in the model for assessment, this conceptualization is not meant to portray categories as mutually exclusive, nor interventions as having effects on only one component.

Sensory Component

The sensory component of a chronic pain problem can be affected by various methods of psychophysiological self-regulation. The patient who learns the relaxation response can counteract the physiological effects of the stress reaction. It has been well documented that relaxation is associated with de-

TABLE 14.2

INTERVENTION STRATEGIES FOR STRESS MANAGEMENT OF CHRONIC PAIN

Sensory Component
- Relaxation Training
- Biofeedback
- Distraction
- Hypnosis

Affective Component
- Reassurance
- Social Support
- Anxiety Management
- Depression Management
- Imagery Training
- Psychotropic Medication

Cognitive Component
- Education in Conceptual model
- Threat Reappraisal
- Monitoring Procedures
- Stress Inoculation

Sociocultural Components
- Pain Classes
- Coping Models

Behavioral Components
- Contingency Management
  - Fixed Interval Medications
  - Gradual Medication Withdrawal
  - Family Counseling
  - Rewards For Well Behavior
  - Activity to Quota vs. Tolerance
- Conflict Resolution
- Skill Training (assertion, sexual, communication)
- Environmental Change

creased arousal to aversive stimuli and increased pain tolerance in chronic pain patients (Turk, Meichenbaum, and Genest, 1983; Feuerstein, Labbé, and Kuczmierczyk, 1986). In addition, if the patient can learn to control the noxious stimulus in the pathophysiology of the pain problem (e.g., muscle spasm, vasomotor spasm), he is likely to experience significant relief. Specific methods by which this psychophysiological self-regulation is accomplished include progressive muscle relaxation training, autogenic training, and various forms of biofeedback training (e.g., electromyographic, thermal).

Obviously, psychophysiological self-regulation affects more than the sensory component of pain. Successful experience in self-control affects perceived control and feelings of helplessness, and thus has both affective and cognitive consequences in the management of pain.

Another intervention aimed at the sensory component consists of attention diversion and distraction strategies. Just as the instruction to "not think" about a pink elephant is likely to be ineffective, one cannot "ignore" pain on command. However, a patient can substitute other imagery, attend to environmental cues, engage in mental arithmetic, and so forth. In fact, the distraction techniques that require more attentional processes tend to be more effective in pain control (McCaul and Malott, 1984). Hypnosis training can also be utilized to focus attention in a manner which blocks sensory pain signals from awareness.

Affective Component

Reassurance and social support are two time-honored methods for promoting health and wellness but are often insufficient in dealing with complex chronic pain problems. Nevertheless, this author has found the social support and social learning aspects of chronic pain groups to be very helpful in promoting change. Reassurance that the clinician does not believe the pain is "imaginary" is mandatory.

Specific interventions for the purpose of anxiety management and depression management are often necessary in dealing with affective components of pain. These may include psychological therapies or pharmacologic methods, or combinations thereof. It is now well accepted that antidepressant medication can relieve some chronic pain, but the mode of action is as yet unclear. Recent studies do suggest an analgesic rather than an antidepressant effect in this phenomenon (Feinmann, 1985).

Strategies which involve positive or neutral imagery can block anxiety and facilitate coping with, or reduction of, pain. For example, the patient can train himself to imagine a nonpainful or pleasant experience (e.g., being on the beach, a time in history prior to pain onset), or to redefine the painful sensation (e.g., trivial versus catastrophic). The preparation-to-cope stage of stress inoculation procedures (Turk et al., 1983) helps reduce feelings of helplessness and lack of control. These strategies have obvious cognitive and sensory effects as well.

Cognitive Component

As indicated before, an educational theme is common to all stress management programs. Specifically, the patient needs a conceptual model by which to understand the relationships among sensory, affective, cognitive, and behavioral components of pain. Face validity of the model is perhaps more important here than scientific validity. We utilize the one described in this chapter, but modify its presentation depending upon the health belief model of the patient.

Monitoring procedures (e.g., pain diaries) can also promote understanding. These procedures, in addition to biofeedback and relaxation training, can promote "physiological insight" in patients who tend not to be psychologically minded. Moreover, they involve concrete, fairly nonthreatening behaviors which facilitate patient involvement in the treatment process as well as monitor treatment progress.

Misattributions of the source or meaning of pain must be corrected. Sometimes simple information provision is sufficient to accomplish this. In other cases, psychotherapy techniques are necessary to work through a long history of maladaptive prior conditioning. Hypnosis procedures can be utilized to facilitate elicitation of the placebo effect.

Stress inoculation procedures as described by Turk and his colleagues (1983) involve both direct action (e.g., preparation for the stressor, relaxation) and cognitive coping components (e.g., positive self-statements), and thus have direct effects upon expectations concerning pain.

Sociocultural Components

While the clinician is powerless to change the culture within which the patient lives, pain classes facilitate patient interaction, exposure to other cultural values, and the opportunity for reexamination of values which may hinder treatment progress. In addition, the use of coping models has been found to be very effective in pain management. One strategy is to have previous patients return to participate in peer counseling—a strategy that reinforces the gains of the individual treatment strategies.

Positive Reinforcement

Policy systems interventions are required to change many of the contingencies between money and pain behavior, and are thus outside the scope of individual treatment programs. It has already been noted that if the treatment program is expected to compete against the potential windfall resulting from liability litigation, success is less likely. Family, friends, and significant persons in the health-care system can be counseled to change contingencies for attention and nurturance from pain behavior to well behavior. In many cases the patient himself can be trained to provide this counseling.

If analgesics are not to be withdrawn entirely, then prescriptions can be urged on a fixed interval versus a PRN basis. Activities can be based on quota systems rather than having the patient "work to tolerance." Pacing is a fundamental principle in pain management programs, and one which many patients report is the most useful in their own self-management.

Negative Reinforcement

To deal with problems of avoidance learning affecting chronic pain, the patient may need to learn new skills (e.g., assertion, sexual functioning, body mechanics, communication) or work through psychological conflicts (i.e., reappraise threat value). In some cases, maintenance of a chronic pain role syndrome may be appropriate, for there is little effective treatment to offer for problems that may become apparent once the avoidance learning is deconditioned.

In other cases, if an environmental stressor is viewed as a problematic source of negative reinforcement, strategies for avoidance other than illness, a change in an aspect of the environment, or a change of environment itself might be recommended.

Rewards for Well Behavior

Nearly all stress management programs involve an increase in activities which compete with pain behavior. This may involve counseling of employers and family members with respect to providing rewards for well behavior. It also involves developing the skills and body conditioning necessary to be "eligible" for such rewards, (although development of appropriate "complaint behavior" can be a first step).

Obviously not all interventions are utilized for each patient. As indicated previously, stress management programs are individually designed. To illustrate the heterogeneity of chronic pain patients, the following case examples are provided.

Case Examples

Case 1. A Seventy-One-Year-Old Woman With Chronic Back Pain

Mrs. A. was seventy-one years old and married, with a three-year history of marked paravertebral muscle spasm in the interscapular area (Belar and Cohen, 1979). This problem began three years prior to treatment, when she sustained multiple compression fractures of the thoracic spine after lifting a rock. Previous treatments had included novocaine injections, use of a brace, and transcutaneous nerve stimulation, all without significant relief. On intake she reported that she could not stand on her feet to accomplish household chores, and that her husband completed most of the housework. She experienced at least one severe muscle spasm per day which sent her to bed for at least one hour. Emotional upset increased her pain. Psychological evaluation (which included diagnostic interview, pain diary, and MMPI) did not reveal significant problem areas in affective or cognitive components, nor was there evidence of substantial sources of positive or negative reinforcement for pain behavior. Electromyographic (EMG) recordings revealed highly variable muscle tension activity.

The decision was made to utilize an intervention designed to directly modify the noxious stimuli arising from the pathophysiology involved (i.e., the muscle spasms). Other interventions were not thought to be necessary. Mrs. A. was given seventeen sessions of EMG biofeedback, with recording site being just below the right inferior scapular angle. Progressive relaxation training was also employed. Backache activity dropped from an average of 1.17 backaches per day per week to 0.43 backaches per day per week during the same period in which her activity level actually increased. Mean EMG level and EMG variability also significantly dropped from the baseline to follow-up period. She believed that she was able to anticipate a backache by attending to muscle tension cues, and to abort its onset by practicing the relaxation response. At one-year follow-up Mrs. A. continued to remain active; she was driving, shopping, doing housework, entertaining, and sewing (an activity she had avoided for three years prior to treatment). Two years later her neighbor, having witnessed a "remarkable change" in Mrs. A., presented for treatment for herself. Unfortunately her problems were not so amenable to such a focal treatment.

Case 2. A Fifty-Five-Year-Old Male With Chronic Back Pain

Mr. J. was a fifty-five-year-old truck driver who injured his back lifting boxes approximately five years prior to treatment. He had subsequently undergone two surgical procedures, including one laminectomy and one spinal fusion. He complained of chronic low back pain, and pain which radiated down into his left leg. Neurosurgical evaluation did not reveal the need for further surgery. Psychological evaluation revealed that Mr. J. was anxious and depressed. He experienced fitful sleep, crying spells, loss of libido, and early morning awakening. Previously a sociable individual, he had withdrawn almost completely from friends and family. Family members were oversolicitious, yet increasingly frustrated. Mr. J. felt guilty about his lack of ability to sustain employment, and believed that he had no right to participate in hobbies or recreational activities if he could not work to earn money for his family.

Multiple targets of intervention were chosen for this patient. He was referred to a physical therapist for exercise planning and body mechanics training. He saw a psychiatrist who prescribed antidepressant medication, and he joined a coping with pain class which met once a week for ten weeks. Classes included information about the sensory, affective, cognitive, and behavioral components of pain. Specific application of these principles to individual patients was emphasized. Patients were encouraged to help each other identify behavior patterns that may exacerbate pain problems. Goal setting and pacing were underscored. Homework assignments were made weekly. Patients were taught how to train significant others in principles of pain management; relaxation training, imagery training, or biofeedback was practiced the last half-hour of each session.

By the end of treatment Mr. J. lost fifteen pounds; he no longer used his cane for routine activity; he was involved in social and recreational activities; he had investigated retraining in small appliance repair; he noted an improvement in mood, sleep, and self-esteem; and he had resumed sexual functioning with his wife. His pain remained about the same, but he reported increased ability to cope with it. He stated that he did not seem to "suffer" as much with his pain problem, and in general felt more in control of his life.

Case 3. A Twenty-Three-Year-Old Male With Chronic Neck and Shoulder Pain

Mr. G. was a twenty-three-year-old medical student. He suffered from neck and shoulder pain, made worse by studying. Medical workups were negative other than to suggest "muscle tension." Mr. G. was on the verge of dropping out of medical school because of his health problems, but had no other vocational plans. He denied interpersonal or emotional problems, nor did he admit to any relationship between stressors and his pain (other than studying). He was quite defensive about having been sent to see a psychologist, but was willing to "try anything if it made scientific sense." Except for some defensiveness on MMPI, psychological evaluation was not remarkable, although there was a paucity of information concerning interpersonal relationships available. Electromyograph (EMG) recordings suggested mildly elevated trapezius muscle tension.

Treatment began with bilateral EMG biofeedback of trapezius muscle tension, plus home relaxation training and a consultation regarding body mechanics. The treatment rationale was described in rather technical and circumscribed terms (initially utilizing a specificity model of pain!) in keeping with the patient's health belief model. As treatment progressed, the therapist made nonthreatening casual inquiries as to other areas of functioning, commented on increased levels of muscle tension when noted, and raised "hypotheses" for the patient to test concerning his own behavior. The patient soon began to recount "pressures" from his father to become a physician, and his own concerns as to whether he could "shoulder this task." As he reexamined the relationship with his father, reappraised perceived threats in his environment, and mastered self-management of muscle tension in the laboratory, he became more confident about his ability to make decisions for himself rather than in an effort to please his father. He decided that he could indeed drop out of medical school, but chose not to. Generalization of his self-management skills was practiced via his reading tedious journal articles while his trapezius muscles were monitored.

Case 4. A Forty-Five-Year-Old Woman With Postmastectomy Pain

Ms. B. was forty-five years old and divorced. She suffered from severe postmastectomy pain along the site of the incision, for which her surgeon could not account. An interpersonally skilled woman, with good social support, she was having difficulty accepting the loss of her breast and was fearful that she would never find a partner who would accept her given that she was "less than a woman." She viewed the incision scar as lasting evidence of her dreaded cancer. While her physician had mentioned the possibility of reconstructive surgery, her focus on cancer had precluded her ability to plan for the future.

Ms. B. was referred back to her surgeon to obtain more information about reconstructive surgery. In addition, she was referred to a postmastectomy support group. This group provided not just social support, but examined issues of body image, what it meant to be feminine, and brought in role models of women who had coped with this procedure in the past. In addition, Ms. B. was trained in two kinds of imagery techniques. In one kind she relived times from the past in which she was pain-free and felt "feminine" (with a strong focus on aspects other than body traits); in the second kind she redefined the meaning of her scar as evidence of having successfully coped with an illness, with a focus on the degree of comfort that this would afford her. Ms. B. experienced a complete remission of pain symptoms within three months. At six months she had her first date.

Case 5. A Thirty-Two-Year-Old Woman With Migraine Headaches

Mrs. C. was a thirty-two-year-old woman who suffered from "lifelong" migraine headaches which had been uncontrolled by trials of Inderal, Cafergot, and Sansert. Some headaches were triggered by red wine and chocolate, but she noted no other identifiable pattern in headache activity. Headaches occurred on the average of twice per week, and resulted in her taking a good deal of sick leave. Mrs. C. was a middle management department head in a large corporation. Her job required long hours, presented conflicting pressures, and provided little support. Her husband was in upper management with another firm. She described marital tensions associated with her husband's frequent travel, but noted that he was always there when she "really needed" him (i.e., when she was sick). She was "hurt" that he never invited her on any of his business trips, and that he never encouraged her to quit her job to become a full-time housewife, which she would have preferred. She was either unable, or unwilling, to initiate discussion of this matter with him, as it might make her appear "weak" in his eyes.

It was hypothesized that in addition to the vascular processes related to migraine headache, significant interpersonal and intrapersonal concerns were exacerbating headache activity, specifically poor marital communication, unmet dependency needs, and inability to deal effectively with negative affect. It was thought that pain behavior was being reinforced by an avoidance of job stress, by attention and nurturance from her husband, and by avoidance of the experience of anger at her chosen source of dependency gratification. Treatment included relaxation training, assertiveness training, communication training, and conjoint sessions with her husband. Mrs. C. subsequently left her job, engaged in full-time work as a housewife, and accompanied her husband on more of his business trips. Headache frequency dropped to one per month. Both partners reported an increase in marital satisfaction.

These cases clearly underscore the heterogeneity of chronic pain patients (both medically and psychologically), the need for careful evaluation before undertaking treatment, and the variety of components that might be included within a treatment program. Case 1 needed to learn a specific physiological self-regulation skill. Contingency management, psychotherapy, and/or information alone would not have been sufficient to produce change. Case 2 needed a multifaceted treatment program, covering the breadth of pain components previously described. Case 3 required an increased sense of *self*-management, and entry into treatment via a technical biofeedback route in order to later develop "physiological insight." Case 4 needed to redefine the meaning of her pain problem and to deal with anxiety about the future. Case 5 needed to learn more direct methods for solving interpersonal and intrapersonal problems, and to have the reinforcement for her avoidance behavior terminated.

It is important to note that the report of pain may not always be the best outcome measure of these treatment programs. Case 2 is doing well, although still experiencing pain. If he had reported marked decrease in pain, but the depression had not improved and his life had not become more fulfilling, we would not have considered it a successful outcome. In addition, not every patient is suitable for the procedures mentioned, and certain patients require special monitoring when utilizing these techniques (borderlines and diabetics, respectively).

Guidelines for Practice

1. When possible, have medications prescribed in a fixed interval versus a PRN schedule. If patients beg for painkillers while asserting that they don't really work, try aspirin.
2. Encourage activity on a quota basis versus working to tolerance. Quotas should initially be set below tolerance level and gradually increased.
3. Contract for specific goals in the areas of occupational recreational, social, and family functioning.
4. Be prepared to provide sexual counseling and information concerning positions and activities for persons with various medical disabilities.
5. Interview family members as necessary, especially when the patient blandly denies family concerns.
6. When needed, facilitate retirement without shame or guilt, while encouraging the development of rewarding activities and hobbies.
7. Become comfortable with the biopsychosocial model of assessment and treatment, which involves the inseparability and interdependence of psychosocial and biologic components.
8. Reassure the patient that his or her pain is not "imaginary." Explain how bodily systems can become con-

ditioned and how pain can be affected by various components. Agree with some specificity aspect of pain if possible, given the prevalence of this model in the general population. Use the patient's language whenever appropriate.

9. Facilitate patient involvement in treatment via assignment of homework tasks, maintenance of diaries, responsibility for graphing own treatment data, becoming a peer counselor, making individual relaxation tapes.
10. Involve significant others in treatment as necessary.
11. Have the patient overlearn the relaxation response.
12. Don't attempt to "cure" the chronic pain patient. Take the attitude of a consultant or teacher who may be of use to the patient, who is ultimately responsible for behavior change.

In general, it should be remembered that while tender loving care is mandatory for acute pain patients, for chronic pain patients it may be destructive if made contingent upon pain behavior and suffering. Health professionals working with this population need to maintain genuineness and empathy, but also respect for the patient's integrity, and responsibility for his or her own self-management.

References

Beecher, H. K. (1959), *Measurement of Subjective Responses*. Oxford University Press.

Belar, C. D., & Cohen, J. L. (1979), The use of EMG feedback and progressive relaxation in the treatment of a woman with chronic back pain. *Biofeed. & Self-Reg.*, 4:345–353.

Blumetti, A. E., & Modesti, L. M. (1976), Psychological predictors of success or failure of surgical intervention for intractable back pain. In: *Advances in Pain Research and Therapy*, Vol. 1 eds. J. Bonica & D. Albe-Fessard. New York: Raven Press.

Bradley, L. A., Prokop, C. K., Margolis, R., & Gentry, W. D. (1978), Multivariate analyses of the MMPI profiles of low back patients. *J. Behav. Med.*, 1:253–272.

Feinmann, C. (1985), Pain relief by antidepressants: Possible modes of action. *Pain*, 23:1–8.

Feuerstein, M., Labbé, E. E., & Kuczmierczyk, A. R. (1986), *Health Psychology: A Psychobiological Perspective*. New York: Plenum Press.

Fordyce, W. E. (1976), *Behavioral Methods For Chronic Pain and Illness*. St. Louis: C. V. Mosby.

Geer, J. H., Davison, G. C., & Gatchel, R. (1970), Reduction of stress in humans through nonveridical perceived control of aversive stimulation. *J. Pers. & Soc. Psychol.*, 16:731–738.

Gentry, W.D., Shows, D., & Thomas, M. (1974), Chronic low back pain: A psychological profile. *Psychosom.*, 15:174–177.

McCaul, K. D., & Malott, J. M. (1984), Distraction and coping with pain. *Psycholog. Bull.*, 95:516–533.

Melzack, R. (1973), *The Puzzle of Pain.* New York: Basic Books.

Sternbach, R. A. (1974), *Pain Patients: Traits and Treatment.* New York: Academic Press.

Turk, D. C., Meichenbaum, D., & Genest, M. (1983), *Pain and Behavioral Medicine: A Cognitive–Behavioral Perspective.* New York: Guilford Press.

Wiltse, L. L., & Rocchio, P. D. (1975), Preoperative psychological tests and predictors of success of chemonucleolysis in the treatment of the low back syndrome. *J. Bone & J. Surg.*, 57:478–483.

15

Group Experience as Healing Process

EDITH W. M. HERMAN, PH.D., M.C.P.A.

Man is distressed not by things but by the view he takes of them.

—Epictetus

Nearly 500 years ago, Paracelsus, the Swiss-born alchemist and physician, said that in all of us reside powers of healing, and to promote health was to find means to rally them and to support them with therapy (Shontz,1975). With this statement, he pronounced the first holistic principle in the healing of man. During the last two decades, group approaches to chronic pain problems have been found to be effective in kindling and supporting these inherent mechanisms of "healing" to bring about therapeutic change in chronic pain patients refractory to traditional interventions.

The underlying philosophy of group work with chronic pain patients is to create a process which helps the patient to help himself as a sine qua non of achieving and maintaining therapeutic gains.

Within the last two decades, scientific and clinical interest in pain has been growing at an accelerating rate. Yet, despite considerable progress in our understanding of pain mechanisms, clinical interventions for pain states, and exciting new discoveries, it is not yet clear how all the pieces fit together. It is well recognized that pain perception is complex and not merely a function of noxious sensory input. One of the essential features of sensory pathways is the modulation of incoming pain messages and their elaboration and interpretation against a background of "noise" of other signals such as ongoing thoughts, hopes, fears, expectations, and past memories (Melzack, 1973, 1984). Signals that threaten the integrity of the organism, such as hunger (deprivation) and pain (tissue damage), result in motivational arousal (Mayer, 1979). Motivational states are invariably accompanied by arousal of the autonomic nervous systems, and in humans, by cognitions that are consistent with the perception, not the reality, of the problem. As a result, the behavior will be in accordance with the meaning that the individual attaches to the emotional arousal, not the event itself.

The threatening pain message derives its meaning from integration of neural messages at the cortical level. Its significance is then evaluated by associating it with stored memories of past experience and with the social environment. Once the threat of pain is cognitively appraised, available means to control it are selected from the options the environment offers (Chapman, 1976) and from the patient's adaptive repertoire (Bellissimo and Tunks, 1984). Pain, therefore, is not only determined by sensory input and the arousal of the sympathetic nervous system, but, and most importantly, by brain activities which can diminish or enhance pain signals. The brain has the ability to organize information by selection, elaboration, analysis, and abstraction from the total sensory input (Melzack, 1984). Despite great individual variation, these processes involve the whole individual and his total life experience: biological, psychological, social, and existential aspects are inseparably entwined and interactive (Melzack, 1973). In chronic pain states, the normative interaction between various biological systems has been disrupted, and an imbalance exists from the cellular (Terenius, 1978) to the social level (Payne and Norfleet, 1986).

There is compelling evidence to suggest that the experience of pain can be modified by interventions in each of the contributing dimensions: the sensory, affective–motivational, cognitive, and psychosocial component. The aim of any pain therapy is to ultimately restore homeostasis within a patient and between the patient and his environment. Whatever the treatment approach, it is prudent to remember that it is not the pain that requires treatment but the whole human being who suffers the pain (Lampe and Mannheimer, 1984).

The reason for successful outcomes of therapy in pain states of recent onset and of organic etiology is that pain is predominantly a function of sensory input from a discernible cause while the motivational and cognitive components of pain are adaptively engaged in restoring homeostatic balance. In acute pain states (as well as in experimentally induced pain), the patient (or subject) has a more or less clear meaning for his discomfort and full expectation of controlling it (contingent on his compliance with medical regimens). Acute pain states, therefore, usually respond favorably to traditional somatic interventions, and the patient's perception of "getting better" reinforces the adaptive spiral. Most clinicians also feel most comfortable to treat a condition within the biomedical model for which they were trained. This approach, however, is frequently inadequate for pain states that persist for longer than six months (Bonica, 1977; Bergman and Werblun, 1978). In chronic pain, physiological changes are manifested in alterations of the activity of levels of neurotransmitters (Sternbach, 1976; Yaksh, Howe, and Harty, 1984); psychologically, the patient lacks the main ingredients for successful therapy: meaning and control (Frank, 1978). Disenchanted with medical expertise after various specialists have given him numerous interpretations of the cause for his pain (which are frequently incomprehensible to him, or even contradictory), the patient's "hopelessness" is reflected in the high failure rate of his treatments. Having neither meaning for pain, nor the expectation of ever controlling it, jeopardizes the efficacy of treatments. Thus, although medical treatments may sometimes be a necessary condition for improving chronic pain states, they are frequently not a sufficient one. In chronic pain states, psychological interventions take on greater importance (Bellissimo and Tunks, 1984). In order to alter the pain perception, it is imperative that its "modifiers" be addressed, such as anxiety, behavior, motivation, cognitions, psychosocial distress, and even cultural factors (Wolff and Langley, 1975; Tursky and Sternbach, 1975; Bellissimo and Tunks, 1984). To address all components of the abnormal functional state "pain" requires combination therapies. The question of how to optimally rehabilitate a patient with chronic pain, however, has no simple formula answers, and rehabilitation techniques are as multivariate as pain is multifactorial (Turk and Flor, 1984; Oxman, 1986).

Since pain perception varies widely between individuals, the challenge lies in integrating the interventions in a coordinated treatment package tailored to the individual needs of the patient (Roy, Bellissimo and Tunks, 1982; Oxman, 1986); the convergent therapies are best provided in multidisciplinary pain clinics (Bonica, 1974, 1977; Newman, Seres, Yospe, and Garlington, 1978; Aronoff, Evans, and Enders, 1983; Moya and Mayne, 1986).

Whatever the etiology, patients referred to pain clinics do not seem to be typical of pain sufferers encountered in a family practice or in the general population (Tunks, 1987). When Pilowsky, Chapman, and Bonica (1977) applied the Illness Behavior Questionnaire (Pilowsky and Spence, 1976) to 100 pain clinic patients, the following profile emerged: the pain clinic patients differed from patients attending a family clinic inasmuch as they demonstrated a higher degree of preoccupation with disease conviction, somatic focusing, and denial of psychological problems. This profile is consistent with more recent findings comparing chronic pain syndromes in pain clinic patients with those of pain sufferers in the community. After Crook, Rideout, and Browne (1984) had conducted a survey to determine the prevalence of acute and chronic pain problems in the community, Crook and Tunks (1985) compared the features that characterized chronic pain sufferers in the community with those who were referred to the pain clinic. Although the two groups did not differ on demographic variables or etiology of pain, they were distinctly differentiated on psychosocial and behavioral variables. In pain clinic patients, pain seemed to interfere more with the patient's life-style (at home and by the loss of jobs), they reported a higher number of pending litigations and demonstrated more addictive behavior to alcohol and drugs. Clearly more depressed and socially alienated than their comparison group, they used health-care services more frequently and with less successful treatment outcomes (Tunks, 1987). For this patient group, traditional medical treatments as the sole approach seem to be ineffective (Turk and Flor, 1984); at best, they provide ephemeral relief of pain; at worst they aggravate the problem (multiple surgeries and iatrogenic effects of drugs). Rather than specific *treatment,* these patients require *management* of their multiple problems to effect therapeutic change.

The art of designing an effective treatment package for individual pain patients is to adapt the program to the patient, not the patient to the program (Kielhofner, 1986). A treatment combination which benefits one patient is not necessarily effective for another, despite identical diagnostic categories. Although treatment combinations present methodological problems for the researcher (as will be discussed later), from a clinical viewpoint, they enhance the probability of therapeutic success. Favorable treatment outcome also depends on a good therapist–patient relationship (Yalom, 1975; Bellissimo and Tunks, 1984; Oxman, 1986) and the amount of time and empathy the clinician offers the patient (Black, 1986).

What a patient thinks and how he behaves while in pain profoundly affects the pain he feels. The patient's thought patterns and behavior are, therefore, primary targets of psychological interventions to modify pain, and lend themselves well to being addressed in group approaches. Group strategies now employed have developed from a blend of the conceptual frameworks of cognitive and learning theories which will be briefly outlined in the following sections.

Group Programs for the Management of Chronic Pain

Current pain programs are mostly based on group approaches because the latter appear to be extremely suitable to address a diversity of problems with a variety of therapeutic procedures. Shared suffering becomes the basis for an adaptive learning process. In groups, a process can be created in which the maladaptive cycle of "abnormal illness behavior" (Pilowsky and Spence, 1976) and helplessness (Seligman, 1975) is reversed into an adaptive spiral. The patient's reconceptualization of his problem, effected by clear and comprehensible explanations of factors that contribute to his pain (Pilowsky and Basset, 1982), is followed by the learning of strategies to control these factors. Ensuing "well behavior" is the reward for learned resourcefulness. Group experience in pain management programs, therefore, involves foremost a learning process.

Not only can the group be used as a vehicle for education and the teaching of pain control strategies, it can also provide the curative factors of human contact, interpersonal learning, mutual support, and thus a corrective emotional experience (Yalom, 1975). Besides offering a means to integrate educative and other rehabilitative approaches, treatment in groups also encourages interaction, communication, and the development of socializing skills.

The ever-increasing use of pain management programs in groups seems to attest to their empirical effectiveness. Attendance of a pain management program in addition to conventional therapy seems to augment the latter's efficacy (Cameron, 1982), and various strategies seem to complement each other (Roy, Bellissimo, and Tunks, 1982). Methodologies of various group programs vary with the underlying conceptual model. Current pain programs fall into three major types: (1) behavioral; (2) cognitive; and (3) multimodal approaches.

The distinction between behavioral (operant) and cognitively oriented group programs lies mainly in the respective goals of the two approaches. In programs based on operant models (Fordyce, Fowler, Lehmann, DeLateur, Sand, and Trieschmann, 1973), the patient's behavior is the target of intervention. Mental processes, although acknowledged (Fordyce, Roberts, and Sternbach, 1985), are not addressed. Behaviorists hold the position that both increased activity and decreased use of medication are accompanied by a decrease of perceived pain, besides having the advantage of being observable and measurable variables (Fordyce et al., 1985).

In contrast, cognitive approaches (Turk, Meichenbaum, and Genest, 1983) address the "suffering" of the patient, attempt to change the patient's perceptions by providing him with coping skills, but do not change his environment. *Cognitive therapy* is a broad term including various methods under its umbrella (Tan, 1982) and is rarely used as the sole approach (Linton, 1986). The basic premise of cognitive theory is that cognitions precede, accompany, and follow the individual's behavior (Meichenbaum and Turk, 1976).

Both approaches share common features: the focus is on mobilizing the patient's own efforts in his rehabilitation. With active involvement, he is less likely to see himself as a passive recipient of specialized health care, overdependent on the medical profession. Since cognitions and behavior are likely to undergo simultaneous changes, a conceptual marriage seems to have occurred between cognitive and behavioral clinical applications, loosely defined as cognitive–behavioral modification. Meichenbaum and Turk (1976) consider cognitions pieces of behavior that lend themselves to manipulation and in turn alter cognitive structures.

Multimodal programs offer a combination of convergent therapies, such as group therapy, biofeedback, relaxation training, transcutaneous electrical nerve stimulation (TENS), counseling, physical and occupational therapy. At present, they appear to be the most popular approach in most multidisciplinary pain clinics. From published reports of comprehensive rehabilitation programs (Newman et al., 1978; Gottlieb, Koller, and Alperson, 1982), it would appear that in a group of chronic pain patients with dissimilar backgrounds and proclivities, the synergistic effect of combined interventions appears to be more effective than the added effects of component methods. Evidently, each strategy may modify other parameters and thereby exert an influence on the total pain experience. Although it has been argued that patient compliance diminishes with an increasing number of strategies (Linton, 1986), this has not been found to be the case in the author's experience with a multimodal group program (described later) which offers the patient a multifactorial learning experience (Herman and Baptiste, 1981; Baptiste and Herman, 1982).

It is not the intention of this chapter to provide an exhaustive review of pain programs, nor to critically examine the advantages and limitations of each approach. The reader is referred to critical reviews by Turner and Chapman (1982), Cameron (1982), Tan (1982), Aronoff et al. (1983), Turk and Flor (1984), and Linton (1986). Taken together, the analyses presented by these authors provide a comprehensive overview of the approaches in pain programs and point out some inherent limitations. The principal elements and specific techniques of each approach, as well as the link to their "parent" theories and a summarized critique, are discussed in greater detail below.

Behavioral Approaches

The Learning Paradigm of Operant Conditioning

The treatment of chronic pain within a framework of operant conditioning developed from learning theory and behavioral psychology based on animal training in the laboratory. (In the literature, *operant* and *behavioral* are frequently used interchangeably.) The central idea (Skinner, 1953) is that an individual continuously emits behavior. If a particular behavior results in pleasant consequences, a person will likely repeat it. If rewards are only forthcoming when the behavior is emitted, that is, reinforcement is contingent upon a specific behavior (the operant), these behaviors can be elicited by discriminative cues. (Discriminative cues are stimuli in the environment that suggest to the individual that behaving in a certain way will be profitable.) Each time the behavior is rewarded (reinforced), it is strengthened and less likely to extinguish, that is, to diminish in strength when the contingent reinforcement is withdrawn.

People are very susceptible to social rewards: praise is a powerful positive reinforcer, while aversive or neutral consequences (ignoring the behavior) will make the occurrence of the behavior less likely. Thus, man has been shaped to perform on cue and, with a low level of awareness, learns to discern and respond to environmental cues.

Operant Conditioning Procedures

The proliferating use of behavioral approaches in group programs (Fordyce et al., 1973; Cairns, Thomas, Mooney, and Pace, 1976; Seres and Newman, 1976; Anderson, Cole, Gullickson, Hudgens, and Roberts, 1977; Swanson, Maruta, and Swenson, 1979; Malec, Cayner, Harvey, and Timming, 1981) can be credited to the publication of Fordyce's work (e.g., Fordyce et al., 1973, 1985; Fordyce, 1976, 1978). In behavioral programs, the etiology of the medical illness is relatively unimportant (Oxman, 1986); instead, chronic pain is conceptualized as a learned behavior which is maintained by reinforced practice during extended periods of time. Pain behavior is the way pain and suffering are communicated to the world, such as by grimacing, posturing, complaining, medication intake and so on. The reinforcements (rewards) that maintain and strengthen pain behavior are of three kinds: (1) direct reinforcement by sympathy, attention, or financial reimbursements; (2) indirect reinforcement by legitimate avoidance of potentially stressful situation (like work); and (3) the nonreinforcement of well behaviors. Chronic pain has come under the control of external reinforcement. The price for immediate reinforcement (secondary gains) is high: abject helplessness, abrogation of personal responsibility, and dependency are the long-range consequences.

Behavior modification is a process of positive reconditioning: in order to establish new behavior in a situation, the desired response (coping) has to be elicited and immediately reinforced, while undesirable responses (behavioral indicators of pain and invalidism) are consistently nonrewarded. Just as the complaint of pain can be maintained by positive consequences, it can be reduced by changing this contingency structure and reinforcing well behavior (Block, Kremer, and Gaylor, 1980a). Praise appears to be the most effective source of reinforcement. Graphic reinforcement, verbal reinforcement, and both conditions combined were compared in nine chronic low back pain patients by Cairns and Pasino (1977). The authors found that only verbal reinforcement was effective in increasing activity levels appreciably.

Social reinforcement and principles of operant conditioning methods, typically not used in group therapy, are applied in all pain groups, even if the program is not strictly behavioral. Demonstrated pain behaviors such as squirming on sitting, grimacing, or stiff postures should be consistently ignored while display of well behaviors (laughing, participating, reports of improvement) should be noticed and rewarded with verbal compliments.

The general goals in behavior-modification group programs for chronic pain patients are to (1) increase activity and exercise tolerance; (2) decrease dependency on drugs and health care services; (3) decrease pain behavior and increase well behavior; and (4) return the patient to a satisfactory life-style with positive family interactions. The achievement of these goals has been documented in several follow-up studies (Fordyce et al., 1973; Seres and Newman, 1976; Cairns and Pasino, 1977; Roberts and Reinhardt, 1980).

The effectiveness of behavioral approaches can be enhanced by objective goal-setting in the following way: after baseline data of the patients' functional abilities have been collected, the patients identify their own long-range goals (e.g., walking for longer distances, increasing social activities). Intermediate goals, with a high probability of eventual attainment, are then negotiated with each patient, and monitored on a weekly basis. It has been found that the patients' own confidence ratings and expectancies increase after achieving these goals, and that activities increase with the development of self-efficacy (Cameron, 1987).

The importance of setting specific behavioral goals has also been emphasized by other researchers (Tunks, 1987). In an evaluation of the inpatient unit at the Chedoke–McMaster Pain Program, three different treatment approaches were compared: operant conditioning, group milieu, in which patients supported each other but were left to set their own goals, and a group-milieu condition with negotiated objective weekly goals. Although on discharge no significant differences in the patients' activity levels were noted, reduction of medication intake differed significantly between the groups. The "milieu plus goals" condition resulted in the most drastic reduction of drug intake (50 percent of the patients had discontinued their medication entirely), while the cohort in the "group-milieu without set goals" condition fared the poorest (only 9 percent completely eliminated medication).

To determine maintenance of therapeutic gains following completion of an inpatient behavioral program, Malec et al. (1981) sent forty patients follow-up questionnaires six months to three years after discharge. Questions referred to activity level–employment, use of pain medication, and the management of pain. Thirty-two patients responded (although not all patients completed the entire questionnaire). Of thirty responders, 57 percent were drug-free, 75 percent of twenty-eight responders were active and/or employed, and of twenty-nine patients 86% reported that they managed their pain well. These follow-up data indicated an overall success rate of 37 percent among the twenty-seven patients who had completed the entire questionnaire. The authors recommended a multivariate criterion to assess maintenance of life-style changes.

Cognitive Approaches

Conceptual Foundation of Cognitive Therapy

In contrast to behavioral theories which associate the individual's (re-)actions with external antecedents, cognitive and self-theories take a more philosophical view of man by placing the focus of his perceptions and behavior within the individual (Kelly, 1955). Self-concept, that is, how an individual perceives himself, is crucial not only during the development, but throughout life as a frame of reference with which he evaluates his actual experience. Experiences that are inconsistent with the way he sees himself (such as suffering chronic pain) are perceived as threat; the greater the threat, the more defensive and rigid the self-structure becomes in order to maintain itself.

> Don Quixote, Cervantes' (1547–1616) valiant knight, knew that what he thought was the absolute truth, and no force on earth could shake that belief. Thus, inns became castles, ladies of easy virtue were revered as maidens of high rank, soggy bread tasted like troutlets, and windmills were attacked as giants. Attributing misfortunes to others, success and glory to himself, our hero even considered himself fortunate to suffer pain and deprivation, for it was all part and parcel of being a "knight errant" [Miguel de Cervantes, *Don Quixote de la Mancha.*]

The way things appear to the individual is called his phenomenological world and is of his own making (Kelly, 1955). Cognitive theory (Mahoney, 1974) posits that thoughts and beliefs intervene not only between the external event and the reaction to it, but also between the individual's adaptive or maladaptative transactions with his environment and his emotions, including physiological changes (Lazarus, 1977). Personal meaning of one's experience is thus derived from its cognitive appraisal (Meichenbaum and Turk, 1976; Genest and Turk, 1979). Cognitive therapy, which grew out of this theory, has as its aim to change a patient's perception of himself and the world around him. Specific strategies will be discussed subsequently.

A note seems appropriate at this point regarding the gap between theoretical foundations and the diversity of their clinical applications. Bellissimo and Tunks (1984) eloquently emphasized this point: "For the critical clinicians, what stands out in this diversity is the gap between fundamental research conclusions and the use of these conclusions as rational and guiding principles for clinical practice (p. 145).

Patient Education

Group therapy traces its roots to a cognitive approach (Baptiste and Herman, 1982). At present, group programs for pain patients are almost invariably initiated with the imparting of knowledge and answering of the patients' questions. Since uncertainty in itself is a source of anxiety and fear (we fear most what we do not understand), replacing it with understanding will reduce fears, especially irrational ones. Didactic persuasion, used in the beginning, appears to be the least stressful mode of instruction and communication for anxious patients (Swanson, Swenson, Maruta, and Floreen, 1978) and most suitable for individuals whose beliefs are consistent with an "external locus of control" (Liberman, 1978). As patients begin to feel more comfortable in the group, discussions replace didactic lectures. Patients ventilate emotions, perceive similarity of problems, express their concerns, thus working through their problems. Pain derives a new meaning.

The acquisition and integration of new relevant information, frequently inconsistent with previously held opinions and beliefs, results in looking at one's problems from a different perspective and promotes problem solving. Erroneous beliefs are frequently covertly mediated for fear of "not being understood" or appearing ridiculous; they can present one of the most powerful obstacles to recovery by engendering anxiety (Bellissimo and Tunks, 1984). The following example may illustrate this problem.

> An immigrant laborer was referred to the pain clinic because of irremediable problems following a whiplash injury sustained two years prior to his attendance of the program. Very reluctant to communicate at first, he admitted after lengthy probing, that he fully expected to "end up in a wheelchair". When asked for the reasons for this assumption, he said that his neighbor (of the same age as he) was now in a wheelchair after a very similar accident. On further questioning, it turned out that this neighbor also suffered from multiple sclerosis, a fact that had seemed irrelevant to the patient.

Because of faulty conceptions, this patient had withdrawn into a chronic illness posture. Resultant anxiety jeopardized a favorable response to treatments directed toward the biological causes of pain. After new information and debates corrected his erroneous beliefs and dispelled his myths, he began to respond to appropriate therapy. His case illustrates the importance of reinterpretation of the patient's pain experience (discussed below).

Cognitive Restructuring

Maladaptive cognitions may contribute significantly to pain problems (Cameron, 1982). The basic assumption underlying cognitive approaches is that pain can be altered by cognitive mediation (Meichenbaum and Turk, 1976). Unlike the operant model, cognitive approaches do not ignore the pain but use various strategies to modify the pain experience. Several cognitive techniques, such as the use of imagery or attention–diversion, have been subjected to experimental investigations (Tan, 1982).

Rybstein-Blinchik (1979) investigated the effectiveness of different cognitive strategies on forty-four pain patients. When compared with attention-diversion and concentration on the sensation of pain, reinterpretation, and relabeling the pain experience resulted in significantly greater pain reduction as measured by the McGill Pain Questionnaire (Melzack, 1975).

The method employed in the McMaster group program is based on Meichenbaum and Turk's "stress-inoculation training" (Meichenbaum and Turk, 1976). This model posits that what the patient says to himself, his "internal dialogue," has a profound effect on his behavior and the perpetuation of his pain. Since these self-statements are for the most part automatic and unrecognized, the first step of cognitive restructuring is to make the patient aware of these thoughts and their self-defeating nature ("educational phase"). Pain is unrealistically appraised within negative thought patterns ("it feels like my fusion is coming apart"), and results in an emotional reaction to the meaning of pain, not its severity. The patient, therefore, has to learn to substitute the negative "self-talk" with incompatible, more positive statements ("rehearsal phase") and immediately reinforce the change by "self-congratulation." At the same time, patients are provided with a variety of suitable coping techniques, such as relaxation, systematic desensitization, assertiveness training, and modeling. These techniques are practiced during the "application phase" and generalized across various situations in daily life ("home assignment"). Different patients will, of course, benefit from different coping strategies (Meichenbaum and Turk, 1976). Table 15.1 illustrates the procedure by which this model is applied in the pain control classes.

TABLE 15.1

COGNITIVE RESTRUCTURING

Situation	Internal Statement	Revised Statement	Reinforcing Statement
Evening preceding first day back to work after two years' rehabilitation	My back is killing me! I won't be able to work tomorrow. . . .	I will not allow myself to become panicky. . . . I can control my pain. . . . I have learned it. . . . Let's start with deep breathing	Good! Just concentrating on breathing eases the pain.
	But it's still too bad to stay on my feet for eight hours.	Let's take one hour at a time, not eight. Tomorrow things will look different. I just let myself relax some more. I feel free of all sensations. Tomorrow will be all right. I feel an inner quietness.	I am already calming down. I can control my mind. Relaxing feels good! I can control my body. I've done it!

The first phase is often the most difficult as patients seem rigidly defended against recognizing (or admitting) negative thoughts.

A fifty-year-old baker, father of five children, who had lost his job because of intractable low back pain, related to the group how he spent a good part of each night pacing the floor since he found himself unable to sleep "because of pain." Asked what went through his mind during those hours, he replied "nothing." When it was pointed out to him that some thoughts always occupied the mind, he professed to be concerned with the fact that he could not sleep. Pressed a little further, he admitted that he compared his

> present state with his healthy condition prior to the onset of pain. When asked what "being fit" meant to him, he observed that he could work and, therefore, was useful to his family. Finally, after further questions from group members, he admitted that he thought his family would be better off without him, and realized (or admitted) that it was suicidal thoughts, not the pain itself, that kept him awake night after night. It took the group's remarks (especially from females!) to convince him that his family might see more in him than a bread-winner, and that his wife and children would prefer a father without employment to losing a loved one. Seemingly for the first time, he took a realistic look at the consequences of suicide on his wife and children. Again, it took a reinterpretation of his predicament to confront his stressor and find an incompatible self-statement. Initially hesitant to "self-congratulate" himself for thoughts, he found that with practice his outlook on life changed. Improved family functioning followed, and a more favorable response to physical treatments ensued. (No antidepressants were required in this case.)

Since cognitive strategies are typically used in combination with other interventions it is difficult to assess their specific effects. In a component analysis study, Kendall, Williams, Pechacek, Graham, Shisslack, and Herzoff (1979) compared coping-skill training with educational information giving and two control groups prior to a stressful cardiac catherization procedure. Both the cognitive–behavioral and educational groups had lower anxiety ratings than the controls, the cognitive–behavioral intervention group showing better adjustment ratings than the educational intervention group. There were, however, no significant group differences in subjective pain ratings.

To bring about behavioral changes in different life situations, various cognitive behavioral techniques are employed. One of these methods is self-monitoring (Eisler, 1976), a home task which requires the patient to record his overt and covert (cognitions) behavior during various activities and events of daily living. Despite validity problems when the reports are used as measurement data (Lipinski and Nelson, 1974), the technique can be used to advantage in self-regulation programs. Not only does the patient become aware of the link between the types of environmental cues that trigger pain and elicit pain behavior, these stimuli become the occasion for practicing self-control strategies. Recorded progress serves as reinforcement over time. Improvement is typically discussed in the group and verbally rewarded by both therapists and group members. Patients who successfully apply self-control practices set up models for underachievers.

Occasionally, patients who do not seem to do well with self-regulation at home benefit from role-play; they have to *pretend* to have overcome their difficulties and give advice to the others as to the means by which this success was achieved. To give an example, a female patient, initially very reluctant to engage in this exercise, became so carried away with acting an unbelievable part, that (to her great surprise) she found herself without pain when the role-play was over. It seems unlikely that this type of reinforcement did not register in her memory.

Not surprisingly, social skills and assertiveness are typically impoverished in chronic pain patients. Toomey, Ghia, Mao, and Gregg (1977) studied the effect of psychosocial factors on the response to somatic treatment (acupuncture). Forty patients with chronic pain were assessed with regard to personality, affect, and stress. The results indicated a significant link between refractoriness to treatment and passivity, depression, social stress, and chronicity of pain. During the program sessions, the deficient behavioral repertoires of patients in coping with the stress of social situations are addressed in various scenarios of assertiveness training. More assertive behavior usually follows the altered cognition of perceived self-worth.

Case Report

A clinical case is presented to illustrate that a combination of various strategies can alter treatment outcome in patients refractory to interventions when efforts are made to understand the patient's personal meaning of pain. Changing the patient's perception of his problem can alter the maladaptive way in which he evaluated and responded to his experience.

> E.W., a sixty-two-year-old former auto mechanic with an eighth-grade education, had suffered a heart attack two years

> prior to his referral to the pain clinic. He presented at the clinic with steadily worsening cardiac "pain attacks" which occurred with increasing frequency and rendered him progressively incapacitated. Feeling unable to work, he had given up his job in a garage, and adopted a passive attitude. His "pain attacks" (for which he required an increasing amount of nitroglycerine) became the focus of his life. In great distress, he appeared two to three times a week at the emergency room of the local hospital. On these occasions he was usually kept overnight for observation, hooked up to sophisticated monitors, surrounded by concerned and competent staff—and sent home the next morning with the assurance that "nothing was wrong." He became so dependent on these visits that he never ventured out of the radius of a nearby hospital. Yet, extensive investigation had not revealed any findings to account for his increasing malaise. All interventions remained totally ineffectual. Gradually, during group discussions, the way things appeared to him emerged. It became apparent that he had taken great pride in his work. At home, his solicitous wife curtailed his functional activities. His only pleasurable moments appeared to be his visits to his former place of work where he met his "old buddies." These visits, however, seemed to accentuate his growing bitterness of no longer being "useful."

Interestingly, self-monitoring revealed that E.W.'s pain attacks never occurred while he was at the garage but most frequently at night. The double-bind position in which this man found himself was obvious: on one hand, he was told he was okay, on the other hand he experienced the very impressive concern he generated on each hospital admission. One message was given verbally, but canceled out by another, which had more impact, since experience usually speaks louder than argument. Although both messages came from credible sources, the patient could not reconcile them. In order to make sense out of the two conflicting pieces of information, he confabulated the "missing pieces" and construed his predicament in his own way: the seriousness of his heart condition had to be kept from him because his worry could prove fatal. With this rationale he lived—and lived up to it.

> Since E.W. was highly defended and psychologically illiterate, reasoning with him proved to be useless, and the dilemma was

> approached with a role-play: E.W. played the role of a garage mechanic, the therapist that of a customer who brought her car to the garage repeatedly after it had been appropriately repaired. Yet, on each occasion—and against his better judgment—he decided to keep the car on the chance of "having overlooked something" and thus compromise his reputation. Suddenly he paused and smiled in astonishment: "Do you think they have to keep me in the hospital for the same reasons?" he asked. It seems more than coincidental that from then on he began to improve and respond to previously ineffective treatment methods. During relaxation training he learned to counteract physiological cues for anxiety; he began to take on small tasks at home. Self-monitoring indicated that his activities (even shoveling snow) increased while his medication intake and hospital visits dropped off (he had to chart both graphically). More importantly, he learned to congratulate himself for his accomplishments. Two months later, he was back at his former working place where he held a part-time job, planned his first vacation in three years, and discontinued treatments for which he had "no more need."

What happened to this patient can be generalized to a great number of chronic pain syndromes in which psychological factors play an important role in perpetuating the problem. Once he reconceptualized his predicament and challenged the erroneous assumption of "being doomed," he opened up to new experience. Gradually he perceived himself as regaining control. Just as once upon a time he had learned helplessness, he now learned resourcefulness and the pride in his self-therapy provided the fuel to reverse the vicious spiral and sent it spinning in the opposite direction.

Behavioral changes are invariably accompanied by a redirection in thinking. Most important, a process has to be created in which the patient assumes responsibility for his own rehabilitation and eventually all outcomes he encounters. To achieve the patient's independence, opportunity for mastery has to be provided by setting small intermediate goals with high probability of a success experience. If expectation of failure (the antecedent of helplessness) can become a self-fulfilling prophesy, so can success.

Modeling

Learning without direct reinforcement, simply by observing others, is mediated by perceptual–cognitive processes. Based on social learning principles (Bandura, Blanchard, and Ritter, 1969), modeling can have a powerful effect in groups. New response patterns may be developed by watching others and the behavioral outcomes they encounter.

Craig and Best (1977) investigated the relative influence of modeling and perceived locus of control (the belief in one's capacity to control external events) on pain perception. Fifty volunteers were assigned to five groups (one control group) according to locus of control beliefs (Rotter, 1966), then exposed to models who exhibited differential tolerance to electric shocks. As expected, the subjects' level of tolerance changed in the expected direction in the presence of more or less tolerant models; that is, the subjects exposed to tolerant models increased their pain tolerance significantly. These effects were durable and, unexpectedly, independent of perceived locus of control. The authors suggest that the combined effects of cognitive–behavioral rehearsals and modeling might potentiate each other.

In the McMaster pain program (Baptiste and Herman, 1982), the influence of modeling is utilized by inviting successful alumni from previous groups to speak to the beginners of new groups. One would, of course, expect that the degree of modeling depends on perceived similarity (salience) to the model. For example, therapists who have experienced and successfully overcome a chronic pain experience can serve as extremely salient models.

On occasion, modeling processes can also exert their influence in the opposite direction. Not all chronic pain patients benefit from group experience. Lack of incentive, a passive and dependent attitude, depression, and reinforcement contingencies at home not conducive to well behavior have been related to deterioration after initial treatment gains in a pain management program (Painter, Seres, and Newman, 1980). Some patients are a priori poor candidates for group approaches. Unrealistic goals, poor insight, lack of motivation, and/or ability to learn new habits, as well as great social distress have been found to be prognosticators for poor results (Tunks, private communication, 1985). Not only are these patients refractory to most interventions, they can also exert a detrimental influence on other group members; with constant complaints and negative comments they undermine the group's progress. These individuals seem strikingly similar to the patient profile Swanson et al. (1978) compiled from thirteen patients admitted to the pain program at the Mayo Clinic. Seemingly angry with their physicians and the administration, they sent letters of complaint to the institution and refused to pay for services. They appeared to be more accident-prone, had a longer duration of pain and of time away from work, a greater number of hospitalizations and surgeries, and reported higher levels of pain. On comparison of the MMPI profiles with those of other chronic pain patients, they demonstrated a higher degree of psychopathology. Twelve of the thirteen were females, more than half of them unmarried. Irritable, demanding, and querulous, this type of patient frequently shows little insight and seems to be unwilling to relinquish pain. Frequently pain serves to gratify dependency strivings (Pilowsky, 1978) as the most reliable method to command attention from others (Craig, 1978). Since the negativism displayed by these patients encourages the pain complaints of others and impedes group cohesion, it seems advisable to avoid "group contamination" by negative models. In the Chedoke-McMaster inpatient program, for instance, a staggered intake of admitted patients and early discharge of patients unsuitable for group milieu ensures exposure of all group participants to appropriate models (Tunks, private communication, 1985).

Relaxation Training

A valuable and indispensable part of pain control programs is the use of relaxation techniques as tools of autogenic control. Relaxation methods are based on the learning paradigm of classical conditioning. Classical or pavlovian conditioning (Pavlov, 1928) refers to a procedure during which an originally neutral stimulus, by being paired with an unconditioned stimulus, is "conditioned" to result in the same (unconditioned) response as the stimulus with which it was paired. Indeed, classical conditioning is the simplest form of learning, and forms the basis for emotional responses and avoidance learning. Classical conditioning principles account for the finding that neutral stimuli in the patient's environment have become discriminatory cues for the initiation of pain behavior.

Wolpe's (1958) systematic desensitization procedure (as used in relaxation training) is based on "reciprocal inhibition"; that is, the weakening (inhibition) of old (undesirable) responses when they are replaced by new (desirable) ones which are incompatible with the previous ones.

While other cognitive–behavioral techniques facilitate the recognition of *external* cues that trigger pain, during deep relaxation the patient learns to discriminate *internal* cues for bodily tension on a nonintellectual level of consciousness. With continued practice of relaxation techniques, control can be gained over responses to stressful situations.

Progressive muscular relaxation is incompatible with anxiety (Jacobson, 1944). By employing principles of counterconditioning, systematic desensitization, and reciprocal inhibition (Wolpe, 1958), arousal and psychophysiological responses to stressors and pain are voluntarily reduced (Patterson, 1979). As the patient learns to emit a response inhibitory of anxiety in the presence of pain (an anxiety-evoking stimulus), the link between pain and anxiety is systematically weakened. Perceived control reduces anxiety (Merskey, 1965).

During the altered state of consciousness induced by deep relaxation, the individual learns to recruit and control inherent homeostatic self-healing mechanisms which are normally inhibited during states of pain, anxiety, and tension (Luthe, 1979). With mastery of relaxation techniques, the patient can consciously sustain the feeling of mental relaxation during stressful situations of daily life, and reduce pain to a purely sensory event, unembellished by anxiety and fear. As pointed out before, "suffering pain" is not a direct function of nociceptive stimulation, and pain and nociception can exist independently

(Fordyce, 1978). As new behavioral patterns in response to stress are adopted, the patient learns to "unstress" himself.

The relaxation process of "passive concentration" (Luthe, 1979) is enhanced by the use of imagery. Instead of focusing on pain and stressful events, attention is directed to neutral feelings of body awareness, breathing rhythms, and sensory details of self-generated pleasant scenes (Bellissimo and Tunks, 1984).

Although it could be argued that the pain-reducing effect of deep relaxation is due to a placebo effect, the latter appears to be an inseparable component of any successful therapy (Frank, 1978; Andersson, 1979). There is experimental evidence that placebo analgesia is physiologically mediated via endorphin release, as suggested by the reversibility of placebo analgesia by the opiate antagonist naloxone (Levine, Gordon, and Fields, 1978).

Autogenic control can also be achieved by biofeedback procedures. Relaxation training, however, has several advantages over biofeedback procedures: a more cost-effective method of promoting physical health and wellness through self-regulation, it appears to be no less effective than biofeedback (Jessup, Neufeld, and Merskey, 1979; Turner and Chapman, 1982). Relaxation training in groups also offers the advantages of "modeling": by witnessing the positive outcome of others, patients are more likely to ascribe success and mastery of this procedure to personal learning which provides incentive to practice. Rather than creating dependence on sophisticated electronic equipment, mastering the art of relaxation renders a patient self-reliant by teaching him that the power of self-healing resides within himself.

Family Issues

The impact of family dynamics on chronic pain problems is increasingly recognized. Because research in this field is of recent origin and beset with methodological problems, the underlying mechanisms are not yet clearly understood (Payne and Norfleet, 1986). Yet, numerous reports in the literature draw attention to the contribution of family factors to chronic pain (Payne and Norfleet, 1986). The results of these investigations support empirical evidence which strongly suggests that close family members, especially spouses, play a significant role in the etiology, perpetuation, and rehabilitation of chronic pain (Roy, 1982).

Shanfield, Heiman, Cope, and Jones (1979) found a significant correlation in highly distressed pain patients between their own psychiatric distress scores and those of their spouses. In an investigation of the spouse's influence on pain reports, the work of Block, Kremer, and Gaylor (1980b) demonstrated that reported pain levels varied as a function of whether the spouse was perceived as relatively solicitous or relatively unsolicitous. After rating their spouses on this dimension, the pain patients had to judge their pain levels in the presence of (1) the spouse and (2) that of a neutral observer. Pain reports changed with the perceived spousal response to pain behavior: patients with solicitous spouses reported higher levels of pain in the presence of the spouse than when observed by a neutral person, while patients with nonsolicitous spouses demonstrated the opposite tendency. Spousal perceptions and attitudes may also affect treatment outcome. Swanson and Maruta (1980) administered identical questionnaires concerning pain problems to 100 chronic pain patients and their spouses (or a close family member). The highest congruency between the patient's and the spouse's interpretation of the pain experience was positively related to problems encountered during rehabilitation and poor treatment results.

Block et al. (1985) investigated how emotional and cognitive factors affected spouses' estimates of the pain patient's functional achievement. The spouses of thirty chronic pain patients who participated in an outpatient rehabilitation program had to complete questionnaires concerning their attitude and response tendencies toward the patient's pain problem and their estimation of the patient's physical capacity; the paper and pencil measures were obtained under differing instruction conditions before and after viewing a videotape of physiotherapy exercises. The authors found that two relatively independent dimensions were underlying spousal perceptions: the belief that the patient's activities ought to be restricted (empathy dimension), and the belief that the patient had major psychological problems (the dimension of negativism). Not surprisingly, spouses rating low on negativism anticipated higher functional achievement of their partners than the pessimistic spouses; it seems reasonable to expect a greater degree of support for the patient's efforts from optimistic than pessimistic family members.

The need to involve family members in pain rehabilitation programs and group interventions is obvious when chronic pain is conceptualized as a learned behavior, reinforced by significant others. Viewed from a biopsychosocial perspective, the family provides the social context in which pain behavior occurs, and the social environment has a profound effect on pain complaints. Spouses can provide discriminative cues for pain behavior. The following patient example illustrates the necessity to modify the spouse's response to pain and well behavior.

> Mrs. B.D. was a seventy-six-year-old lady who would come regularly every few months for a course of treatments (not referred from the pain clinic). The diagnosis of cervical spondylosis was confirmed by X ray. She was nearly blind, but exceptionally well dressed and groomed, and always accompanied by her touchingly concerned husband. Extremely attentive to his wife's requests, he used to almost tenderly undress and dress her and sit by her side during treatment. When on one occasion the therapist had the opportunity to speak to B.D.'s husband alone, she inquired about what the couple was talking about all day at home. "Why, her pain, of course" was his answer. Asked whether his wife also talked to other people, he assured me that his wife had many friends and each day would receive several phone calls. To the question what she was discussing on the telephone, the answer was the same as before "Why, her pain, of course." He continued to say what mental anguish it was to see her suffer so much pain. Asked what he did about it, he answered that he brought her flowers whenever the pain was severe. When I suggested to him that in order to help his wife, he might try to give her the flowers when she did *not* complain, he looked at me rather skeptically and found the idea "a bit absurd." Here the report unfortunately ends, because the nice couple discontinued treatment soon afterwards. Somehow, however, the author doubts that the carefully explained suggestions

> regarding behavioral management were followed; it seems more likely that B.D.'s pain behavior continued to be reinforced and, therefore, to flourish.

Following rehabilitation in an environment with strictly controlled reinforcement contingencies, the patient, on his return home, finds himself surrounded by numerous environmental cues associated with the sensation of pain and "secondary gains." Because family members are considered powerful reinforcers of learned behaviors, their participation in group programs seems essential to long-term success (Fordyce, 1976; Roberts and Reinhardt, 1980).

Evidence of linkages between spouse involvement and treatment outcome is not unequivocal. Moore and Chaney (1985), in a seven-month follow-up study of forty-three pain patients who had completed an outpatient program, found that spouse participation did not enhance treatment outcome. It is noteworthy, however, that this group program was not based on operant principles but emphasized cognitive–educational approaches. Considering the myriad of interacting variables in the family context, it is apparent that their relationship remains yet to be explored.

Limitations of Group Programs

Not surprisingly, the evaluation of the benefits of pain management programs is complicated by a multitude of problems. It is one thing to accept a logically plausible (and experimentally verified) theory on philosophical grounds; it is quite another to provide empirical evidence of its clinical tenability that would permit drawing confident conclusions. Given the kaleidoscopical interaction of the plethora of factors potentially affecting outcome, it seems a nearly impossible task to isolate the variables in order to determine which strategy proved most useful for what type of patient. Some of the major criticism of published reports, pointed out in review of group programs (Cameron, 1982; Tan, 1982; Turner and Chapman, 1982; Aronoff et al., 1983; Turk and Flor, 1984; Linton, 1986), may be summarized as follows.

Difficulties Assessing Outcome

The most frequent shortcoming of group program evaluations is the lack of controls. For obvious practical and ethical reasons, clinicians are reluctant to conduct double-blind prospective studies in a deterministic manner by assigning pain patients randomly to experimental and "placebo" groups. Unintentional therapist-bias and experimenter effects are nearly always present as therapists inevitably influence their patients in subtle ways to respond to the interventions in ways that will confirm the therapists' beliefs (Quinn, 1979). Outcome data frequently include self-reports that are often colored by what the patient perceived a trusted therapist may want to hear. Further, adequate baseline and follow-up measures over an extended period of time are frequently missing, and some studies report the results of small numbers of selected patients. Thus, it remains yet to be determined which specific ingredient within hybrid techniques is most effective for what type of patient. Component studies using multivariate analyses and single subject designs have, therefore, been suggested in order to obtain selection criteria for patients suited for specific approaches (Turner and Chapman, 1982; Linton, 1986). Added to the list of factors that make comparison of nonequivalent studies difficult are problems of self-selection, compliance, and attrition, lack of standardization in measurement, operationalization of theoretical concepts, and criteria of what constitutes "success." These methodological problems tend to cloud issues and limit confidence in the conclusions drawn from the studies.

Nevertheless, despite these drawbacks the overall results of pain management programs are encouraging: group management programs have established their pragmatic effectiveness as a valuable adjunct to the patient's total treatment package. On the positive side, one might also argue that the collective findings of numerous investigations, despite flawed methodology of single studies, may generate new hypotheses and, therefore, have heuristic value. Even if the results of each study have to be interpreted with caution, the pieces of experimental data put together contribute to the mosaic of prevailing knowledge, offering hope to find a means to ease suffering.

THE MCMASTER PAIN CLINIC

The university-based Pain Clinic of Chedoke-McMaster Hospitals in Hamilton, Ontario, Canada, is organized as an outpatient and inpatient facility. Since its inception in 1977, the number of chronic pain patients seen yearly at the pain clinic has been growing at an accelerating rate. Directed by a psychiatrist, the multidisciplinary nature of the clinic is reflected in the specialized personnel and consultants who meet in bimonthly pain conferences. Epidemiological research is carried out on a continuous basis. The range of modalities provided by the pain clinic in the management of referred patients with chronic pain includes physiotherapy, occupational therapy, TENS applications, acupuncture, nerve blocks, neurosurgical interventions, pharmacological management, biofeedback, relaxation training, psychotherapy, hypnotherapy, psychosocial interventions by individual and family counseling, and group therapy.

As part of the outpatient rehabilitation, a group program referred to as Pain Control Classes, has been developed (Herman and Baptiste, 1981; Baptiste and Herman, 1982). The following is a brief account of its operation. Initially intended as an educational program with lectures about the patients' common medical problems and biomechanical instructions, the sessions were conjointly organized by the Rehabilitation Departments of Physiotherapy and Occupational Therapy. It soon became apparent, however, that the imparting of information was a necessary but not sufficient ingredient in an adaptive learning process of self-modification. Patients did not just want to "tune in," they wanted to "broadcast" as well; they showed indications of the truism that "misery loves company." They wanted to share their "suffering" experiences, and requested advice beyond merely understanding the reasons for ongoing pain. From these pragmatic observations evolved the eclectic framework of the present group format. A nine-week program, the Pain Control Classes are designed for patients with pain of longer than six months duration which is refractory to conventional treatments and the cause of dysfunction. In order to assure a measure of homogeneity in groups, individuals with psychiatric etiologies are not accepted (Tunks, 1982).

At present, each session (twelve to fourteen patients and two therapists) consists of three parts. Didactic but participatory lectures about various pain-related topics (the educational part of the program) are followed by group discussions during which the patients interact and the feeling of "belonging" develops. Most of the aforementioned techniques are employed with emphasis on cognitive strategies. During the last segment of each group session progressive relaxation training for self-regulation is taught and practiced. The overall goal of the group sessions is to replace learned helplessness with learned resourcefulness. The patients have already demonstrated some measure of motivation for change by mere virtue of their presence. To foster realistic expectations, the rationale for group participation is stated clearly at the beginning: the program does not offer a "cure" for pain, but rather the means for learning to control it. Assured of unconditional support (Rogers, 1952), the patient's own responsibility for the outcome is emphasized. A voluntary "contract" commits the patients to the group's goals and rules.

In a climate of honesty, mutual influence, and support, a "therapeutic milieu" (Tunks, 1982, p. 189) is created. A positive outlook on the prognosis is enhanced by relating previous successful experiences with the program. Confidence in the patient's ability to master the challenge of pain control is communicated and mobilizes expectations for a positive outcome. Frank (1978) refers to this essential ingredient of successful therapy as the "power of expectant faith" (p.4).

The results of a study to assess the benefits of this program to group participants are reported and discussed in the following section.

Evaluation of the McMaster Outpatient Group Program

The effectiveness of the program was evaluated in a pilot sample of the first seventy-five patients who attended the pain control classes. The results are presented elsewhere (Herman and Baptiste, 1981) but will be summarized here: Of the seventy-five patients, 61 percent were female, 39 percent male; 73 percent were married. The ages ranged between twenty-one and seventy-one years; the average age was forty-six years. Twenty percent were gainfully employed, 32 percent received Workman's Compensation Board benefits or had litigation pending; the remainder were either unemployed or housewives. The most frequent pain complaint was low back pain (61%), 25 percent had head and neck pain, the remaining patients presented with pain of various etiologies. The duration of pain ranged from six months to thirty years; while the most frequently reported chronicity was three years, patients with low back pain had, on the average, suffered pain for longer than five years. The number of pain-related surgeries ranged from one (most commonly) to four in 37 percent of the sample. Psychosocial problems were present in 87 percent of the patients, for which the majority had received either psychiatric or family interviews and/or counseling. Fifty-four percent of the group attendants received psychopharmacological treatment or psychotherapeutic intervention.

Multiple baseline measures in several categories (pain at best and worst times, its impact on mood, locus of control, depression, activity level, and drug intake) were obtained on consecutively admitted patients (no matched control group) and compared with ten posttreatment measures at discharge in order to calculate the final score (based on percentage improvement). The scores in three evaluation categories were derived from validated instruments (Visual Analogue Scale, Beck's Depression Scale, Strickland's Locus of Control Scale), the remainder from self-reports or self-designed questionnaires (mood, attitude, cognitive control, group participation, and patient's belief in the benefit of the program). The patient's overall improvement was determined by converting the points totaled across the ten evaluated categories to a percentage basis.

A change of more than 39 percent was deemed successful. The final scores were recorded on a standardized form and sent to the patient's case manager for completion after examination of the patient.

The results of comparing pre- and postprogram scores indicated that 79 percent of the patients demonstrated improvement in different (but not necessarily the same) areas. Most strikingly, successful patients appeared to have altered their reported thought patterns; they had assumed a more self-reliant attitude, seemed to manage their lives successfully despite pain, and used the adopted coping strategies to advantage.

The most marked improvement was observed in the measures of depression ($p = 0.001$) and perceived level of pain ($p = 0.001$). The shift toward internal locus of control ($p = 0.06$) appeared to be correlated with positive attitudinal changes. Decreased use of pain medication did not reach the set level of significance ($p < 0.05$), possibly because analgesic intake is routinely reduced on admission to the pain clinic. Twenty-eight percent of previously unemployed patients returned to work within six months after termination of the program.

Despite reports of improved life-styles by the majority of patients, their activity levels were not significantly increased. The lack of correlation between perceived pain intensity and physical measurements has been noted previously (Brena, Wolf, Chapman, and Hammonds, 1980). When "successes" were compared with "failures," it was noted that the highest failure rate occurred in the forty-one to fifty age group and was twice as high in males (14%) than in females (7%). This finding is consistent with the report of substantially higher failure rates among males in a follow-up study of 500 patients following completion of a pain program (Painter et al., 1980).

Psychosocial distress was more prevalent in the failure group (75%). Ten of the sixteen "failures" had participated only marginally in group activities and somatized the stress they were experiencing. Successful outcome of the program was significantly related to the absence of financial gains ($p = 0.003$), female gender ($p = 0.008$), and to married status ($p = 0.01$).

Unfortunately, approximately one-fourth of initially successful patients do not seem to maintain the improvement and regress to pretreatment levels within a few months after termination of the pain program (Swanson et al., 1979; Painter et al., 1980). A six-month follow-up telephone survey was conducted to determine the changes within this period of time. Questions referred to drug intake, uptime per 24 hours, employment status, perceived pain level, coping ability, and the use of health services. The responses of fifty patients who could be reached revealed that of forty-one patients rated as "successes," twenty-four (58%) continued to improve in the six areas of inquiry, eleven (27%) had maintained their level of improvement, while six (15%) had regressed. In their review of follow-up studies, Aronoff et al. (1983) pointed out that the same instruments should have been used in the follow-up as in the initial assessment. Although this criticism is well taken, requiring patients to return to the clinic would have resulted in an even higher attrition rate at follow-up.

Fifty percent of the "failures" received financial reimbursement for pain, compared to 32 percent in the total sample. Congruent with other reports of group programs (Roberts and Reinhardt, 1980; Painter et al., 1980), the outcome of patients who received Workmen's Compensation benefits or had litigation pending was poorer than that of other patients. In fact, three patients who voluntarily disclaimed benefits and returned to work demonstrated significant improvement following their decision. At first impression, this observation would seem to confirm the contention that patients on entitlement programs are less likely to benefit from treatment. In a recent study, however, a more complex relationship between compensation, litigation, and employment was disclosed. Dworkin, Handlin, Richlin, Brand, and Vannucci (1985) assessed short-term and long-term treatment outcome in 454 chronic pain patients as a function of compensation benefits, employment status, and pending litigation. Teasing these variables apart, the authors found that pending litigation was not associated with poorer outcome. While both employment and compensation benefits predicted poorer treatment outcome in univariate analyses, when using multiple regression analyses, only employment, but not compensation benefits, emerged as a significant predictor of the criterion. Since beneficiaries of compensation and individuals with pending litigation are less likely to be working, these variables are typically confounded. These observations, contradictory to traditional opinion, are consonant with other reports of the strong relationship between work and pain problems (Newman et al., 1978; Shanfield et al., 1979). Catchlove and Cohen (1983) retrospectively examined the data of forty-seven work-injured patients, referred by the Quebec Workmen's Compensation Commission. Twenty of these patients (earlier admission) received a multidisciplinary treatment package; the other twenty-seven patients were treated with the same approach but with the additional instruction that return to work was an essential part of getting well. A return-to-work contract committed them to resume work within a few months. Twenty-five percent of the noninstructed group and 59.3 percent of the instruction group returned to work. On follow-up (19.9 months for the noninstruction group and 9.6 months for the instruction group), a greater proportion of the instructed group than the noninstructed group continued to work.

Comparing the results of the McMaster outpatient group program (with a foremost cognitive–educational orientation) to the outcomes of behavioral programs, it appears that programs based on operant principles achieve superior results regarding activity levels and medication intake. The effects of cognitive strategies do not lend themselves well to objective assessment measures.

Taken together, despite some controversy on the most effective ingredients of group programs, there appears to be agreement on the importance of all those factors that contribute to a patient's independence, functional abilities, and a positive self-percept.

Conclusion

Although the underlying conceptual frameworks may vary, group programs are designed to help chronic pain sufferers to help themselves. Obviously, the above described methods for learning self-control are strongly interrelated, complement each other, and can be adapted to the individual needs of patients in manifold combinations by an astute therapist. One final point demands attention. The acquisition of coping strategies does not ensure successful mastery of pain; it requires *competence* to select a certain combination of those skills, and apply them effectively in different and novel situations.

The challenge for rehabilitation remains the durability of the therapeutic gains in the absence of continued input from the health services. Just as no particular approach can assure positive treatment outcome, no professional expertise can bestow on a patient the means to maintain newly adopted coping strategies and behavioral changes in an environment with different contingency structures.

Quality of life can only be self-determined and attained through one's own efforts. With continued self-control, patienthood is replaced by personhood, nurtured by a sense of functional "wholeness."

References

Anderson, T. P., Cole, T. M., Gullickson, G., Hudgens, A., & Roberts, A. H. (1977), Behavior modification of chronic pain: a treatment program by a multidisciplinary team. *Clin. Orthop.*, 129:96–100.

Andersson, S. A. (1979), Pain control by sensory stimulation. In: *Advances in Pain Research and Therapy.*, Vol. 3, eds. J.J. Bonica, J.C. Liebeskind, & D.G. Albe-Fessard. New York: Raven Press, pp. 569–585.

Aronoff, G. M., Evans, W. O., & Enders, P. L. (1983), A review of follow-up studies of multidisciplinary pain units. *Pain,* 16:1–11.

Bandura, A., Blanchard, E. B., & Ritter, B. (1969), Relative efficacy of desensitization and modeling approaches for inducing behavioral, affective, and attitudinal changes. *J. Pers. Soc. Psychol.*, 13:173–199.

Baptiste, S., & Herman, E. (1982), Group therapy: A specific model. In: *Chronic Pain, Psychosocial Factors in Rehabilitation,* eds. R. Roy & E. Tunks. Baltimore: Williams & Wilkins, pp. 166–178.

Bellissimo, A., & Tunks, E. (1984), *Chronic Pain. The Psychotherapeutic Spectrum.* New York: Praegar.

Bergman, J. J., & Werblun, M. N. (1978), Chronic pain: A review for the family physician. *J. Fam. Pract.*, 7:685–693.

Black, R. G. (1986), Evaluation of the patient with the complaint of pain. In: *Practical Management of Pain,* ed. P. P. Raj. Chicago: Year Book Medical Publishers, pp. 123–133.

Block, A. R., Boyer, S. L., & Silbert, R. K. (1985), Spouse's perception of the chronic pain patient: estimates of exercise tolerance. In: *Advances in Pain Research and Therapy,* Vol. 9, eds. H. L. Fields, R. Dubner, & F. Cervero. New York: Raven Press, pp. 897–904.

———Kremer, E., & Gaylor, M. (1980a), Behavioral treatment of chronic pain: variables affecting treatment efficacy. *Pain,* 8:367–375.

——— ——— ———(1980b), Behavioral treatment of chronic pain: the spouse as discriminative cue for pain behavior. *Pain,* 9:243–252.

Bonica, J. J. (1974), Organization and function of a pain clinic. In: *Advances in Neurology,* Vol. 4, ed. J. J. Bonica. New York: Raven Press, pp. 433–443.

———(1977), Basic principles in managing chronic pain. *Arch. Surg.,* 112:783–788.

Brena, S. F., Wolf, S. L., Chapman, S. L., & Hammonds, W. D. (1980), Chronic back pain: Electromyographic, motion and behavioral assessments following sympathetic nerve blocks and placebos. *Pain,* 8:1–10.

Cairns, D., & Pasino, J. A. (1977), Comparison of verbal reinforcement and feedback in the operant treatment of disability due to chronic low back pain. *Behav. Ther.,* 8:621–630.

———Thomas, L., Mooney, V., & Pace, J. B. (1976), A comprehensive treatment approach to chronic low back pain. *Pain,* 2:301–308.

Cameron, R. (1982), Behavior and cognitive therapies. In: *Chronic Pain, Psychosocial Factors in Rehabilitation,* eds., R. Roy & E. Tunks. Baltimore: Williams & Wilkins, pp. 79–103.

———(1987), 'Self-efficacy' manipulation. Paper presented at Pain Research Retreat Chedoke-McMaster Hospitals, Chedoke Division, Hamilton, Ontario, February 20.

Catchlove, R., Cohen, K. (1983), Directive approach with Workmen's Compensation patients. In: *Advances in Pain Research and Therapy,* Vol. 5, eds. J. J. Bonica, U. Lindblom, & A. Iggo. New York: Raven Press, pp. 913–918.

Chapman, C. R. (1976), Psychologic aspects of cardiac pain. Paper presented at National Conference on Cardiac Pain, Princeton, New Jersey, May 15, 16.

Craig, K. D. (1978), Social modeling influences on pain. In: *The Psychology of Pain,* ed. R. A. Sternbach. New York: Raven Press, pp. 73–109.

———Best, J. A. (1977), Perceived control over pain: Individual differences and situational determinants. *Pain,* 3:127–135.

Crook, J., Rideout, E., & Browne, G. (1984), The prevalence of pain complaints in a general population. *Pain,* 18:299–314.

———Tunks, E. (1985), Defining the 'chronic pain syndrome': An epidemiological method. In: *Advances in Pain Research and Therapy,* Vol. 9, eds. H. L. Fields, R. Dubner, & F. Cervero. New York: Raven Press, pp. 871–877.

Dworkin, R. H., Handlin, D. S., Richlin, D. M., Brand, L., & Vannuci, C. (1985), Unraveling the effects of compensation, litigation, and employment on treatment response in chronic pain. *Pain,* 23:49–59.

Eisler, R. M. (1976), Behavioral assessment of social skills. In: *Behavioral Assessment,* eds. M. Hersen & A. S. Bellack. New York: Pergamon Press, pp. 369–395.

Fordyce, W. E. (1976), Behavioral concepts in chronic pain and illness. In: *The Behavioral Management of Anxiety, Depression and Pain,* ed. P. O. Davidson. New York: Brunner/Mazel, pp. 147–188.

———(1978), Learning processes in pain. In: *The Psychology of Pain,* ed. R. A. Sternbach. New York: Raven Press, pp. 49–72.

———Fowler, R. S., Lehman, J. F., DeLateur, B. J., Sand, P. L., & Trieschmann, R. B. (1973), Operant conditioning in the treatment of chronic pain. *Arch. Phys. Med. Rehab.*, 54:399–408.

———Roberts, A. H., & Sternbach, R. A. (1985), The behavioral management of chronic pain: a response to critics. *Pain,* 22:113–125.

Frank, J. D. (1978), Expectation and therapeutic outcome—the placebo effect and the role induction interview. In: *Effective Ingredients of Successful Psychotherapy,* eds. J. D. Frank, R. Hoehn-Saric, S. D. Imber, B. L. Liberman, & A. R. Stone. New York: Brunner/Mazel, pp. 1–34.

Genest, M., & Turk, D. (1979), A proposed model for group therapy with pain patients. In: *Behavioral Group Therapy: An Annual Review,* eds. D. Upper & S. M. Ross. Champaign, IL.: Research Press.

Gottlieb, H. J., Koller, R., & Alperson, B. L. (1982), Low back pain comprehensive rehabilitation program: A follow-up study. *Arch. Phys. Med. Rehab.*, 63:458–461.

Herman, E., & Baptiste, S. (1981), Pain Control: mastery through group experience. *Pain,* 10:79–86.

Jacobson, E. (1944), *Progressive Relaxation,* 2nd ed. Chicago: University of Chicago Press.

Jessup, B. A., Neufeld, R. W. J., & Merskey, H. (1979), Biofeedback therapy for headache and other pain: An evaluative review. *Pain,* 7:225–270.

Kelly, G. A. (1955), *The Psychology of Personal Constructs.* New York: W. W. Norton.

Kendall, P. C., Williams, L., Pechacek, T. F., Graham, L. E., Shisslack, C., & Herzoff, N. (1979), Cognitive-behavioral and patient education interventions in cardiac catherization procedures: The Palo Alto medical psychology project. *J. Cons. Clin. Psychol.*, 47:49–58.

Kielhofner, G. (1986), Enhancing clinical practice through theory. Paper presented at an educational session, McMaster University, Hamilton, Ontario, Canada, June 12.

Lampe, G. N., & Mannheimer, J. S. (1984), The patient and T.E.N.S. In: *Clinical Transcutaneous Electrical Nerve Stimulation,* eds. J. S. Mannheimer & G. N. Lampe. Philadelphia: F. A. Davis, pp. 219–238.

Lazarus, R. S. (1977), A cognitive analysis of biofeedback control. In: *Biofeedback: Theory and Research,* eds. G. E. Schwartz & J. Beatty. New York: Academic Press, pp. 67–87.

Levine, J. D., Gordon, N. C., & Fields, H. L. (1978), The mechanism of placebo analgesia. *Lancet,* 2:654–657.

Liberman, B. L. (1978), The role of mastery in psychotherapy: Maintenance of improvement and prescriptive change. In: *Effective Ingredients of Successful Psychotherapy,* eds. J. D. Frank, R. Hoehn-Saric, S. D. Imber, B. L. Liberman, & A. R. Stone. New York: Brunner/Mazel, pp. 35–72.

Linton, S. J. (1986), Behavioral remediation of chronic pain: a status report. *Pain,* 24:125–141.

Lipinski, D., & Nelson, R. (1974), The reactivity and unreliability of self-recording. *J. Consult. Clin. Psychol.*, 42:118–123.

Luthe, W. (1979), About the methods of autogenic therapy. In: *Mind/Body Integration,* eds. E. Peper, S. Ancoli, & M. Quinn. New York: Plenum Press, pp. 167–186.

Mahoney, M. J. (1974), *Cognition and Behavior Modification.* Cambridge, MA.: Ballinger.

Malec, J., Cayner, J. J., Harvey, R. F., & Timming, R. C. (1981), Pain management: Long-term follow-up of an inpatient program. *Arch. Phys. Med. Rehab.*, 62:369–371.

Maruta, T., Swanson, D. W., & Swenson, W. M. (1979), Chronic pain: Which patients may a pain-management program help? *Pain*, 7:321–329.

Mayer, D. J. (1979), Endogenous analgesia systems: neural and behavioral mechanisms. In: *Advances in Pain Research and Therapy*, Vol. 3, ed. J. J. Bonica, J. C. Liebeskind, & D. G. Albe-Fessard. New York: Raven Press, pp. 385–410.

Meichenbaum, D., & Turk, D. (1976), The cognitive-behavioral management of anxiety, anger, and pain. In: *The Behavioral Management of Anxiety, Depression and Pain*, ed. P. O. Davidson. New York: Brunner/ Mazel, pp. 1–34.

Melzack, R. (1973), *The Puzzle of Pain.* New York: Basic Books.

———(1975), The McGill Questionnaire: major properties and scoring methods. *Pain*, 1:277–299.

———(1984), Neuropsychological basis of pain measurement. In: *Advances in Pain Research and Therapy*, Vol. 6, eds. L. Kruger, & J. C. Liebeskind. New York: Raven Press, pp. 323–339.

Merskey, H. (1965), The characteristics of persistent pain in psychological illness. *J. Psychosom. Res.*, 9:291–298.

Moore, J., & Chaney, E. (1985), Outpatient group treatment of chronic pain: effects of spouse involvement. *J. Cons. Clin. Psychol.*, 53:326–334.

Moya, F., & Mayne, G. E. (1986), Organization of a pain clinic. In: *Practical Management of Pain*, ed. P.P. Raj. Chicago: Year Book Medical Publishers, pp. 20–27.

Newman, R. I., Seres, J. L., Yospe, L. P., & Garlington, B. (1978), Multidisciplinary treatment of chronic pain: Long-term follow-up of low pack pain patients. *Pain*, 4:283–292.

Oxman, T. (1986), A psychosomatic approach to the diagnosis of chronic pain. In: *Practical Management of Pain*, ed. P. P. Raj. Chicago: Year Book Medical Publishers, pp. 134–145.

Painter, J. R., Seres, J. L., & Newman, R. I. (1980), Assessing benefits of the pain center: Why some patients regress. *Pain*, 8:101–113.

Patterson, D. M. (1979), Progressive relaxation training: Overview, procedure, and implications for self-regulation. In: *Mind/Body Integration*, eds. E. Peper, S. Ancoli, & M. Quinn. New York: Plenum Press, pp. 187–200.

Pavlov, I. P. (1928), *Lectures on Conditioned Reflexes.* New York: International Publishers.

Payne, B., & Norfleet, M.A. (1986), Chronic pain and the family: A review. *Pain*, 26:1–22.

Pilowsky, I. (1978), Psychodynamic aspects of the pain experience. In: *The Psychology of Pain*, ed. R.A. Sternbach. New York: Raven Press, pp. 203–217.

———Basset, D. (1982), Individual dynamic psychotherapy for chronic pain. In: *Chronic Pain. Psychosocial Factors in Rehabilitation*, eds. R. Roy & E. Tunks. Baltimore: Williams & Wilkins, pp. 107–125.

———Chapman, C. R., & Bonica, J. J. (1977), Pain, depression, and illness behavior in a pain clinic population. *Pain*, 4:183–192.

———Spence, N. D. (1976), Illness behaviour syndromes associated with intractable pain. *Pain*, 2:61–71.

Quinn, M. (1979), Beliefs and attitudes. In: *Mind/Body Intergration*, eds. E. Peper, S. Ancoli, & M. Quinn. New York: Plenum Press, pp. 201–205.

Roberts, A. H., & Reinhardt, L. (1980), The behavioral management of chronic pain: long-term follow-up with comparison groups. *Pain*, 8:151–162.

Rogers, C. R. (1952), 'Client-centered' psychotherapy. *Sci. Amer.*, 187:66–76.

Rotter, J. B. (1966), Generalized expectations for internal versus external control of reinforcement. *Psychological Monographs*, 80, No. 609.

Roy, R. (1982), Marital and family issues in patients with chronic pain. *Psychother. Psychosom.*, 37:1–12.

———Bellissimo, A., & Tunks E., (1982), The chronic pain patient and the environment. In: *Chronic Pain. Psychosocial Factors in Rehabilitation*, eds. R. Roy & E. Tunks. Baltimore: Williams & Wilkins, pp. 1–9.

Rybstein-Blinchik, E. (1979), Effects of different cognitive strategies on chronic pain experiences. *J. Behav. Med.*, 2:93–102.

Seligman, M. E. P. (1975), *Helplessness.* San Francisco: W. H. Freeman.

Seres, J. L., & Newman, R. I. (1976), Results of treatment of chronic low-back pain at the Portland Pain Center. *J. Neurosurg.*, 45:32–36.

Shanfield, S. B., Heiman, E. M., Cope, D. N., & Jones, J. R. (1979), Pain and the marital relationship: psychiatric distress. *Pain*, 7:343–351.

Shontz, F. C. (1975), *The Psychological Aspects of Physical Illness and Disability.* New York: Macmillan.

Skinner, B. F. (1953), *Science and Human Behavior.* New York: Macmillan.

Sternbach, R. A. (1976), The need for an animal model of chronic pain. *Pain*, 2:2–4.

Swanson, D. W., & Maruta, T. (1980), The family's viewpoint of chronic pain. *Pain*, 8:163–166.

——— ———Swenson, W. M. (1979), Results of behavior modification in the treatment of chronic pain. *Pschosom. Med.*, 41:55–61.

———Swenson, W. M., Maruta, T. & Floreen, A. C. (1978), The dissatisfied patient with chronic pain. *Pain*, 4:367–377.

Tan, S. Y. (1982), Cognitive and cognitive-behavioral methods for pain control: A selective review. *Pain*, 12:201–228.

Terenius, L. (1978), Significance of endorphins in endogenous antinociception. In: *The Endorphins: Advances in Biochemical Psychopharmacology*, Vol. 18. ed. P. London. New York: Raven Press, pp. 321–329.

Toomey, J. N., Ghia, J. N., Mao, W. & Gregg, J. M. (1977), Acupuncture and chronic pain mechanisms: The moderating effects of affect, personality, and stress on response to treatment. *Pain*, 3:137–145.

Tunks, E. (1982), Psychiatric management of chronic pain. In: *Chronic Pain. Psychosocial Factors in Rehabilitation*, eds. R. Roy & E. Tunks. Baltimore: Williams & Wilkins, pp. 179–212.

———(1987), Psychological treatment: The importance of objective behavioral goals in pain management. In: *Advances in Pain Research and Therapy*, Vol. 10, eds. M. Tienga, J. Eccles, A.C. Cuello, & D. Ottoson. New York: Raven Press, pp. 45–58.

Turk, D. C., & Flor, H. (1984), Etiological theories and treatment for chronic back pain. II. Psychological models and interventions. *Pain*, 19:209–233.

———Meichenbaum, D., & Genest, M. (1983), *Pain and Behavioral Medicine: A Cognitive–Behavioral Perspective.* New York: Guilford Press.

Turner, J. A., & Chapman, C. R. (1982), Psychological interventions for chronic pain: A critical review. II. Operant conditioning, hypnosis, and cognitive–behavioral therapy. *Pain*, 12:23–46.

Tursky, B., & Sternbach, R. A. (1975), Further physiological correlates of ethnic differences in responses to shock. In: *Pain. Clinical and Experimental Perspectives*, ed. M. Weisenberg. St. Louis: C. V. Mosby, pp. 152–157.

Wolff, B. B., & Langley, S. (1975), Cultural factors and the response to pain: A review. In: *Pain. Clinical and Experimental Perspectives*, ed. M. Weisenberg. St. Louis: C. V. Mosby, pp. 144–151.

Wolpe, J. (1958), *Psychotherapy by Reciprocal Inhibition.* Stanford, CA: Stanford University Press.

Yaksh, T. L., Howe, J. R., & Harty, G. J. (1984), Pharmacology of spinal pain modulatory systems. In: *Advances in Pain Research and Therapy*, Vol. 7, eds. C. Benedetti, C. R. Chapman, & G. Moricca. New York: Raven Press, pp. 57–70.

Yalom, I. D. (1975), *The Theory and Practice of Psychotherapy*, 2nd ed. New York: Basic Books.

16

The Psychology and Psychotherapy of the Chronic Pain Patient

ROBERT LAKOFF M.D., F.R.C.P.(C)

There can be little doubt that patients suffering from pain which is unresponsive to medical management represent a therapeutic challenge of the highest order. Not only do they often reject the psychological model for their pain, which they resent, believing it to disregard their symptoms, but they tend to cling tenaciously to the physician or surgeon who has treated them in the past, albeit without success. The therapist attempting to use a psychological approach often finds himself faced with a bewildering array of defense mechanisms which may include: (1) conversion (Merskey, 1978); (2) denial (Gross and Gardner, 1980); (3) splitting; (4) projection of the bad (painful) parts of the self; and (5) regression (from mild to severe in degree) (Gross and Gardner, 1980). Treatment personnel may be angrily rejected because they are perceived as persecutors. Although rare, depersonalization may occur in an attempt to cope with persistent, severe pain.

The integrative and synthetic functions of the ego may become overtaxed resulting in severe distortions of the body image (Schilder, 1957). Ritualized behaviors to cope with pain often have an obsessive tinge in these patients, and the theories they develop about pain mechanisms reflect primary process thinking. Excessive withdrawal of libidinal cathexes back upon the ego may lead to psychosis (Freud, 1914). This highly undesirable outcome is usually avoided, however, by excessive restrictions of the personality imposed by the variety of defense mechanisms described above.

In recent years there has been increasing recognition of the psychological aspects of pain; however, the trend has been toward the development of behavioral management rather than psychotherapy, which, practiced in isolation, was usually ineffective. Enquiries into the psychic mechanisms of pain, such as those by Rangell (1953), Szasz (1957), and Ramzy and Wallerstein (1958), have not focused on treatment, and interest in this type of study has diminished. There has been little written on psychotherapy with chronic pain patients, possibly because until the recent development of multimodal therapeutic approaches, these people remained inaccessible to psychotherapy.

There appears to be a growing consensus (Rangell, 1953; Smith and Duerksen, 1980) that chronic pain patients often show the following psychological characteristics: (1) infantile dependency needs; (2) marked passivity; (3) masochism; (4) denial; (5) regression; (6) repressed anger or overt hostility; and (7) feelings of guilt, anxiety, and depression. Chronic pain patients are known to score higher on Minnesota Multiphasic Personality Inventory (MMPI) scales measuring hypochondriasis (HS), depression (D), and hysteria (Hy) (Bond, 1979). They verbalize emotions poorly, tend to to be concerned with somatic experiences rather than psychic conflict, and show a marked inability to mourn.

Psychotherapy

Contrary to Blumer (1980), who has indicated that these patients are poor candidates for psychotherapy because of their tendency to think operationally, their lack of fantasy, and impoverished imagination, these patients can be imaginative and do respond positively to interpretive psychotherapy. Hunter and Ross (1960) found that 94 percent of migraine patients treated with psychotherapy showed significant improvement which lasted up to six to twelve months in the majority of cases. They conclude:

> Though it is usually assumed that psychiatric illness associated with migraine is due to the migraine, and therefore to cure the migraine is to eliminate the psychiatric disturbance, our results show the reverse—namely, that frequency and severity of attacks may be influenced for better or for worse by psychological factors. It seems almost as if it was more important to ask patients "who or what is your headache?"—rather than "when or where?" [pp. 1088].

Ruttick and Aronoff (1983) also found psychotherapy useful in the treatment of chronic pain but cautioned that:

> [A]n undue focus on psychodynamics can be countertherapeutic when patients either blame their problems on the past or find explanations irrelevant. It becomes more important to explore how the patient's dependency needs were met when he was functioning well—and how the injury upset this balance—than to focus on the origin of his dependent personality [pp. 60R].

Clinical Vignettes

Case 1

Mr. M., a thirty-seven-year-old plumber, abandoned by his parents as an infant, and brought up in a series of foster homes, had as an adolescent, felt exploited by his foster parents for the social welfare checks they received for his care. His young adulthood was characterized by hard work, a happy marriage, two children, and social and financial success. A work accident in his middle thirties necessitated an unsuccessful back operation. He claimed compensation for an injury which he said prevented him from engaging in his customary occupation. A five-year history of repeated neurological and orthopedic investigations ensued. He had begun drinking excessively. Interpretive work during his stay in a pain unit centered around bitter memories of rejection and exploitation by foster families whose unqualified love he craved, but never felt he received. His pain elicited the concern and protectiveness of his wife who previously had admired his apparent independence and productivity. Careful exploration of his fantasy life led to the interpretation that because of his pain he felt he had paid his dues, and now expected compensation from society along with the indulgence of those close to him (i.e., there was a regression to oral dependency needs with strong narcissistic cathexis of the painful part). This man improved in the hospital setting; however, he failed to return to work, preferring a semicompensated life-style which featured private contracting to augment his disability payments.

Case 2

Mrs. H., a sixty-four-year-old teacher, was referred to the pain unit with a five-year history of continuous pain which began with the prolapse and surgical removal of two lumbar disks. Shortly thereafter she developed a severe postherpetic neuralgia which was treated by rhizotomy of the fifth to ninth thoracic nerve roots. Numerous physical therapies including transcutaneous nerve stimulation were unsuccessful. An intelligent woman, highly stoical, in character, she continued working throughout, and resisted the use of analgesics for fear of becoming addicted.

The initial interview revealed her to be depressed and anxious. She had had to stop work because of her inability to concentrate due to the pain. Her complaint was that she was unable to enjoy life. She blamed herself for giving in to the pain, but was willing to do anything to get rid of it, even to accept admission to a psychiatric ward for psychological management of her condition, although she had little faith that this would help her.

Her treatment on the ward consisted of: (1) cognitive behavior therapy; (2) relaxation therapy; (3) physiotherapy; (4) occupational therapy; and (5) analytically oriented psychotherapy. Interpretive work in psychotherapy was done based on the following account of her life:

The patient was born in London and emigrated to Canada at the age of three years. Her father, a veteran of the First World War, was severely alcoholic. He worked as a game warden and would take the patient along with him into the forest, forcing her to have sexual relations with him on a regular basis when she was between twelve and fourteen years old. When her mother learned of this, she returned to England with the patient and her younger brother. There had been no further contact with the father, who died in a mental institution in Canada when the patient was twenty years old.

Subsequently the patient became a nurse and served in the British Army in World War II and was discharged for psychiatric reasons in 1945 (migraine, jitters). She married an alcoholic man at the age of thirty-three and after seven miscarriages adopted two children, a boy and a girl. The marriage lasted thirteen years, ending in divorce. Her husband is currently in a mental institution. Her two children are well. Her son, age twenty-three, is married and her daughter, twenty-one is single and living on her own.

Psychotherapy was done concurrently with other forms of therapy. Pharmacotherapy included the use of small doses of nonnarcotic analgesics. No antidepressants were used. The patient's angry feelings toward doctors who had "assaulted" her were explored in the light of her incestuous relationship with her father. Her present life crisis had awakened strong dependency needs, for which there was much guilt.

In a most revealing document the patient wrote down her internal experience of a confusional state lasting three weeks after her rhizotomy. Among numerous hallucinatory experiences, she was accused of turning her mother's home into a brothel. The interpretation of her guilt at the childhood "Oedipal victory" was shocking to the patient. She remembered, with shame, that she had enjoyed sexual intercourse with her father, but was also disgusted with herself and hated him for having taken advantage of her.

Following considerable abreaction, an interpretation of the transference was made: "Your pain allows you to need me without guilt." During the working through period of several weeks she showed markedly less pain behavior and reported much subjective improvement.

These and other interpretations were discussed with the treatment team so that a dynamic understanding of the patient was integrated with the entire treatment approach. It was felt by the patient and the staff that the interpretive work greatly enhanced the efficacy of the program.

Case 3

Mr. S., a twenty-seven-year-old textile cutter from Punjab, India, was admitted for a pain in the vertex of his head which had lasted seven years. His quest for a "cure" had led him to specialists in ears, nose and throat (ENT) and neurology, and hospitalization for correction of a deviated nasal septum, which was thought to be responsible for the pain. Chiropractic treatments, acupuncture, and homeopathic prescriptions were all ineffective. He described the pain as deep and localized, and it seemed to be alleviated briefly by pressure on the area. He was certain the pain was related to the redness of his eyes, and produced a series of drawings to show this, which revealed a severely distorted image of his own body.

Exploration of his developmental history revealed that the pain had begun shortly after his arrival in Canada. He was of the Sikh religion and had worn a turban all his life, until then. Initially the interpretation of guilt relating to the removal of the turban was flatly denied; however, as treatment progressed, he was able to express considerable conflicts relating to the rigid, authoritarian attitudes of his parents ("all Sikhs are supposed to wear beards and turbans"). His envy of a favored brother who was serving in a Sikh regiment in India was quite evident.

The patient's behavioral program was designed to treat the phobic anxiety with which he was accustomed to meet new situations; for example, the arrival of his new wife from India. Interpretive psychotherapy centered around the defense mechanisms of denial and conversion. Although the degree of insight achieved was judged by the therapist to be minimal, symptoms alleviation was complete. On seven-month follow-up, the patient stated that he did not want to return to the clinic because he feared that this would remind him of his pain.

Case 4

Mrs. R., a sixty-two-year-old real estate agent, was referred for the treatment of ischemic pain resulting from thrombotic emboli to her legs. The pain was of two years' duration. A sudden decompensation of her chronic heart disorder had severely damaged her self-confidence in addition to placing limitations on her physical endurance. She blamed her previous physicians for blunders in treatment, and this carried over to the therapist, whom she suspected of not believing she was physically ill.

History revealed that her father, a fur salesman, died when she was an infant, leaving her mother, an energetic, hard-working woman, to bring up the family of four. The patient suffered hardships throughout life, but was always the one upon whom others relied. Her younger brother, whose birth followed her father's death, was dependent upon her even as an adult. Her husband of twenty years had been a chronic cardiac invalid.

This fiercely independent woman, upon becoming an invalid herself, reacted with intense anxiety and angry depression. She related to her doctors with ambivalence. They were "uncaring and "unfeeling" (absent fathers), on the one hand, and overidealized healers on the other.

Upon admission to the hospital, she complained about every feature on the ward; the fact that there was no elevator, that there were teenagers and "crazy people" there, that she was in a four-bed room and could not open the window, that she was not given her laxative at the right time, that the nurses and doctors were uncaring, the food was unhealthy for her, and so on. A behavioral program was instituted and frequent communication among staff members helped the tension caused by the manipulation of this very unpleasant, complaining patient.

Within two weeks the complaints had ceased, the patient had relinquished the cane she had used to walk with, and negotiated the stairs without great difficulty. Her pain had mostly gone.

From this high level the patient regressed after one month, following a recrudescence of physical illness (an eye infection). She blamed her therapist: "I am depressed because you made me depressed. I wasn't before I met you and you began telling me I was." The sessions were a litany of complaints. Acting out occurred in the form of arguments with other patients and a refusal to cooperate in her program. At a staff meeting the defensive nature of her complaints was discussed (i.e., that it was a defense against deep depressive affect). This permitted the staff to work through a strong countertransference engendered by the patient and to continue working with her in a consistent manner.

Recently her angry defiance has abated and she has been able to accept that she has sad feelings about her illness and to express these more openly without alienating staff, patients, family, and friends as she had been doing. She continued to improve within the program and had maintained this improvement on follow-up one year later.

Case 5

S., a thirty-six-year-old divorced woman, was referred for analytic treatment as a "last resort." She had undergone numerous treatments and investigations for a variety of ailments including chronic pain of her jaw, which had been given the label temporomandibular joint syndrome (TMJ). She also complained of pain in her eyes, nose, head, neck, shoulder, knee, and rectal pain due to hemorrhoids. In spite of her high anxiety, she had been able to function in her profession until one year prior to her referral to the analyst. At that time she had become obsessed with the idea that the motorcyclist boyfriend of a dissatisfied client of hers might follow her home and rape her. After changing jobs she became preoccupied with the smell of gas in her basement, necessitating frequent calls to the gas company, and she eventually changed her furnace although no leak was ever detected. Gradually, in the months preceding her referral to the analyst, her focus shifted to her own body.

She became aware of "bulging veins" on her abdomen and in her groin. A normal venogram and reassurance from her doctor seemed insufficient to allay her anxiety. She developed pain in her left knee which was investigated radiographically, revealing no observable pathology. This pain alternated with one in her neck and shoulder, which in the beginning of the analysis prevented her from lying comfortably on the couch. The weekends were long and desperate. She would wake up at night certain that she was about to exanguinate via her nose which, due to the dryness of the air in her home, occasionally bled. She would feel compelled to examine her nostrils with a flashlight. In addition, she was plagued by pain in her jaw for which she was given a retainer by her dentist. This caused sores in her mouth which increased her discomfort enormously. After several unsuccessful adjustments of the retainer she stopped wearing it. During this period she was a regular visitor at the local clinic and was followed by a very supportive general practitioner who eventually referred her to the analyst. The patient, during this period and in the early part of her analysis, was involved with many health professionals, including medical specialists, physiotherapists, dentists, a chiropracter, and an acupuncturist. She initially blamed the chiropracter for causing the pain in her neck by his "therapeutic manipulations."

History revealed her to be the oldest of two sibs born to an obsessional mother and an alcoholic father. Her parents never showed affection to each other or to the children. She remembers father as being disinterested and withdrawn and mother as being domineering and more interested in her younger brother than herself. Her wish as a teenager was to ride horses, but this was frustrated at seventeen by the sale of the land upon which they lived. She developed anorexia nervosa for which she was hospitalized several times in her late teens and early twenties. She was amenorrheic during this period and off and on over several years. She had not menstruated in ten years. Her marriage, at twenty-six, failed after two years. She could not meet the sexual demands of her husband who insisted that she initiate sexual contact. She had briefly enjoyed sexuality but the experience had left her with a profound sense of inadequacy. Over the years she became increasingly isolated socially and her dependence on mother increased. She was unable to mourn her father's death two years earlier. She now lives alone but in close proximity to mother, who lives with the patient's brother and sister-in-law. When she was anxious, the patient frequently called her seventy-two-year-old mother to come over. Mother, who had little understanding of psychological treatment, was initially very disparaging of the patient's visits to the analyst. As the symptoms became more numerous, bizarre, and frequent, however, mother began to show a somewhat grudging support of the treatment which she believed to be a "last resort" for her ailing daughter.

It was at this point in the analysis that the patient began to associate, albeit cautiously, to the analyst. The sessions hitherto had been filled with endless descriptions of symptoms, doctor's visits, and theoretical propositions about the origin of her symptoms. Dream material and increased fantasy in the sessions permitted some working through of conflicts relating to her symbiotic relation with mother, some mourning for the father she never had, and the recognition of angry, jealous feelings toward her brother. After eight months of analysis, symptoms were rarely mentioned in the sessions and visits to doctors had greatly diminished. Pain behavior both within and outside of the sessions had been markedly reduced for at least two months at the time of writing of this paper.

Discussion

The cases presented here are typical in that dynamic conflicts were identified in all of them. Cases one to four were treated in an inpatient setting where the dynamics were discussed with the treatment team within the context of multimodal therapy. The fifth case is currently undergoing psychoanalysis without a coordinated team approach. The working through of these conflicts helped the first four patients adapt to and utilize other treatment modalities in the program. Interpretive (analytic) psychotherapy is useful in conjunction with other forms of treatment (behavior modification, relaxation therapy, occupational therapy, group and family therapy, etc.)

combined in a multimodal approach (Catchlove, 1979). The cornerstone of interpretive psychotherapy is a sound knowledge of the patient's developmental history, upon which a psychogenetic model of the patient's behavior may be formulated. This may then be shared with the other members of the team helping to shape the overall management of the case.

The fifth case serves as a basis of comparison. A greater intensity of individual treatment may compensate for the lack of the team approach. As noted, the analyst found that the patient, in the early stage of treatment, required other points of reference than himself until the transference was firmly established.

Psychological Models of Pain

Although one does not become habituated to severe pain (Jones, 1957), one may, however, evolve ego adaptations in order to live with chronic pain. The converse is that chronic pain may accentuate neurotic trends with consequent ego distortions and restrictions of the personality (Engel, 1959; Merskey, 1980). There have been a number of significant attempts to understand pain as an aspect of ego psychology. Freud (1926) noted the similarity of physical pain to the experience of the loss of an object. The concept of pain as "the affect referring to ego-body orientation," as opposed to anxiety, which refers to ego-object orientation, was proposed by Szasz (1957). Schilder (1957) noted that pain must be localized and therefore brought into connection with the organization of the body image, a concept which is germane to the understanding of how the body integrates and copes with painful stimuli.

Seen in the light of ego functions, pain need not be as uncompromising as Jones (1957) believed it to be. Interpretive psychotherapy links pain with affective experience and strengthens the ego by bringing about insight. The working through of neurotic conflicts in this group of patients is greatly facilitated by the multimodal program, and symptom alleviation is often dramatic. Interpretation also has the effect of enhancing the therapeutic relationship by reducing countertransference. The patient's angry resistance, seen as a defense against disturbing affects, is less threatening to the therapist's narcissism. Analytic psychotherapy, by creating a bridge with the past, helps the patient utilize previous more adaptive ego resources.

Chronic pain may thus be viewed as a continuing life crisis in which ego functioning is impaired in several ways. Freud (1914) described a hypercathexis of the painful part accompanied by regression to narcissism. Schilder (1957) discussed distortions in body image, perception, and object relations resulting from pain. Work impairment, inability to concentrate, sexual dysfunction, and depression with suicidal ruminations are also common features.

Bastiaans (1977) describes psychosomatic patients as neurotics who pretend to be mentally healthy and well adapted. He states: "as a result of their increased and chronic efforts to maintain this pretention (sic) they must pay a high price in the form of the bodily symptom" (pp. 87). This is particularly true of pain patients whose focus on the sensory quality of the pain experience serves as a defense against deeper underlying conflicts. Ramsay (1977) noted that they often, to their detriment, have succeeded in convincing physicians that "the peripheral components of the pain experience should [receive] first attention" (pp. 58). In the past, surgical measures such as anterolateral chordotomy, brain stem trachotomy, thalamic resection, and leucotomy were frequently performed on patients whose pain had been labeled as intractible prior to any consideration of psychological investigation and treatment. Although the pain clinics of the 1970s became increasingly aware of the delicate balance between physical and psychological factors in the experience of pain (Catchlove and Ramsay, 1978), spinal fusions and dorsal fusions were often performed without prior psychiatric consultation. Successful alleviation of pain in this group of patients with psychologically oriented multimodal therapy (Bonica, 1974; Maline and Crue, 1975) convincingly highlights the need for earlier recognition and utilization of the psychosomatic approach to pain.

The accident or illness which initiates the pain career may be viewed by the therapist as a nidus around which many conflicts are congealed. These conflicts originate in early developmental fixations and arrests which have, prior to the accident, been compensated for by rigid adaptations and character distortions.

BEHAVIORAL CHARACTERISTICS OF CHRONIC PAIN PATIENTS

The success or failure of any treatment for chronic pain must be judged from the vantage point of a good understanding of the goals of treatment. Brena and Chapman (1983) point out that:

> [S]ome 30 percent of all patients who go through a pain control and rehabilitation programme will deny any positive result. An analysis of these *failures* shows four inter-mixed groups of subjects. One group includes patients who went through the motions of pain rehabilitation treatment with no real interest, obsessed by the idea that something *must be wrong in their body* and needs to be diagnosed and removed to provide a *permanent cure.* A second group comprises what Szasz (1968) called the experts in *painmanship.* These patients wish to maintain their sick role while pretending the contrary. A third group includes a few patients who feel compelled to deny all results from any treatment modality in order to justify their continuing disability compensation. A fourth group includes patients with inadequate personalities who lack the skills to cope with daily living. In a medical milieu that relies heavily on biomedical interventions, these groups of unfortunate patients may be expected to float from hospital to hospital and from one specialist to another with no result other than astronomical increase in medical costs [pp. 116]

Morse (1983) described the Loss, Anger, and Depression syndrome (LAD) in which a cycle of these emotions is "expressed through pain and becomes the predominant factor in the patient's life." He states:

> [B]ecause the patient's pain is a representation of an inability to handle loss, anger and depression, the patient's actual recovery cannot be measured through verbal pain behavior. Indeed, the relationship may be inverse. The more verbal pain behavior is exhibited regardless of its disgruntled content, the less the physiological, non-verbal or other manifestations of pain. It is often heard from the astute referring physician that the patient has appeared in the physician's office in an angry and verbal manner, debunking all treatment efforts, but had never looked better. Similarly, patients often express ingratitude toward the pain therapist, yet, paradoxically, are recovering and becoming more independent [pp. 53].

Steger, Fox, and Feinberg, (1980) classified chronic pain patients into doloric, stoic, and assimilated types. Doloric patients show operant pain behavior which is contingent on situations such as the performance of a task which the patient finds unpleasant. They respond to behavioral modification programs. Stoic patients are those who "exhibit little overt pain behavior, tend to underutilize health care services and medication, and, so far as possible, deny that they have a pain problem" (Johnson, 1983). These individuals often have conditioned respondent pain. They are active and refuse to modify their life-style in response to pain. Unlike the doloric patients, stoic patients do not show pain behavior in response to environmental rewards. Their condition may be exacerbated by stress and high activity levels. They respond to instruction, education, and counseling, coupled with transcutaneous electrical nerve stimulation (TENS), biofeedback, nerve blocks, and medication, all of which are often ineffective with doloric patients. Johnson (1983) cautions that "ill-advised surgery, drastic curtailling of activities or habit forming medication may move stoic patients to a doloric state" (pp. 88).

The third category of assimilated patients have managed to adjust their life-style in order to remain as active as possible in spite of their pain problem. The goal in treatment with these patients is to maintain the assimilated pain state through education. According to Johnson (1983), "problems can occur if assimilated patients are misdiagnosed and inappropriately treated because of a desire on the part of the health care providers to *do something* for the chronic pain problems" (pp. 89).

PAIN AND PERSONALITY

Engel (1959) has noted that chronic pain patients conform to a guilt-ridden, masochistic personality type with an excessively punitive superego. These patients regularly regress, becoming irritable, demanding, and egocentric, eventually placing themselves beyond the empathy of those around them. They are unloving and, as such, become unloved. Freud (1914) states:

> It is universally known, and we take it as a matter of course, that a person who is tormented by organic pain and discomfort gives up his interest in things of the external world, insofar as they do not concern his suffering. Close observation also teaches us that he also withdraws libidinal interest from his love object; so long as he suffers he ceases to love [pp. 82].

Thus, the patient suffering from continuous pain loses interest in family, friends, and treating personnel. Often those in contact with him begin to feel they are being used, eventually lose their sympathy, and begin to withdraw.

Mr. A., an inpatient whose continual complaint of back pain was the focus of an intensive behavior therapy program, would not tolerate hearing Mr. G., his roommate, complain of his chronic leg discomfort. Very little empathy developed between these two chronic pain patients, and eventually they had to be separated. Mr. A., fearing even less understanding from the nonpain patients who were to be his new roommates, discharged himself. His sense of isolation had remained unabated throughout his admission.

Mr. G., who had always repressed his anger and disappointment with doctors and others who had failed to cure his pain, had attempted suicide prior to admission. His demanding behavior toward his wife had driven her to consider separation.

It was extremely difficult for Mr. G. to relate to the treatment team in any other way than by complaining. He feels that when his complaints are not responded to, it is because the listener does not believe him. When he is unable to project his anger, it is turned against him in the form of depression.

Mr. C., a twenty-six-year-old amputee suffered chronic phantom limb pain following a motorcycle accident in which he suffered an avulsion of the brachial plexus. His injury followed the breakup of a turbulent seven-year relationship with a woman. The pain was associated with his inability to mourn the loss of his arm, with its attendant threat to his fragile sense of masculinity. He drank excessively both before and after the accident. His continual complaints of pain and alcoholism served as a screen for conflicts related to low self-esteem, guilt over passive homosexual longings, and poor verbal skills. Treatment focused on these conflicts rather than on the palliation which the patient demanded. Although the patient continued to experience pain, a marked improvement was noted in his attitude. He was less depressed and suicidal, less paranoid in his relations with treating personnel, and had cut down his dependency on codeine by two-thirds.

In their desperation, many patients turn to alcohol and drugs, further increasing their isolation from others. Object cathexes are given up in preference for the relief provided by the drug. Pain, by this time, may have caused such severe distortions in the ego that the behavior has become ego-syntonic and extremely resistant to change. Alternate solutions must be provided, and may only be successful through an understanding of both the physiology and the psychology of pain.

The Relationship of Pain, Fear, and Anxiety

Freud's earliest concept of pain (Freud, 1895) is that the phenomenon of pain (here he does not make the distinction between affect and sensation) is regularly associated with a breach in the continuity of a protective barrier between the physical self and the outer world. Later, in "Inhibitions, Symptoms and Anxiety" (1926), he enlarges the concept by pointing out the similarity of physical pain to the experience of loss of an object. This brings it closer to the definition of an affect.

Szasz (1957) elaborates the theme that pain is a specific affect which pertains to the body in a manner analagous to the way in which anxiety refers to external objects. He states "pain is . . . the affect referring to ego-body orientation, anxiety to ego-object orientation" (pp. 77). Schilder (1957) integrates the concept of pain with the concept of the body image. He compares the sensation of pain with other sensations such as vision, and states that, whereas, in optic perception we concentrate on the object and we are hardly aware of the sensation, "in pain, the object becomes comparatively unimportant. When we suffer pain we care less for the quality of the object than for the sensation. At the same time object and subject come so close together that differentiation becomes difficult" (pp. 99). He also makes the point that pain has to be localized and, therefore, brought into connection with the organization of the body image, a concept which is germane to an understanding of how the ego integrates and copes with painful stimuli. Pain, according to Schilder (1957), "helps us to decide what we want nearer to our personality, to the center of our ego, and what we want further away from it" (pp. 105). He continues:

> The effect of pain on the body-image has not hitherto been sufficiently studied. The part of the body in which pain is felt gets all the attention. Libido is concentrated on it (Freud) and other parts of the body image lose in importance; but at the same time the painful part of the body becomes isolated. There is a tendency to push it out of the body-image. When the whole body is filled with pain, we try to get rid of the whole body. We take a stand outside our body and watch ourselves. When one has a toothache and one is near to falling asleep, one may have the feeling that one is watching oneself and that the pain belongs to another body [pp. 104].

Schilder's observations are strikingly illustrated by a fifty-two-year-old woman who during her analysis described a beating administered by her husband as follows: "I then had an out-of-the-body experience. I was floating on a silver cord while that woman (myself) was being beaten down there in the garden. I came to [consciousness] in the hospital." History revealed that she had been repeatedly beaten by her mother as a child. She had developed the defensive ability of taking a stand outside her own body. On this occasion she had calmly watched herself being beaten. An example of the opposite kind of projection is of a psychotic patient who upon being asked where his pain was, pointed to the top of a nearby flagpole (W.M.C. Scott, personal communication).

The mechanism of projection implies that a portion of the ego has become split off. Splitting without projection may also occur. Mr. G. hated to go out in the cold as this would aggravate the pain in his legs. He, nevertheless, derived much pleasure in activities which required that he leave the hospital (part of his behavioral modification program). On his return from one of these outings, he told the therapist: "The top half of my body enjoys it, but not the bottom half." In a later interview he referred to his body as being only one third painful and two thirds pain free. When asked to describe where the pain was, however, its distribution had not changed. Thus, splitting had helped the ego free itself from a larger portion of the hyper-cathected painful area.

The ego has many ways of adapting to continuous pain of which we are all familiar. In the following patient's statement pain is personified: "I guess It stopped because It decided I had had enough". The use of the word *It* refers to the primary process. In the terminology of the Lacanian school of psycho-analysis, "It" is a signifier but the thing signified lies deeply within the unconscious and relates to the very personal meaning of pain for each person.

Pain and Hypnosis

Hypnosis has long made use of the processes of dissociation (splitting and projection) in order to produce analgesia. It has been described by D. L. Scott (1974) as follows:

> The dissociative method of producing analgesia . . . may be described as "projection of the body image." The principle can be explained to the patient that if the body is (projected) "elsewhere", it cannot be "here" and that it will thus have no sensation. In other words, analgesia of the projected part will occur. . . . The patient can be told that his arm is going to float up and up and finally away from his body. A physical arm levitation may occur, in which event it can be suggested that when the projected image of the arm leaves the body and floats away, the physical arm will drop. . . . The analgesia produced is profound, and the method is very suitable to patients with burned extremities who require regular burn dressings, and also in obstetrics [pp. 55].

Scott describes the case of a young dental assistant who was stricken with Hodgkin's disease.

> He was aware of the diagnosis and prognosis. However, the cytotoxic drugs used created an intense and widespread pruritis. He put his . . . problem simply, "I know the score, and one of the few pleasures I have left is to enjoy a glass of beer at my local. But I cannot help scratching all the time, and people will think I am lousy. If I take anti-histamines, then the irritation goes but I cannot drink alcohol without going asleep" [pp. 102–103].

Knowing of no orthodox medical solution to such a problem, Scott hypnotized him, and under hypnosis it was suggested that the irritation would nearly all disappear.

> A small area on his cheek still itched, this he could easily remove by fresh hypnosis or he could scratch. He determined this, which did not matter anyway. . . . The effect wore off, of course, but he soon learned autohypnosis and was able to reproduce this freedom from irritation. He was becoming a master of this situation. As his disease progressed he became less able to do this himself, so rapport was passed over to his wife [pp. 102].

When asked about the shift in therapists, he replied, "I felt rather like a small child who was being told a story I knew well, and I realized the story-teller got it muddled. It didn't matter really" (pp. 102).

The patient had permitted himself to regress in the service of the ego. His dyspnoea diminished considerably under hypnotic relaxation and in the posttrance period, although the main site of the glandular involvement was mediastinal. He died at the age of thirty-one from anoxia.

Relief of chronic pain without hypnosis can be achieved through an undoing of global self-perception and a resynthesis at a different level of organization. This can be achieved only if the patient can learn to split his consciousness. He must take himself as an object (this is the basic goal of all cognitive and analytic therapies) and study his own behavior and perception. He must then learn to pay attention to separate parts of himself, to relax, to defocus his attention, to realign his body image, and reconstitute his state of consciousness in a way which will leave him pain free. Zeltzer and LeBaron (1986) discussed the use of fantasy in children for similar purposes concluding that "the use of fantasy as a means of communication and intervention for children with chronic disease appears promising" (pp. 197).

Pain, Body Image, and Sleep

Szasz (1957) considers the organic–psychogenic dichotomy of pain as misleading because it creates "numerous pseudo problems in the borderline between medicine and psychology" (pp. 19). That pain is, in fact, a borderline concept has been noted by several authors. "Like similar subjective things [it] is known to us by experience and described by illustration (Lewis, 1942). "Virtually every man has experienced pain, yet so common an experience eludes precise definition, and one could not describe pain to a person who had not experienced it" (Scott 1974, pp. 48). Pain must be referred to the body image (Schilder, 1957), yet it is not limited to it. Pain may be referred or radiated to parts of the body not associated with physical damage. In hypnosis and the phantom limb, pain may be experience as outside the body. In sleep:

> [T]he ego, via the dream, and *within* the sleeping state, converts somatic stimuli into hallucinated images and thoughts (the particular forms of which are associatively linked to the somatic stimulus [pain] of which they are the indirect mental representations in the dream. . . . The opposite transformation can, likewise, occur within the dream. What is perceived while awake as a mental pain may be perceived in the dream as a physical pain—or "dreamed pain" [Ramzy and Wallerstein, 1958, pp. 170–171].

Thus, Mr. G., while complaining of continual pain all day, had no difficulty in falling asleep, and anticipated his sleeping hours with considerable pleasure. Ramzy and Wallerstein also point out, in the same paper, that pain is influenced by the mood of anxiety and fear and cannot be clearly conceptualized without reference to them. It is also well known that pain may not be felt as expected in certain psychotic states such as schizophrenia, whereas it may be experienced where no organic pathology can be found, such as in hypochondriasis and hysteria. In masochism, pain may be experienced as a source of sexual excitement.

Pain and Paranoia

The ancients associated pain with punishment. Eve, for example, was condemned to bear her children in pain as a punishment for her disobedience in the Garden of Eden. The Latin root for pain is *poena*, penalty. Not infrequently, someone suffering chronic pain feels he is being punished either by God for some real or imagined transgression or by some person, usually a loved one, family member, or a member of the medical profession whom he has failed to ingratiate. The pain patient fears abandonment and is quick to accuse those who treat him of impatience or incompetence when faced with therapeutic failure. This, in turn, is a result of childlike and grandiose expectations placed upon the doctor or treating person. When disappointed, these patients may become litigative, focusing upon the doctor as a cause of their suffering. A sense of grandiose entitlement may serve as a defense against the hopelessness and helplessness engendered by the pain experience. Compensation is demanded of employers and insurers when there is scanty if any evidence of any physical impairment. When surgery has been successful, the patient may sue the physician for false promises which, in fact, were based on the patient's own unrealistic expectations. Psychotherapy in these cases must focus on disappointments in development which preceded the pain experience and which set the tone for the patient's current reaction. Painful memories must be uncovered, and abreaction encouraged within the context of an accepting and supportive relationship. The therapist's hopeful and confident attitude can do much to allay fears of rejection and abandonment.

Neurophysiology of Pain

In recent years treatment of chronic pain has hinged on our understanding of the multiple contributory elements of the pain experience, its psychogenic, peripheral–physiologic and neurobiologic components. Although neurophysiological mechanisms cannot fully explain the experience of pain, they have contributed significantly to pain theory. The pathway for pain is up the contralateral spinothalamic tract from where the pain fibers reach the thalamus and upper part of the reticular system. The thalamic fibers project to: (1) the cerebral cortex, where they provide the different components, for example, perception, emotion, and memory of the painful experience; and (2) the hypothalamus, where they produce visceral changes via the autonomic nervous system. The reticular fibers project: (1) upwards to the cerebral cortex, where they alter the level of awareness to the above-mentioned cortical components of the painful experience, that is, the *intensity*; and (2) downwards to the first synapses of the pain fibers in the central nervous system (CNS) where they can alter the number of ascending painful stimuli (i.e., the *input*).

The state of hypnosis may be described neurophysiologically as a state of diminished and restricted awareness produced by a modification of the activity of the reticular system.

> Awareness is 1) *diminished* by a reduction in the facilitory activity of the ascending reticulo-cortical fibers. This would lead to a reduction in the intensity of the pain experience, and 2) awareness is *restricted* by an increase in the inhibitory activity of the descending reticular fibers. In the pain experience this would limit the input of pain stimuli. The summation of these two alters our awareness of pain. This, in turn, would lead to an altered pain experience, decreased emotion and a different memory from that which would have been occasioned by an unmodified pain experience [Scott, 1974, pp. 48–49].

Other theories include those of Melzack and Wall (1955), who have proposed that a gate mechanism is mediated by inhibitory feedback from the cerebral cortex. The gate is closed by a preponderance of large over small fiber input from the peripheral nerves. When a painful area is stroked or rubbed, the touch sensation is carried along large fibers which close the gate on painful stimuli traveling along smaller ones.

Pain Management

Although pain management is best accomplished using a team approach where the mutual support and intercommunication of team members prevents the development of countertransference which may hamper treatment, this may not be available in most cases. Psychotherapy or psychoanalysis can be effective when the external support system of the patient is adequate. A lesson to be learned from Case 5 is that the psychotherapist (or analyst) undertaking treatment of this type of patient should not expect the patient to relinquish all other treatments immediately. The reliance on physical "cures," which is linked to pain behavior, should subside once the therapeutic alliance has been established and there has been some working through of repressed conflict.

For most people "pain as a consequence of thought processes is a particularly hard notion to accommodate" (Merskey, 1980). Because of this, chronic pain patients usually only turn to the psychiatrist as a last resort. Psychiatry has many resources with which to meet this challenge. We must remain open to and convey to our patients the idea that "there can be more to pain than pain" (Scott, 1974, pp. 102). Experience has amply shown that pain is a culturally determined and modifiable by-product of living. The treatment of chronic pain should offer hope and understanding and should not be based on an all-or-nothing approach, which has more to do with the narcissistic needs and omnipotent fantasies of the treater than the requirements of the patient. All too often the physician's statement "there is nothing more *I* can do for you" is taken as "there is nothing more *that can be done* for you." The latter may or may not be a correct perception of what was implied. Chronic pain patients complain loudly, become addicted, develop complications, and otherwise make demands which try physicians' patience and arouse existential anxieties in them which they then project onto their patients. The patient's will to live may hinge on the hope that the physician holds out for him. There are many unanswered questions about pain. It has the qualities of sensation, affect, and drive. Its one universal feature is that it cannot be ignored. Treatment should always be undertaken with the idea that it is a compelling and complex psychic event which is a touchstone for a fuller understanding of the human condition.

References

Bastiaans, J. (1977), Psychoanalytic psychotherapy. In: *Psychosomatic Medicine*, eds. E. Wittkower & H. Warnes. New York: Harper & Row.

Blumer, O. (1980), Psychiatric approaches to chronic pain. *Audio Digest*, 9:20.

Bond, M. (1979), *Pain: Its Nature, Analysis and Treatment.* New York: Churchill, Livingstone Press.

Bonica, J. (1974), Organization and function of a pain clinic. *Adv. Neurol.*, 4:433–443.

Brena, S., & Chapman, S. (1983), An algorithm for decision-making in patients with pain. In: *Management of Patients With Chronic Pain*. eds. S.F. Brena & S. Chapman. New York, S.P. Medical & Scientific Books.

Catchlove, R.F. (1979), La douleur. *42e Congres des medecins français.* Paris, pp. 103–114.

Catchlove, R.F., & Ramsay, R.A. (1978), Psychosocial assessment of chronic pain patients. Paper presented at the Second World Congress on Pain, Montreal, Canada.

Engel, G. (1959), Psychogenic pain and the pain prone patient. *Amer. J. Med.*, 26:899–918.

Freud, S. (1895), Project for a scientific psychology. *Standard Edition*, 1:283–397. London: Hogarth Press, 1966.

——— (1914), On Narcissism. *Standard Edition*, 14:69–102. London: Hogarth Press, 1953.

——— (1926), Inhibitions, Symptoms and Anxiety. *Standard Edition*, 20:77–175. London: Hogarth Press, 1953.

Gross, S., & Gardner, G. (1980), Child pain: Treatment approaches. In: *Pain, Meaning and Management*, eds. W. Smith, H. Merskey, & S. Gross., New York: SP Medical & Scientific Books.

Hunter, R.A., & Ross, I. (1960), Psychotherapy and migraine. *Brit. Med. J.*, 1960:1084–1088.

Johnson, S. (1983), Psychological assessment of chronic pain. In: *Management of Patients With Chronic Pain.* eds. S. Brena & S. Chapman. New York: S.P. Medical and Scientific Books.

Jones, E. (1957), Pain. *Internat. J. Psycho.-Anal.*, 38/3:255–63.

Lewis, T. (1942), *Pain.* New York: Macmillan.

Maline, D., & Crue, B. (1975), Evolution of the pain center at the city of Hague National Medical Center. In: *Pain Research and Treatment*, ed. B. Crue Jr. New York: Academic Press.

Melzack, R., & Wall, P. (1955), Pain mechanisms: A new theory. *Science*, 150:971–979.

Merskey, H. (1978), Pain and personality. In: *The Psychology of Pain*, ed. R.A. Sternbach. New York: Raven Press.

——— (1980), Psychological and psychiatric aspects of pain control. In: *Pain, Meaning and Management*, eds. W. Smith, H. Merskey, & S. Gross. New York: SP Medical & Scientific Books.

Morse, R.L. (1983), Depression and Pain: The LAD Syndrome. Unpublished Dissetation, University of Pennsylvania.

Ramsay, R.A. (1977), Psychiatric considerations in chronic pain states. In: *Psychosomatic Medicine*, eds. E. Wittkower & H. Warnes. New York: Harper & Row.

Ramzy, I., & Wallerstein, S. (1958), Pain fear and anxiety: A study of their interrelationships. *The Psychoanalytic Study of the Child*, 13:147–189. New York: International Universities Press.

Rangell L. (1953), Psychiatric aspects of pain. *Psychosom. Med.*, 15:22–29.

Ruttick, G., & Aronoff, M. (1983), Combined psychotherapy for pain patients, *Hosp. Pract.*, 18/9:60E–60T.

Schilder, P. (1957), *The Image and Appearance of the Human Body.* New York: International Universities Press.

Scott, D.L. (1974), Hypnotic psychotherapy in anaesthesia. In: *Mechanisms of Pain and Analgesic Compounds*, eds. R.F. Beers & E. Bassett. New York: Raven Press.

Smith, W., & Duerksen, D. (1980), Personality and the relief of chronic pain: Predicting surgical outcome. In: *Pain, Meaning and Management* eds. W. Smith, H. Merskey, & S. Gross. New York: SP Medical & Scientific Books.

Steger, H., Fox, C., & Feinberg, S. (1980), Behavioral evaluation and management of chronic pain. In: *Behavior and the Disabled: Assessment and Management.* ed. D. Bishop. Baltimore: Williams & Wilkins.

Szasz, T. (1957), *Pain and Pleasure: A Study of Bodily Feelings*. New York: Basic Books.
——— (1968), The psychology of persistent pain: A portrait of "Homodolorosus." In: *Pain*. ed. E. Soulariac. New York: Academic Press.
Zeltzer, K., & LeBaron, S. (1986), Fantasy in children and adolescents with chronic illness. *J. Dev. Behav. Pediatr.*, 7/3:195–198.

17

Pharmacologic and Nonpharmacologic Approaches to Pain Management

THOMAS W. MILLER
LOUIS L. JAY

INTRODUCTION

When pharmacologic therapy is indicated for chronic pain relief, it may be most prudent to begin treatment with the mildest effective analgesic drug and dose, preferably aspirin or acetaminophen (Fordyce, Roberts, and Sternbach, 1985). Chemotherapy with Stadol (butorphanol), a drug that has been reported to have five times the pain-relieving potency of morphine and a lesser addictive potential, has had great success in bringing relief of severe pain in cancer patients. It is interesting to note that the pain threshold and tolerance toward pain in chronic pain-suffering patients decreases as their condition deteriorates because of a depletion of their endorphin levels. (Table 17.1 summarizes analgesics used in pain management).

Chronic pain drug therapy, among patients suffering from excruciating pain, should be instituted with utmost care and caution. The dosage regimen of these patients must be therapeutically titrated and frequently monitored to check for adverse reactions, drug allergies, drug reactions, side effects, and patient tolerance (Kantor, 1984).

TABLE 17.1

ANALGESIC MEDICATIONS PRESCRIBED FOR PAIN MANAGEMENT

Drug Agent	Usual Adult Daily Dose (mg)	Administration Route	Frequency PRN
Simple Analgesics			
Aspirin (ASA)*	325–650	p.o. or rectal	q 4h
Acetaminophen	325–650	p.o. or rectal	q 4h
Ibuprofen (Mortrin, Advil, Nuprin)	200–600	p.o.	q 4h
Sodium Salicylate	325–600	p.o. or rectal	q 4–8h
Nonnarcotic			
Butorphanol (Stadol)	0.5–2 or 1–4	I.V. I.M.	q 4h q 4h
Nalbuphine HCL (Nubain)	10	s.c., I.M., or I.V.	q 4h
Narcotic Analgesics			
Buprenorphine HCL (Buprenex)	0.3	I.M.	q 6h
Codeine Sulfate	15–60	p.o.	q 4h
Codeine Phosphate	15–60	p.o., s.c., or I.M.	q 4h
Hydrocodone Bitartrate with	5	p.o.	q 6h
Acetaminophen (Zydone)	100	p.o.	
Levorphanol Tartrate (Levo-Dromoran)	2–3	p.o., s.c.	q 6–8h
Methadone HCL (Dolophine)	5–10	p.o., I.M., or IV.	t.i.d.
Hydromorphone HCL (Dilaudid)	1–6 or 3	p.o., s.c., I.M., I.V., or rectal	q 4–6h q 6–8h
Meperidine HCL (Demerol)	50–150	p.o., s.c., I.M., or I.V.	q 3–4h
Morphine Sulfate	5–15 or 30–60	s.c., I.M., I.V. p.o.	q 4h q 4h
Oxycodone HCL (in Percodan)	4–5	p.o. or rectal	q 6h
Oxymorphone HCL (Numorphan)	1–1.5 or 0.5	I.M., s.c. I.V.	q 4–6h q 4–6h
Pentazocine HCL (Talwin)	50–100 or 30	p.o. I.M., I.V., s.c.	3–4h 3–4h
Propoxyphene HCL (Darvon)	65	p.o.	4h
Propoxyphene napsylate (Darvon-N)	65	p.o.	4h

TABLE 17.2

ANCILLARY TECHNIQUES USED IN THE TREATMENT OF CHRONIC PAIN

Technique	Mode of Action	Parameter
Acupuncture	Provides psychological control over perception of pain. Local intense stimulation of large fibers or perhaps specific cellular aggregates by needles rotated rapidly at specific body sites (meridians); may activate an inhibitory pathway, reducing noxious stimuli transmitted to the brain	Acupuncture not widely used or accepted by Western clinicians. Repeated treatments often indicated
Biofeedback	Can condition an individual's control over pain by reduction of anxiety and by developing the ability to control physiological function, such as producing alpha waves in the brain. Distracts person by forcing concentration on inner state and feedback signal until he develops sufficient awareness to describe and generalize the control strategies	Adjunctive treatment. Difficult to generalize biofeedback training to pain control and difficult to maintain control. Requires a high degree of motivation. Different forms of biofeedback for different types of chronic pain
Group and Family Counseling	Encourages sharing of fear and concern, which helps to decrease anxiety. Provides group and family support. Use of cognitive system to develop and implement treatment.	Family dysfunction. Motivation of group or family. Dynamics which promote pain behaviors
Hypnosis	Facilitates tension reduction by decreasing anxiety. Increases control by cortical structures indicating affective behavior. Promotes relaxation. Produces its effect through suggestion and distraction	Requires careful screening and extensive training of patients. Is an adjunct to other treatment
Psychotherapy	Dynamic or cognitive–behavioral programs focus on determination of the underlying cause of maladaptive behavior and on guiding the patient in successful coping with pain	Necessitates a long treatment period and motivation on part of the person. Cognitive–behavioral approaches have had success in treating chronic pain
Relaxation Techniques	Reduces perception of pain through distraction and dissociation of self from pain sensation enhancement of self-control, muscle relaxation and tension reduction	Advanced techniques require practice. Often used as adjunct to other treatments. Use of audiotapes may assist in providing patients with standardized model
Trancutaneous Nerve Stimulation	(1) Electrical stimulus alters electrical potential of nerve to prevent full depolarization and repolarization. (2) Increased sensory input yields increased inhibition. (3) Stimulation of large fibers changes dorsal horn interaction pattern, yields in inhibition of small fiber transmission	Not tolerated by some persons due to tingling sensation produced. Patients may become habituated and require increased stimulus intensity with greater possibility of skin burn. Low success in emotionally disturbed patients

Chronic pain often leads to an endless cycle of anxiety, frustration, and depression (Katon, 1984). Clinical experience suggests early recognition and treatment of an individual's physical and psychological symptoms. In addition to medication, there are numerous strategies that can have a significant impact on chronic pain. Acupuncture as a means of providing pain relief has been used in the Orient for centuries, but the method has not had widespread acceptance in the United States. The mechanism of acupuncture analgesia remains uncertain.

Chronic pain involves cognitions and behavior and is subject to environmental and learning principles. Numerous psychological techniques (Turk and Genest, 1979), such as operant conditioning, biofeedback, progressive muscle relaxation, hypnosis, distraction techniques, and placebo have had varying degrees of success in relieving pain (see Table 17.2).

Categories of Pain

The most common forms of physiologic and emotional pain include the following categories:

Headache Pain

It is conservatively estimated that over 40 million Americans suffer daily episodes of recurrent headaches which disrupt jobs, family peace, and tranquillity, leaving the victims emotionally distressed, physically impaired, and often in severe pain and agony. Headache pain manifests itself in many forms and invades the entire spectrum of our physical and emotional life. In and of itself, it is not a disease but a symptom of a disease, or functional disturbance, a warning that all is not well, and it should be clinically investigated and treated at the earliest possible moment.

Headache disorders have continued to defy a complete understanding of either their pathogenesis, or a universally effective therapy. These impairments are generally caused by acute or systemic intracranial vascular disorders, head injuries, severe hypertension, cerebral hypoxia, dental disease, fever, diseases of the eyes, ears, and nose, or in cranial infection or tumor. It is also associated with patients who suffer from muscle tension headache, migraine, or head pain for which no structural cause can be identified.

The following describe the most common forms of headache.

Simple Headache. Simple headaches may be precipitated by stress, tension, or emotional problems. Many are of short duration and require change of environment, fresh air, and freedom from inciting factors and rest. Symptomatic treatment with plain aspirin, acetaminophen, ibuprofen, or diflunisal are also therapeutic, and are summarized in Table 17.3.

While aspirin has been the cornerstone of simple tension headache pain therapy, it has been clinically documented that its chronic use often results in gastrointestinal pain, irritation, and heartburn. It should be avoided in patients with gastrointestinal bleeding, ulcers, gout, or aspirin allergies. It should also be noted that enteric-coated aspirin tablets may be safely used in patients who can tolerate them.

Tylenol or Datril (acetaminophen) is an analgesic pain drug whose therapeutic activity is said to be equal to, or greater than, that of aspirin. Clinical evidence and experience further indicate that it should be the drug of choice among patients exhibiting strong aspirin allergies, gastric disturbances, or other salicylate toxicities or intolerances.

Headache may occur as a symptom of many disorders, and it may not always be possible to determine the exact cause in a given case without elaborate diagnostic procedures. Conservative wisdom suggests clinical investigation and assessment of the validity of impaired physical, emotional, and psychological integrity of a patient's symptoms and condition before instituting a course of therapy. Furthermore, with long-term treatment, periodic blood counts and blood chemistry analysis are advisable to ensure safety and effectiveness of treatment when necessary.

TABLE 17.3

ANALGESIC MEDICATIONS PRESCRIBED FOR HEADACHE PAIN MANAGEMENT

Drug Agent	Usual Adult Daily Dose (mg)	Administration Route	Frequency PRN	Max. Dose (mg) Daily = d Weekly = w
Analgesics				
Acetaminophen	325–360	p.o., rectal	q 4h	2,600-d
Aspirin	325–360	p.o., rectal	q 4h	2,600-d
Diflunisal (Dolobid)	Initially 1,000	p.o.	500mg in 12h	1,500-d
Ibuprofen (Advil, Motrin, Nuprin)	200–600	p.o.	q 6h	2,400-d
Benzodiazepines				
Chlordiazepoxide (Librium)	5–25	p.o.	3–4xd	100-d
Diazepam (Valium)	2–10	p.o.	3–4xd	40-d
Oxazepam (Serax)	10–15	p.o.	3–4xd	60-d
Barbiturates				
Amobarbital (Amytal)	30–50	p.o.	3–4xd	200-d
Phenobarbital (Luminal)	15–45	p.o.	3–4xd	180-d
Mild Narcotics				
Codeine	15–60	p.o.	q 4h	240-d
Propoxyphene (Darvon)	65	p.o.	3–4xd	260-d
Adrenergic Blockers (Sympatholytics)				
Dihydroergotamine Mesylate (D.H.E. 45)	1mg	I.M. or I.V.	May repeat q 1–2h	3–d; 6-w
Ergotamine tartrate (Ergomar, Ergostat)	2mg	p.o., S.L.	q ½h	6–d; 10-w
Medihaler Ergotamine	One inhalation	Nasally	q 5 min.	6–d
Combinations				
Ergotamine Tartrate 1 mg and Caffeine 100mg (Cafergot, Ergocoff, Wigraine)	2 tabs.	p.o.	1 q ½ h prn	6–d; 10-2
Cafergot Supp.	Initially one	rectal	1 hs	2–d; 5-w
Wigraine Supp.	Initially one	rectal	1hs	2–d; 5-w
Methysergide Maleate (Sansert)	2–4	p.o.	b.i.d. with meals	8–d
Other				
Propranolol (Inderal)	Initially 20	p.o.	q.i.d.	160–240-d
Verapramil HCL (Calan, Isoptin)	80	p.o.	q.i.d.	320-480

Chronic Tension (Muscular) Headaches. Chronic tension headaches are the most common of all headaches. They are induced by stress, tension, emotional problems, and muscular contractions–usually the temporal and occipital muscles in the sides and back of the head. They cause pain by producing muscle spasms and pressing upon pain-sensitive tissues. It has been clinically suggested that Type A individuals (Skevington, 1983), people who are generally overly ambitious, anxious, perfectionistic, worried, resentful, angry, easily frightened and frustrated, and tend to rigidity in their attitudes and ideas, are prime candidates for chronic tension headaches.

Chronic Tension Headache Treatment. While drug therapy is required for the treatment and management of most types of headache, a clinical record of reliability and effectiveness should always be of paramount concern and importance in its selection by a knowledgeable physician. The dosage regimen should always be instituted at the lowest effective level and periodically monitored, adjusted, reviewed, and evaluated to maintain the patient's stability and safety.

Some physicians supplement the use of a mild sedative such as Luminal (phenobarbital), or Amytal (amobarbital), alone or in combination with aspirin or acetaminophen. Care and caution with periodic evaluation of dosage regimen should be exercised with the long-term use of barbiturates in patients with impaired liver or kidney function or with a history of drug dependence or abuse.

Treatment for the chronic tension headache may include neck, shoulder, and back massage, warm bath or hot shower, cold wet cloth over aching areas, muscle relaxation exercises, rest, and relaxation and freedom from emotional stress and environmental stressors (Blanchard, Andrasik, Arena, Neff, Saunders, Jurish, Teders, and Rodichok, 1983). Biofeedback as an adjunct therapy has been discussed earlier (Andrasik, Blanchard, Arena, Saunders, and Barron, 1982). Biofeedback is a technique or tool for which positive outcomes have been reported only when the modality is combined with a passive, nonthreatening, therapeutic alliance. That therapeutic alliance is comprised of components of psychotherapy, behavior therapy, progressive relaxation, autogenic therapy, physical therapy, relaxation training, and hypnotic variants. Nonprescription analgesics such as aspirin, ibuprofen, diflunisal, or acetaminophen often prove therapeutic.

Other clinicians favor the use of mild narcotic agents such as Darvon, Darvon-N (propoxyphene) or codeine. These agents are characterized as drugs possessing moderate analgesic activity, with some potential for tolerance, psychic, or physical dependence. With chronic use, these drugs are further associated with symptoms of nausea, vomiting, constipation, sedation, sleepiness, euphoria, and skin rash. Patients should be cautioned that abrupt withdrawal can induce symptoms of delirium, convulsions, and abdominal and muscle cramps, among others. However, in terms of a benefit-risk ratio, the use of the above agents is on the plus side; upon the discontinuance of these drugs, the dosage regimen should be gradually reduced to zero intake over a period of a few weeks.

Migraine Headaches. Migraine is a recurring vascular headache. It is characterized by a marked increase of symptoms such as severe pain, photophobia (sensitivity to light), and autonomic (involuntary) disturbances during the acute phase which may last for hours or days. This disorder occurs more frequently in women than in men and a predisposition to migraine may be inherited. Statistics indicate that it affects 5 to 10 percent of the population.

The exact mechanism responsible for the disorder is not known. The head pain is related to dilation of extracranial blood vessels, which may be the result of chemical changes that cause spasms of intracranial vessels. Migraine may be triggered by allergic reactions, excess carbohydrates, iodine-rich foods, alcohol, bright lights, loud noises, slow or stalled traffic, drastic changes in the weather, disruption of sleep patterns, hormonal changes or treatment, such as oral contraceptives, or various drug agents including vasodilators.

An impending attack usually manifests itself by visual disturbances such as flashing lights or wavy lines, by a strange taste or odor, numbness, tingling, dizziness, ringing or buzzing in the ear, or a feeling that part of the body is distorted in size or shape. The acute phase may be accompanied by vomiting, chills, excessive urination, facial edema, irritability, and extreme fatigue.

Migraine headache treatment alternatives. During the past several years, it has become apparent that most patients suffering from chronic muscle contraction headaches also have some vascular headaches as well. These vascular events are manifested periodically, usually as migraine attacks, occurring upon a background of daily or almost daily muscle contraction pain. This combination of headache mechanisms is called the mixed headache syndrome, and is thought to reflect a predisposition to exaggerated vascular and neuromuscular reactivity. This syndrome is most frequently characterized by daily pain, depression, and analgesic abuse. It also inflicts more anguish, pain, and tragedy upon its victim than the human mind, body, and spirit can bear.

Medical treatment for migraine usually consists of an abortive (symptomatic), preventative (prophylactic or other), or combined program. The appropriate choice depends upon many factors, including frequency, intensity, and duration of the migraine attacks and the health of the patient and other clinical circumstances. Effective drug treatment for this syndrome is available with the use of the several agents, which are also summarized in Table 17.3. Sansert (methysergide) is characterized as an effective prophylactic prescription drug for migraine, probably exerting its effect by peripheral vasoconstriction. Its utility is limited by its tendency to produce significant adverse reactions with prolonged use, such as cardiovascular complications, gastrointestinal distress, deleterious CNS symptoms, edema, weight gain, and various blood disorders, among others. There must be a medication-free interval of three to four weeks after every six months of treatment.

Some areas of research suggest that abnormalities in the metabolism of serotonin (a complex chemical in the brain which acts as a neurotransmitter) may play a role in the migraine syndrome. Other research indicates that a platelet abnormality may be related to migraine. In any event, it has been clinically reported that as the vasoconstrictor phenomena recede, vasodilator headache commences, and may be eliminated or reduced by vasoconstrictor agents, particularly Cafergot (ergotamine tartrate plus caffeine), or by D.H.E. 45 (dihydroergotamine mesylate).

Cafergot or D.H.E. 45 has been used to prevent or abort acute vascular headache such as migraine variants, and in combination with phenobarbital to abort or prevent migraine complicated by tension and gastrointestinal disturbances. Nonetheless, caution should be exercised with its use since many deleterious side effects, such as numbness and tingling of the fingers and toes, muscle pain in the extremities, weakness in the legs, distress and pain in the region above the heart, and below the thorax, transient increase or decrease in heartbeat, nausea, vomiting, localized edema, or itching may occur.

Traditionally, the vasoconstrictor effect of ergotamine tartrate taken orally, rectally, or sublingually has provided effective treatment for clinically diagnosed migraine patients. It should be noted that promptness is the key to treating migraine attacks as they occur, to avoid having to cope with the devastating oncoming symptoms. In view of the hazards of vasoconstrictive therapy, the most rational approach to sound clinical migraine therapy is treatment with close supervision and individualized dosage regimen within the clinical parameters of therapeutic limits. Some physicians prefer a trial of aspirin, acetaminophen, and/or codeine analgesic therapy to alleviate the painful symptoms of a mild attack prior to initiating stronger drug therapy.

Cluster Headache. Patients afflicted with cluster headaches can experience excruciating pain. It is estimated that one-half of 1 percent of the American population between twenty and fifty years of age, is thought to suffer from cluster headache. It is also 5 to 10% more frequent in men than in women. Cluster headache (a variant of migraine) is characterized by a sudden onset of throbbing, excruciating unilateral pain. The pain is of short duration and subsides abruptly, but may recur several times daily, and attacks occur most frequently during sleep. It is associated with symptoms of dilated carotid arteries (in the neck), fluid accumulation under the eyes, tearing or lacrimation, nasal congestion, and runny nose. The sharp pain involves the orbital area, frequently radiating to the temple, nose, upper jaw, and neck.

Cluster headache treatment. Since cluster headache is a variant of migraine, prophylaxis and treatment by a qualified physician as outlined above under migraine headache treatment may prove beneficial. Additionally, the patient should be advised that prophylatic treatment at bedtime for nocturnal attacks should be given two hours before an anticipated attack. A short course of prednisone, with a gradual tapering off over a three-week period, has also been recommended by some clinicians.

Posttraumatic Headache. This type of headache usually occurs following head injury, or injury to the upper cervical spine or its associated soft parts, such as ligaments, muscles, or intervertebral disks. Resulting head pain is variable in intensity, frequency, and duration and is generally increased by emotional disturbances. It is usually associated with dizziness, irritability, insomnia, and inability to concentrate. Treatment for posttraumatic headache requires both analgesic drugs and sedatives, coupled with psychotherapy, relaxation, and biofeedback as adjuncts to treatment by qualified health professionals.

Psychogenic Headache. Psychogenic headache is usually caused by conversion hysteria and anxiety states. Conversion hysteria is a type of neurosis in which emotional conflicts are repressed and converted into sensory, motor, or visceral symptoms having no underlying organic cause. The person who is afflicted with this disorder is usually indifferent to the symptoms, yet firmly believes the condition exists. Causal factors include a conscious or unconscious desire to escape from, or avoid, some unpleasant situation or responsibility, or to obtain sympathy or some secondary gain. Treatment usually consists of aggressive psychotherapy, coupled with analgesic and sedative drug therapy prescribed by a qualified health professional. Such therapy is essential to alleviate the viselike immobilizing headache or tight muscles causing neck and shoulder problems for the patient.

Sinus Headache. Sinus Headache, also known as congestive headaches, are associated with pain, redness, tenderness, and swelling over the affected sinus, coupled with purulent nasal discharge. Sinus headaches may be relieved by analgesic pain killers such as aspirin or acetaminophen and in some cases with the use of an oral or nasal decongestant to relieve the swelling and congestion.

Rheumatoid Arthritis and Chronicity in Pain

The Arthritis Foundation estimates that symptomatic arthritis currently affects more than 32 million Americans, with over a million new victims added each year. It further estimates that the economic impact of arthritis upon the nation is staggering—more than $15 billion annually. The Foundation's statistics also indicate that over 16 million Americans suffer from osteoarthritis and from 6 to 8 million are afflicted with rheumatoid arthritis (RA), reported to be the number one crippling disease in the United States (Arthritis Foundation, 1985).

Common Forms of Arthritis

There are over 100 specific types of arthritis. Among the most common forms are psoriatic arthritis, rheumatoid arthritis, juvenile rheumatoid arthritis, ankylosing spondylitis, osteoarthritis, acute and subacute bursitis, acute and nonspecific tenosynovitis, acute gouty arthritis, and infectious arthritis.

Rheumatoid Arthritis. Rheumatoid arthritis (RA) is one of the arthritic disease states whose definitive cause is unknown. It is an incurable (but manageable) chronic, progressive, degenerative disease that is associated with pain and swelling, and leads to deformity and crippling of the patient's joints, typically the small hand joints, feet, wrists, elbows, and ankles. Although any joint can be affected, it generally starts in the fingers. Rheumatoid arthritis usually begins with inflammation of the synovial membrane lining of the joint space. Chronic progression of this condition produces bone and cartilage calcification which compromises joint stability and causes dislocation to occur—which in turn produces joint deformities. There are several predisposing and contributing factors in the development of RA. One major factor may be interference with a person's autoimmune system, which adds to the exacerbation of the existing pain, inflammation, and deformities of the disease.

The incidence and prevalence of rheumatoid arthritis increases with age, the onset usually occurring during middle age. Some patients suffer from a monocycle form of the disease which, in its severe form, lasts about two years and then remits. Other patients may suffer from a polycyclic form with exacerbations and remissions throughout life. Still others, unfortunately, suffer from a continuous, progressive, and unremitting from of RA.

There are over 250,000 children suffering from juvenile rheumatoid arthritis in the United States. It generally occurs during early childhood in the systemic or severe form, and is usually associated with high fever, inflammation of the joints and tissues, and destruction of multiple joints. The milder form is characterized by less debilitating joint involvement of the knees and ankles.

Early symptoms. The early warning signals of arthritis are (1) persistent pain and stiffness upon arising; (2) pain and tenderness in one or more joints; (3) swelling in one or more joints; (4) recurrence of above symptoms; (5) tingling sensation in fingertips, hands, or feet; and (6) unexplained weight loss, fever, or weakness.

An arthritic patient's passport to tolerable fair health is a realistic clinical approach to early diagnosis, sound therapeutic drug regimen, and effective supportive measures for the control, treatment, and management of the disease.

There is no known cure for rheumatoid arthritis. However, there are a number of available intervention procedures and techniques aimed at reducing or alleviating pain and inflammation, correcting disabilities and deformities, and maintaining mobility of the joints. It is interesting to note that the pain threshold and tolerance toward pain and inflammation in these patients decreases as their condition deteriorates because of a depletion of their endorphin levels.

Treatment modalities. Among the many modalities of treatment available for patients suffering from RA are any one, or combination, of the following: A comprehensive program of rest, physiotherapy, exercise and heat; medical, radiological, surgical, or pharmacological intervention; and/or psychological rehabilitation.

Because drug therapy is a major component in the control, treatment, and management of rheumatoid arthritis, its selection should always be conservatively approached. Qualified clinical experience and judgment also suggest that dosage regimen should always be instituted at the lowest effective therapeutic level to maintain the patient's safety and stability and to minimize the risk of deleterious side effects and serum level toxicities. Periodic review and evaluation of drug regimen would also be advisable and beneficial for the patient's well-being.

A wide spectrum of pharmacological agents are currently used in the control, treatment, and management of RA disease states. Of those, the most therapeutically effective agents, by category, are as follows:

Salicylates—acetylsalicylic acid (ASA), or aspirin, is the cornerstone of arthritis treatment. When taking aspirin, it is most advisable to take it with meals, with an antacid, in an antacid buffered combination, or in an enteric-coated tablet. It is well documented that long-term ASA ingestion often results in gastrointestinal pain, irritation, or heartburn. The mode of action of ASA is unknown; however, as with some nonsteroids, its activity may result from its ability to block prostaglandin synthesis.

To prevent salicylate toxicity—which can introduce tinnitus, confusion, memory loss, and tremors—patients on long-term aspirin therapy should have their dosage regimen frequently checked and titrated for safe and effective dosage. Aspirin should be avoided in patients with a history of gastrointestinal bleeding, ulcers, gout, or aspirin allergies.

Nonnarcotic analgesic agents—as a single entity or in combination–may be used for arthritic patients. Even though acetaminophen or other nonnarcotic drug analgesic activity is equipotent or greater than ASA, these agents' greatest single dificit is their low level of anti-inflammatory action. This deficiency most often results in a return of joint tenderness, swelling, and stiffness. Chronic use of these drugs may induce lightheadedness, sedation, nausea, vomiting, constipation, pruritus, and photosensitivity.

Nonsteroidal anti-inflammatory drugs (Nsaids) are also very effective alternatives for control of pain and inflammation generally associated with arthritis. Their therapeutic effectiveness usually becomes apparent within a few days after administration, and these drugs possess a lesser incidence of gastrointestinal side effects than aspirin (Table 17.4).

It has been suggested that piroxicam is the most promising nonsteroidal antiarthritic drug to appear on the American pharmaceutical market in some time. It is available in once-daily dosage form, exhibits a lower liability for adverse side effects, and possesses a greater potential for increased compliance and therapeutic effectiveness.

Some of the newer nonsteroidal agents appear to possess a lesser incidence of gastrointestinal side effects than aspirin. However, all of these drugs have been reported to cause some gastrointestinal bleeding, and they fail to halt the progressive nature of rheumatoid arthritis. Other side effects include pruritus, skin rash, leukopenia, allergies, and renal malfunction.

Remissive agents. Remissive agents are used when long-term drug therapy with other agents has failed to effectively control the devastating symptoms of progressive rheumatoid arthritis. They are a diversified group of drugs which share some of the following characteristics: (1) therapeutic response results only after weeks or months of drug administration; (2) they all possess a high potential for toxicities and deleterious side effects; (3) drug therapy should always be instituted at the lowest effective dose; and (4) they require caution and frequent assessment of patient's condition and dosage regimen.

Gold salts are also valuable remissive agents, and are used in severe, progressive forms of arthritis. These agents are effective only against active joint inflammation and are not usually helpful in advanced RA with pronounced joint destruction and residual inflammation. Gold compounds are contraindicated in patients with hepatic or renal disease, blood dyscrasia, or acute systemic lupus erythematosus (SLE). However, maintaining a good remission requires long-term sustained administration coupled with frequent laboratory accumulation tests.

TABLE 17.4

SELECTED NONSTEROIDAL DRUGS USED FOR R-A PAIN MANAGEMENT

Drug Agent	Usual Adult Dose (mg p.o.)	Frequency	Maximum Adult Analgesic Daily Dose
Nonsteroidal			
Choline Magnesium Salicylate Trilisate	1000	b.i.d. or t.i.d.	2000–3000
Diflunisal (Dolobid)	Initially 1000, then 500	q 8–12h	1000–1500
Fenoprofen (Nalfon)	200	q 4–6h	800
Ibuprofen (Motrin)	400	q 4–6h	2400
Indomethacin (Indocin)	25	t.i.d. or q.i.d.	75–150
Meclofenamate (Meclomen)	200–400	Daily	400
Mefenamic Acid (Ponstel)	Initially 500, then 250	q 4h	1000
Naproxen (Naprosyn)	Initially 500, then 250	q 6–8h	1250
Naproxen Sodium (Anaprox)	Initially 500, then 275	q 6–8h	1375
Phenylbutazone (Butazolidin)	100–200	t.i.d. or q.i.d.	400–600
Piroxicam (Feldine)	20	Once daily	20
Sulindac (Clinoril)	150–200	b.i.d.	400

Some of the above agents are also available in other brand names

Among the gold salts' most common toxicities and side effects are pruitus, skin rashes, diarrhea/loose stool, proteinuria, GI disturbances, conjunctivitis, stomatitis, thrombecytopenia, and leukopenia. Auranofin, a gold compound and the first oral from of gold, should prove to be a most welcome and valuable addition to the arthritic group of remissive agents.

Antimalarial agents are also valuable arthritic remissive drugs, and are usually prescribed for patients who have been unresponsive to gold or other agents. They also take two to three months of therapy before any beneficial effects are realized. Antimalarials have a very high potential for inducing toxicities and adverse side effects, making them prime candidates for frequent laboratory testing, monitoring, and evaluation. Among the host of deleterious side effects produced by these remissive agents are skin lesions, nausea, alopecia, gait disturbances, low blood-cell count, photosensitivity, and ophthalmic disorders.

Penicillamine is another effective remissive agent. It is associated with clinical improvement and a reduction of pain, swelling, and morning joint stiffness—characterized by an increased sense of well-being and functional capacity in severe arthritic patients. However, it usually takes a period of three to four months before signs of clinical improvement are experienced by patients. Among some of those common adverse side effects encountered with penicillamine therapy are skin lesions and rashes, oral ulcers, anorexia, bone marrow depression, aplastic anemia, and nephropathy (kidney disease).

Corticosteroids are a group of very potent agents used for symptomatic relief in very severe cases of arthritis. They are most useful when more conventional forms of therapy fail to halt the intractable conditions developed by this crippling disease. However, the corticosteroids' high risk for toxicity and potential for adverse side effects suggest that long-term therapy should be carefully considered, plus dosage regimen should be instituted at the lowest effective level.

Some of the more common adverse effects of corticosteroid therapy are fluid and electroclyte disturbances; musculoskeletal, gastrointestinal, endocrinic, ophthalmic, and metabolic impairments; plus the characteristic "moon face."

Psychological disturbance may also appear with corticosteroid therapy, including euphoria, insomnia, mood swings, personality changes, and depression. Regardless of their shortcomings, short-term use of corticosteroids in acute arthritic flare-ups may be justified by their effectiveness in quickly relieving pain and inflammation, and improving joint mobility.

Cytotoxic (immunosuppressive) agents are used in patients who have become unresponsive and intractable to other modalities of conventional treatment. The use of these potent drugs may be helpful; however, they do not always guarantee complete remission. Because of their potential for hematopoietic (affecting blood) toxicity, infection, and adverse reactions, complete blood counts—including platelets—should be taken frequently. The most common side effects of cytotoxic agents are anemia, leukopenia, thrombocytopenia, oral lesions, stomatitis, nausea, vomiting, alopecia, and possibly cancer.

Psychological pain control. Psychologists and other specialists can provide arthritis patients with adjunct stress management, biofeedback procedures, and behavioral strategies. Several psychological modalities of treatment have been employed to teach patients to cope with arthritic pain. Current methods focus on behavior adjustment and biofeedback. Nursing personnel recognize the value of a behavioral technique used in conjunction with more traditional approaches to pain management.

Pain control techniques provide an individual with the skill to voluntarily cope with, or reduce, the level of pain which he or she experiences. Techniques such as biofeedback utilize instrumentation to augment the training procedure. Visual imagery is also utilized to develop conscious control. The object of pain management training is to establish in the individual the ability to invoke a significant release of tension through the muscle system. Training and practice enable the sufferer to use relaxation techniques in response to both environmental and internal cues.

The most obvious advantage of pain control is that the patient can employ these skills even when reclining in a chair with the eyes closed. Another advantage is its inherent capacity to allow the patient to assume basic responsibility for treatment and self-control. Having a skill which eases pain can greatly increase a patient's confidence.

An important component of pain control involves learning specific steps which are essential to dealing with arthritic pain. In this component, the first step is to think through and carefully evaluate what options one has in dealing with pain. The second step is being able to confront the pain by mentally rehearsing the way in which a person chooses to deal with it when it is experienced. This technique may not eliminate the pain, but reasoning things through and mentally preparing oneself for it means that the person can develop a mental preparedness and patterned response to whatever degree of pain is confronted.

Low Back Pain

Low back pain may be associated with a variety of causes. A careful history and physical examination of such a patient may yield important clues regarding the site and cause of the disorder. The incidence of this condition increases with age, reaching 50 to 80 percent of the population of industrial societies. It becomes a significant problem in the third decade of life and reaches its hightest peak in and after the sixth decade. Most low back pain is related to degenerative joint disease of the lumbosacral area resulting from shear-strain in the lumbosacral junction caused by man's upright posture (Dolce and Raczynski, 1985).

The cause of low back pain may often be established by correlating the findings of a carefully elicited history with a thorough physical examination. When historical and physical findings suggest diseases requiring specific treatment, X rays of the involved area of the spine are often required for diagnostic and legal purposes. X ray findings may provide a convenient basis for the initial differentiation of the causes of back pain (Gottlieb, Strite, Koller, Madorsky, Hockersmith, Kleeman, and Wagner, 1977).

Various forms of low back pain may be caused by: (1) a

ruptured intervertebral disk with subsequent hernition of the nucleus pulposus into the spinal canal, causing inflammatory or direct mechanical nerve root pressure; (2) fracture, infection, or tumor involving the back, pelvis, or retroperitoneum, or traumatic ligament rupture or poraspinous muscle tear; (3) commonly occurring, mild congenital defects of the low lumbar and upper sacral spina (e.g., spina bifida occulata, abnormal intervertebral facets, sacralization of L-5 transverse processes); (4) bilateral loss of substance in the pars interarticularis and subsequent slipping forward of a vertebra upon the one below (spondylolisthesis); and (5) back strain due to stretching of the abdominal muscles by obesity or pregnancy.

Other causes of low back pain include vascular aneurysms, visceral disorders, and psychoeurotic problems which may be simulated on the basis of psychosocial problems and conflicts. These factors regularly alter the patient's perception and reporting of structurally mediated pain, as well as the resultant degree of disability and response to therapy.

Treatment and management of acute low back pain, due to musculotendinous strain, includes relieving muscle spasms with complete bed rest, local heat, a firm mattress or sleeping surface, oral analgesics or sedatives summarized in Table 17.1. After twenty-four hours of pain-free recumbancy without medication, walking activity may be tried, with progression to full activity if symptoms do not recur.

Treatment and management of chronic low back pain is directed toward alleviating the cause. Analgesics may relieve pain; narcotics should be avoided. Intervertable joint arthritis may respond to proper bracing and abdominal muscle-strengthening exercises. A note of caution, lumbosacral flexion exercises may increase symptoms.

Angina Pectoris

Angina pectoris is the clinical manifestation of myocardial ischemia, the result of an imbalance of myocardial oxygen supply and demand. When the pain radiates down the inner aspect of the left arm it is frequently accompanied by a feeling of suffocation and impending death. Attacks of angina pectoris are often related to exertion, emotional stress, and exposure to intense cold. The pain may be relieved by rest and vasodilation by medication. The distribution of the distress may vary widely in different patients. In 80 to 90 percent of the cases, the discomfort is felt behind or slightly to the left of the breastbone. When it begins farther to the left or uncommonly, on the right, it characteristically moves centrally and is felt deep in the chest.

Examination during a spontaneous attack frequently reveals a significant elevation of systolic and diastolic blood pressure; occasionally, gallop rhythm is present during pain only. Carotid sinus massage often causes the pain to subside more quickly than usual if it slows the cardiac rate, and it is a helpful maneuver of abnormal angina.

Types of Angina. 1. Several types of angina pectoris have been identified from their clinical characteristics. Stable angina is often referred to as classic or effort-induced angina. In this type of angina, discomfort is precipitated by physical activity or emotional stress, and is usually relieved by rest. Each episode of symptoms lasts about three to five minutes and is characterized by chest pain or discomfort, with radiation to the neck, jaw, back, shoulders, or arms. Nausea, diaphoresis, palpitation, or shortness of breath may be present. It results from an increase in myocardial oxygen demand beyond that which can bypass narrowed coronary arteries (Basmajian, 1983).

2. Unstable angina describes chest pain occurring with increased intensity and frequency associated with decreasing levels of work and a decrease in the responsiveness to treatment. Unstable angina may signal the prodome of acute myocardial infarction and requires urgent diagnosis and treatment. The mechanism contributing to unstable angina is an increased myocardial oxygen demand in the presence of severe coronary artery stenosis, thrombosis, or spasm (Basmajian, 1983).

3. Variant angina, or Prinzmetal's angina, is characterized by recurrent chest pain at rest and an electrocardiogram showing ST-segment elevation during pain. The pain associated with variant angina differs from that of stable angina in

that it may be of longer duration, it is usually not precipitated by exertion, and it may occur only at certain times of the day. Decreased blood blow in this type of angina results from coronary artery spasm (Basmajian, 1983).

Prophylaxis and treatment of anginal pain. Treatment and prevention of anginal pain has improved markedly in recent years. Nitroglycerine is the drug of choice; it acts in about one to two minutes. This drug, and all nitrates summarized in Table 17.5 decrease arteriolar and venous tone, reduce preload and afterload, and lower the heart's oxygen demand.

Sublingual nifedipine, 10 to 20 mg, may rapidly relieve angina, especially if spasm is the cause (Luce et al, 1979). The patient should be advised that it would be helpful if he or she would stand still, sit or lie down as soon as the pain begins and remain quiet until the attack is over (Luce et al., 1979). Since angina may coexist with, or be aggravated by, left ventricular failure, obvious or incipient, treatment of the cardiac failure with diuretics or digitalis or both, as well as with other methods such as prolonged rest, may be extremely helpful.

Beta-blocking agents such as Inderal (propranolol), 10 to 80 mg, three to four times daily by mouth; Lopressor (metoprolol), 50 mg twice daily, Corgard (nadalol), 40 mg once daily; Tenormin (atenolol), 50 to 100 mg once daily; Viskin (pindolol), 5 to 10 mg twice daily; or Blocadren (timolol) 10 to 20 mg twice daily (each drug then increased to tolerance) has been given with benefit to patients with angina who have never had ventricular failure.

Extreme care and caution should be observed with the use of beta-blocking agents, since the side effects can be either absolute or relative contraindications, such as the development of bronchial asthma in patients who have had allergy in the past; severe bradycardia; atrioventricular conduction defects; left ventricular failure because of the negative iotropic action of the sympatholytic action of the drug; Raynard's phenomenon, especially in women in cold weather; and rarely, CNS symptoms with excitement and confusion. However, combination therapy with long-acting nitrates such as isoride dinitrate has been significantly more effective than single drug therapy.

TABLE 17.5

NITRATES USED FOR ANGINA PECTORIS PROPHYLAXIS AND PAIN MANAGEMENT

Drug Agent	Administration Route	Dosage	Onset of Action (Minutes	Duration of Action
Amyl Nitrate	Inhalant	0.18–0.3 ml	0.5	3–5 min.
Nitroglycerine	I.V.	Variable	1–2	3–5 min.
	Sublingual	0.15–0.6 mg q 3 min. within 15 min.	Within 2	Up to 30 min.
	Spray on tongue or sublingually	1 (0.04 mg) to 3 sprays within 15 min.	0.05	Up to 30 min.
	Oral SR	2.5, 6.5, or 9 mg b.i.d.	30–60	8–10 h
	Topical ointment 2% (15 mg/inch)	1–2 inch q 4h	30	3h
	Transdermal patch	1 q 12–24 h	30	20–24 h
Isorbide Dinitrate (Isordil, Sorbitrate)	Sublingual	2.5–10 mg q 2h	2–5	1–2 h
	Chewable	5–10 mg q 2h	2–5	1–2 h
	Oral	5–40 mg q 4–6h	60	5–6 h
	Oral SR	40 mg q 12 h	30	6–8 h
Erythrityl Tetranitrate (Cardilate)	Sublingual	5–10 mg q 2–3 h	5	2h
	Chewable	5–10 mg q 2–3 h	5	2h
	Oral SR	5–40 mg q 4–6 h	30	Up to 12 h
Pentaerythritol Tetranitrate (Peritrate)	Oral/Chewable	10–40 mg q 6h	30	4–5 h
	Oral SR	30–80 mg q 12h	30	Up to 12 h

Calcium-entry blocking agents, Calan (verapamil) 80 mg and S-R 240 mg, Cardizem (diltiazem) 30 mg, and Procardia (nifedipine) 10 mg, is often helpful, especially if coronary spasm coexists, although these drugs may be effective in the absence of spasm, since they cause vasodilation.

Persantine (dipyridamole) is classified as a coronary vasodilator. It is indicated as "possibly" effective for long-term therapy of chronic angina pectoris. The usual adult daily dose is 50 mg p.o. three times daily at least one hour before meals to a maximum of 400 mg daily. Prolonged therapy may reduce the frequency of, or eliminate, anginal episodes and reduce nitroglycerine requirements. The drug is not intended to abort the acute anginal attack. Psychotherapeutic interventions with the use of mild sedatives or tranquilizers, lowering of obesity to normal levels, smoking should be stopped, and sufficient rest and relaxation are essential measures which, when utilized, may reduce the frequency and severity of painful anginal attacks.

For patients whose anginal pain is related to narrowed coronary arteries, treatment has been advanced with coronary bypass surgery, in which blood flow is routed around areas of restricted flow, and coronary angioplasty in which a small balloon is inserted into a coronary artery and gently inflated and deflated a number of times to compress plaque and increase blood flow.

Dental Pain

Elimination or control of acute and chronic pain is a major problem in dental practice. It can be caused by trauma, disease, or orofacial malfunction, and is often excruciating and unbearable. Dental pain affects the entire spectrum of our population at one time or another during a lifetime.

In some cases, dental pain can begin in infancy, recurring periodically with advancing age, unless effective daily preventive measures are diligently practiced. Effective oral hygiene should include daily brushing and flossing to remove bacterial plaque and food debris from the teeth. The use of a fluoridated or tartar-control toothpaste and mouth rinse are also very therapeutic, especially in the prevention of tooth decay, cavities, and peridontal disease.

Recognition of the significance of pain and apprehension as impediments to dental care has led to development of an array of techniques to overcome these obstacles. The techniques include psychological approaches, local anesthetics, and various types and combinations of sedatives and general anesthetic agents. Use of these techniques helps overly fearful individuals who avoid or postpone dental treatment, as well as normal people undergoing stressful dental procedures. Some of the most painful dental problems are caused by a toothache, an abscess of the tooth or gums, extraction, temporomandibular joint (TMJ) disorders, trigeminal neuralgia, and oral cancer among others.

Toothache

Prudence suggests that prompt professional diagnosis and treatment of a toothache prevents further decay, erosion of tooth enamel, development of a cavity or abscess, and relieves severe pain. Predental relief may be obtained with the use of simple analgesics such as aspirin (325–650 mg q 4h), acetaminophen (325–650 mg q 4h), or ibuprofen (200–600 mg q 4h).

Tooth Extraction. The intensity of pain during tooth extraction is generally eliminated or modified with the injection of a local anesthetic just prior to extraction. Postextraction pain, depending on anticipated severity, may be treated with simple analgesics, as suggested under toothache, or in combination with codeine. The usual adult oral dose of codeine is 30 to 60 mg q 4 to 6h. Various opiates such as morphine and its congeners, summarized in Table 17.1, can also be used in the treatment and relief of postsurgical or postextraction pain.

Periapical Abscess. This condition is characterized as an acute or chronic supportive process of the periapical region. It is secondary to an infection of the dental pulp, usually due to caries. However, it may occur after trauma to the teeth or from periapical localization of organisms, usually ahemolytic or staphylococci.

In the early stage of pulp infection, the symptoms may not be localized to the infected tooth. Intermittent throbbing pain is usually present and is intensified by temperature change. In the later putrescent stage, the pain is extreme and continuous and may be accentuated by heat, but is often relieved by cold. After the infection reaches the bone, the typical syndrome is localization, pain upon pressure, and looseness of the tooth. Symptoms may then disappear completely, and if drainage occurs, a gumboil may be the only finding. When drainage is inadequate, swelling, pain, lymphadenopathy, and fever are often present. At this stage, antibiotics are advisable before local therapy is undertaken. Penicillin V 250 to 500 mg q 6 h is the antibiotic of choice. Analgesics such as aspirin or acetaminophen 650 mg alone or in combination with codeine 30 to 60 mg orally q 3 to 4h is usually needed.

If not eventually treated by root canal therapy or extraction, the abscess may develop into a more extensive osteomyelitis or cellulitis (or both) or may eventually become cystic, expand, and slowly destroy bone without causing pain.

Temporomandibular Joint Dysfunction (TMJ). This problem is also known as myofacial pain dysfunction (MPD) syndrome. This abnormal condition is characterized by facial pain and mandibular dysfunction, apparently caused by a defective or dislocated temporomandibular joint. Some common indications of this syndrome are the clicking of the joint when the jaws move, limitation of jaw movement, subluxation (a partial dislocation), and temporomandibular dislocation.

This disorder occurs more frequently in women than in men. Most cases are psychophysiologic in origin and result from tension-relieving jaw-clenching or grinding habits, or a centrally generated increase in masticatory muscle tones in response to stress. The ensuing muscle fatigue in turn induces spasm of the masticatory muscles, the immediate cause of MPD. Poorly aligned teeth or ill-fitting dentures occasionally contribute to the condition. Secondary degenerative arthritis may involve the joint in the late stages.

Characteristically, the patient complains of unilateral, dull aching preauricular pain that radiates to the temporal region, the angle of the jaw, and the occiput (the back part of the head); tenderness in one or more of the muscles of mastication; and occasional "clicking" or "popping" sounds in the joint. Joint pain on awakening may indicate bruxism during sleep.

Conventional treatment includes a soft, nonchewy diet; limited use of the jaw; hot, moist applications or diathermy; diazepam 2 to 5 mg orally q.i.d. (the last dose taken at bedtime) as a muscle relaxant and tranquilizer; analgesics such as aspirin 650 mg q.i.d. for pain; and the use of a biteplate. Psychological stress counseling may be helpful in chronic cases.

New advanced treatment includes corrective surgical procedures performed by an oral surgeon, preferably in a multidisciplinary clinic setting.

Trigeminal Neuralgia (tic douleureux). This neuralgic condition is characterized by sudden bursts of excruciating pain of short duration radiating along the course of the fifth cranial nerve. The attack is often precipated by touching a trigger point or by activity such as chewing or brushing the teeth. It is characterized by recurrent paroxysms of sharp, stabbing pains in the distribution of one or more branches of the nerve. It generally occurs in people over fifty, and the incidence is higher in the female population. Although each episode is brief, lasting one to two minutes, successive longer episodes may incapacitate the individual. The frequency of attacks varies from many times daily to several times a month or year (Katon, 1984).

Treatment modalities may include: (1) Carbamazepine 200 to 1200 mg/day, which is generally effective and should be carefully monitored for evidence of serious hematologic and cutaneous reactions; (2) phentoin sodium 300 to 600 mg/day is also effective in some cases; (3) massive doses of vitamin B-12, 1 mg intramuscularly daily for ten days, have been reported to relieve the severe pain (4) alcohol injection of the ganglion or the branches of the trigeminal nerve may produce analgesia and relief from pain for several months or years; (5) surgery may be required when medical treatment brings no relief of intractable pain. Percutaneous electrocoagulation of the preganglionic rootlets under local anesthesia is also an effective modality of treatment of resistant cases of trigeminal neuralgia.

Phantom Limb and Phantom Pain

The sensation that an amputated part of the body is still attached occurs normally after most amputations. Painful phantom sensations are rare, but may arise from abnormalities in stump nerve endings or more centrally located nerve endings. Causalgia, a posttraumatic pain syndrome, occurs in 2 to 5 percent of patients after nerve injury and may contribute to phantom pain. The psychological reaction and degree of adjustment to the amputation may also affect the degree of pain experienced.

Oral Cancer

Chronic irritation of the oral cavity, such as that caused by sharp jagged teeth, projecting fillings, or ill-fitting dentures may often lead to the development of oral cancer. Excessive drinking of alcohol with or without tobacco use also appears to play a role in the development of mouth cancer. Certain noncancerous mouth conditions that tend to become malignant include leukoplakia of the mouth, some tumors, and a tissue-wasting disease called Plummer-Vinson syndrome.

Early detection, diagnosis, and corrective treatment of chronic irritation, pain, disease, or dental malfunction in the early stages, have the best patient survival and cure rates. Surgery, radiation, and chemotherapy are the principal methods of treatment, the choice depending on the site and stage of the disease. Sometimes either form of treatment may be used effectively, and often one is used to supplement the other. For example, radiation is sometimes used to shrink tumors of the cheek or floor of the mouth before surgery. Various analgesic agents used to treat acute and chronic pain of oral cancer are summarized in Table 17.1. Appropriate radiation and chemotherapy treatment measures are outlined in the following section.

Oncology Pain Management

Clinical research to address, control, and alleviate oncology-related pain has long been a major goal of research scientists and clinical cancer specialists. The American Cancer Society estimates that this year over 910,000 people will be diagnosed as having some form of cancer. They also estimate that 35 percent of the 470,000 who will die this year might have been saved by early screening, detection, and prompt treatment. Fortunately, as our knowledge of cancer grows through pharmacologic and molecular research and development, so does the creativity and sophistication of diagnosis and treatment in cancer prevention, control, and pain management.

Until a cure is achieved, living with oncology pain continues to afflict all levels of our society and is physically, emotionally, and spiritually devastating. During such a critical period in their life, patients need all the compassion, empathy, and understanding of family, friends, and significant others, including counseling, treatment, and management by a professional oncology health care team.

The variety and complexity of available cancer treatment modalities suggests that the multidisciplinary concept and approach is most appropriate and beneficial for the integration of medical care, treatment, and management of pain relief for the patient. The team approach can also help fulfill the patient's social, emotional, and psychological needs, including a strong desire and hope for prolonging and maintaining a reasonable quality of life.

Clinical issues related to treating the cancer pain patient have gained considerable attention in the medical and health care literature (Hendler, 1982; Brena, 1983). Addressed are the management strategies which focus specifically on psychotherapeutic, radiological, and pharmacologic approaches to treating the oncology pain patient. Each strategy possesses unique qualities that can benefit the care and management of the cancer patient and provide a better understanding of the disease entity, and the patient's ability to develop coping strategies that may be effective in understanding and confronting pain associated with cancer.

For the oncology patient, pain is all-pervasive, manifests itself in many forms, and invades the entire spectrum of physical and emotional life. Cancer pain management is becoming increasingly individualized, both with respect to diagnostic procedures and to care and treatment. Detection and diagnosis of the disease and accompanying pain are usually followed by more than one kind of therapy, and often in combination. As surgery alone does not always improve the cure rate of some cancers, follow-up adjunctive chemotherapy or combined modality therapy given soon after surgery appears to significantly increase the cure rate of cancer. Since the discovery of nitrogen mustard, many new compounds have been proposed as chemotherapeutic agents. The usefulness of many chemotherapeutic drugs for use with cancer patients depends on their therapeutic to toxicity ratio. The oncologist is concerned primarily with the incidence, predictability, and severity of the potential side-effects and the possibility of reversibility in utilizing such chemotherapeutic agents. A myriad of considerations must be taken into account, including the age, nutrition, and preexisting organ damage, as well as the impact of said therapeutic agents on the simultaneous use of other drugs.

The management of pain in the oncology patient generally follows similar principles that are applied throughout the adult age group. There are, however, some special considerations which cover the use of pharmacological interventions that have psychological implications and must be carefully considered as a part of the psychosocial aspects of cancer. A health care professional must be cognizant of the fact that the patient complaining of pain may well be utilizing a language of pain to describe distress from an ideology other than the disease entity, while the complaint of pain may well be the result of an incipient or organic condition or an expression or attention-seeking mechanism. The health care professional attempting to treat the pain appropriately must establish the correct diagnostic entity and be certain that the complaint of pain is responsible for the pain experienced.

Among some of the common treatment modalities and techniques being currently utilized in the war against cancer pain are: (1) cancer surgery, which is used to remove a tumor and nearby tissue and is one of the most effective procedures; (2) radiation therapy with computerized controlled CAT scans and Magnetic Resonance Imaging (MRI) machines which can precisely locate the tumor, allowing these tools to specifically aim radiation doses into it and selectively destroy tumors while sparing normal tissue; (3) chemotherapy, a treatment modality which scientists are diligently working on to limit the deleterious side-effects. Some are searching for new toxic agents to kill cancer cells while others are synthesizing less toxic versions of existing drugs. Clinical experience indicates that the combinations of radioisotopes have proven to be more effective than single treatment drugs.

The following are among some of the new exciting developments in chemotherapy:

1. Gamma Interferon is a member of the same family of proteins as the more familiar Alpha Interferon. The gamma variety is produced mainly by T-cells, important in cellular immunity. Successfully synthesized in the laboratory, it appears to make tumor cells recognizable to the immune system and therefore more vulnerable. It may also be used in conjunction with monocytes, the largest of the white blood cells, in an adaptive immunotherapy. Clinical trials of Gamma Interferon have recently begun and studies of adaptive immunology are underway.

2. Monoclonal antibodies are produced by animals inoculated with substances specific to the surface of cancer cells.

Other promising treatment modalities and/or diagnostic techniques developed or in various experimental stages of development are:

1. Interleukin-2 (IL-2), called adaptive immunotherapy, is a growth factor that enables doctors, using a complex technique, to turn some of a patient's own leukocytes into anticancer warriors that attack some tumors. Dr. Steven Rosenberg and his National Cancer Institute colleagues who have devel-

oped IL-2 suggest that this treatment, which is tailormade for each patient, is a promising step in a significant approach to use the body's own immune system against cancer. It should be noted, however, that in its present form of development it is not a specific cure and is only one of several lymphokines and related substances showing promise in the immunological treatment of cancer. Further experimentation indicates that when "low" doses of interleukin-2 are combined with "high" doses of the anticancer drug cyclophosphamide, within therapeutic parameters, the cure rates for lung tumors are increased. About 200 of these antibodies have been produced in the laboratory so far. They could work in various ways; for example, by "directing" toxic substances to a tumor or by attacking a growth factor on which the tumor is dependent.

2. Other treatment modalities may include Tumor-Necrosis Factor (TNF), Colony-Stimulating Factor (CSF), laser beam diagnosis and treatment, Cytosin and Leukoregulin, and specific anticancer dietary programs.

Pharmaceutical Approaches. There are several cancer-fighting drugs which have been used effectively in the course of treating a variety of carcinoma conditions. Retinoids, a synthetic analog of Vitamin A, has shown promise in combating cancer of the lung, esophagus, and pancreas. Over the past three decades, many cancer-fighting drugs have been introduced into the commercial pharmaceutical market and have proven to be very effective in the treatment of many forms of cancer. Among the most successful and popular are Mustargen, Oncovin, Procarbazine, Prednisone (MOPP), and Adriamycin, Bleamycin, Vinblastine, Decarbazine (ABVD). The two groups are used in a cyclic manner if/or as needed, also Fluorouracil, Methodthrexate, and many others.

Pain associated with cancer conditions often involves acute and/or chronic pain. Acute pain is produced by unpleasant emotional experiences, such as disease, injury, and excessive exposure to heat or chemicals. It is generally characterized by increased heart rate, excessive sweating, and muscle tension. These conditions most often may benefit from a regimen of tranquilizers, muscle relaxants, or analgesic medications, alone or in combination. The most popularly used drugs in this category are carisoprodol, chlorpromazine, diazepam, meprobamate, methocarbamol, and many of the nonprescription analgesic agents.

Chronic pain is a more complex and difficult pain to treat, manage, and control, especially in the oncology patient. It not only imposes great physical and emotional pain, but also causes social stress and other complications in victims. It further creates the potential for addiction as a result of long-term narcotic drug therapy (see Table 17.1 for the most popular narcotic analgesic drugs used in the treatment of chronic pain).

Chronic drug pain therapy, among patients suffering from excruciating pain, should be instituted with the utmost care and sensitivity. The dosage regimen for these patients must be therapeutically titrated and frequently monitored to check for adverse reactions, drug allergies, drug reactions, side-effects, and patient tolerance.

When pharmacological therapy is indicated for pain relief, it is prudent to begin treatment with the mildest effective analgesic drug and dose, preferably aspirin or acetaminophen. Chemotherapy with Stadol (butorphanol), a drug that has been reported to have five times the pain-relieving potency of morphine and a lesser addictive potential, has had great success in bringing relief of severe pain in cancer patients. It is interesting to note that the pain threshold and tolerance toward pain in chronic pain-suffering patients decreases as their condition deteriorates because of a depletion of their endorphin levels.

Psychotherapeutic Treatment Modalities

Cognitive. There are several modalities of treatment available to patients suffering from pain. Among the most prominent are surgery, chemotherapy, behavior therapy, and stress management, acupuncture, local and systemic anesthesia, radiology and hypnosis. The most prudent and cost-effective approach to the control, treatment, and management of chronic pain is the interdisciplinary health-related professional approach. Thus it is essential that the channels of communication and cooperation among health care professionals be kept open with mutual acceptance, professionalism, and respect.

Several alternative modalities of treatment have been employed to alleviate, control, and teach patients to cope with pain. Earlier efforts focused on more analytic approaches. More contemporary approaches have focused on behaviorally oriented treatment approaches and biofeedback. Nursing personnel have recognized the value of a behavioral technique that has been used separately and in conjunction with more traditional approaches to pain-related problems. The development and use of cognitive-oriented muscle relaxation is principally employed to reduce sensory input. By tensing and relaxing various muscle groups that receive intense stimulation, and combining this with deep breathing and cognitive imagery, individuals can develop appropriate skills for coping with the conceptualization and sensory input in the pain experience.

Perhaps one of the most useful coping strategies involved with sensory alteration of pain experiences involves the process of focusing. Focusing directs the attention of the individual experiencing the pain to that part of the body where the intense sensations are realized. The individual analyzes sensations in that specific area of the body and compares them to the less intense stimulation experienced in another part of the body. One might even conceptualize that area of the body where the pain experience is the greatest as having been filled with an injection of novocaine, or imagine a part of the body made of a pliable substance that absorbs and numbs the pain. The use of cognitive coping strategics involving vivid visual imagery can provide an effective element in the control and management of pain. When combined with muscle relaxation, sensory input can be controlled, managed, and sometimes relieved for the individual with chronic pain conditions. Turk, Meichenbaum, and Genest provide a more detailed presentation of cognitive coping strategies in relieving the sensory stimulation to pain (Turk, Meichenbaum, and Genest, 1983).

Pain Management Techniques. Pain management techniques refer to a variety of techniques that provide an individual with the skill to voluntarily cope with, or reduce, the level of pain being experienced (Butler, 1978; Miller 1980; Gaarder and Montgomery, 1981). Some techniques use instrumentation to augment the training procedure referred to as biofeedback (Olton and Noonberg, 1980). Occasionally visual imagery is used to make development of conscious control easier. The object of pain management training is to establish in the individual the ability to invoke a significant release of tension through the muscle systems in response to his or her desire to do so. Training and practice are designed to habituate the relaxation response to identifiable environmental and internal cues.

Pain management training has also been useful as a tool in helping patients learn control of affective arousal that causes or exaggerates symptomatic events, including pain (Orne, 1980). This has helped professionals to more effectively treat anxiety impulse control and related problems of a psychiatric nature. The techniques provides several ways the patient can voluntarily control the response to pain and produce a state of coping with chronic pain. The most obvious advantage is that the patient can employ pain management techniques even when reclining in a chair with eyes closed. Having a skill that can be employed to ease the pain state can greatly increase the patient's confidence. Another advantage of the training is its inherent capacity to allow the patient to assume basic responsibilities for treatment, particularly as it may reduce the need for some pharmaceutical control. Once the patient has learned the skill, the patient retains it as he or she would any skill and its efficiency is directly related to practice.

Behaviorally oriented pain management is integrally related to how the patient processes stress (Peper, Ancoli, and Quinn, 1979). The pain management training program for chronic pain patients involves four components, each with specific therapeutic tasks and expected outcomes.

Behavioral assessment. The initial component is one of behavioral assessment (Turk et al., 1983). The assessment phase involves the careful analysis of the variety of components of pain experienced by the patient. Significant life events cause stress reactions mainly because the events have some direct impact on individuals' lives; this may intensify pain. Because of this, it is essential that the patients take responsibility for the pain and stress that they are experiencing by carefully evaluating the circumstances that led to the stressful situation. They must evaluate how they are processing the information related to the stressful situation, and the extent to which they can cope with it. Thus, pain management becomes stress management. Stress management training teaches an individual how to evaluate and develop coping mechanisms that can relieve the anxiety experienced as a result of the stress.

Cognitive appraisal. The second component of pain management training involves a cognitive phase that aims to assess the specific process of cognitively interpreting stressful events (Turk et al., 1983). The cognitive phase recognized that individuals perceive life events in a variety of different ways. The way in which life events are communicated and the way in which individuals have learned to perceive them, tie into each person's own anticipatory anxiety, his or her aspirations, and the threats to satisfactory coping with life stress events and pain. The process of appraising a situation in life events has the potential to cause anxiety. The self-statements that individuals make emphasize their ability or inability to cope with that situation. While cognitive appraisal is functioning, the body, including muscles, salivary glands, and blood pressure, produces comparable physiological responses. Some of these responses are in the form of muscle tension, perspiration, or a variety of other somatic concerns. They result in a self-fulfilling anxiety response and thus become the focus of control.

Education. The third component of pain management training involves education (Turk et al., 1983). This educational component teaches four specific steps that are essential to anyone's preparation for coping with stress and pain. The first step, or phase, is to prepare for the pain. In preparing for the pain, an individual thinks through and carefully evaluates what triggers pain. Preparing for the triggering event allows the individual to think through the options that he or she has in coping with it. There is also an anxiety-reducing effect in visually imagining role-playing about the particular situation for which one is anticipating a great deal of anxiety. As part of preparing for this pain-producing situation, an individual can call on the use of muscle relaxation skills, which can be used in conjunction with the visual imagery one uses as a way of coping with the anticipated stressful situation.

The second phase concerns being able to confront the pain by cognitively rehearsing (in the mind) the way that has been chosen to deal with this significant life event. Once this rehearsal phase has been completed, one is ready to face the triggering event and to use both the cognitive imagery and relaxation skills that will allow the individual to see him or herself through this stressful life event.

The third phase of the education component emphasizes coping with painful situations based on the preparation and cognitive–rehearsing phases. Reasoning things through and mentally preparing oneself for stressful life events means that an individual can develop a mental preparedness for whatever situation is confronted.

The fourth phase is the evaluation of the level of satisfaction one has realized in coping with this particular pain experience. In particular, this should involve self-statements that support the individual's efforts to be in control and to manage the level of control he or she has realized in the use of pain management skills.

Relaxation exercises. The fourth component of training is one of relaxation exercises (Turk et al., 1983). Relaxation exercises become the physical response experienced in conjunction with cognitive appraisal and coping skill. Relaxation exercise involve tensing and relaxing all the different muscle groups as summarized in Table 17.6. As a part of muscle relaxation training, individuals are asked to listen to an audiotape that leads the individual through the sequential phase of muscle relaxation training. Muscle relaxation recognizes that anxiety, stress, and tension are stored in the various muscle groups of the body. These same muscle groups that one deliberately tenses are the muscle groups that become tense and tight when anxiety, stress, and tensions are experienced. The tensing and relaxing phase of muscle relaxation allows one to learn a physiological method of coping with pain.

TABLE 17.6
PAIN MANAGEMENT TRAINING UTILIZING MUSCLE RELAXATION SKILLS

Muscle Group	Directive
Breathing Exercises	Slowly inhale, hold, and release. Repeat two or three times
Right Hand and Forearm	Tense by making a tight fist. Hold and release
Left Hand and Forearm	Tense by making a tight fist. Hold and release
Biceps and Triceps	Tense by bringing elbows in toward body. Hold and release
Forehead	Tense by raising eyebrows upward. Hold and release
Facial Muscles	Tense by squinting and wrinkling nose. Hold and release
Mouth and Jaw	Tense by clenching teeth and lips. Hold and release
Neck	Tense by pushing the head back, rolling in one continuous motion
Shoulders and Chest	Tense by pressing shoulder blades back and together
Abdomen	Tense by tightening stomach muscles. Hold and release
Lower Back	Tense by arching back. Hold and release
Thighs	Tense by raising leg (left, then right) off ground. Hold and release
Calves	Tense by pointing toes toward head. Hold and release
Feet and Toes	Tense by curling the toes and pointing feet inward. Hold and release

Once the individual has had an opportunity to learn the progressive muscle relaxation sequence, a period of conditioning and reinforcement of both the cognitive and relaxation exercises is necessary for pain management to be effective. A cue-controlled response can be obtained by the patient in a matter of seconds simply by using the pain management skills learned, both cognitively and from the relaxation training. The body systems, which are often vulnerable to stress-related concerns, will respond effectively, assuming a conditioned response cued by the experience already gained from practicing the longer, more complete relaxation therapy.

The Role of the Health Care Professional

The health care professional who is training chronic pain patients in pain management skills can enhance the patient's competencies in coping with anxiety producing situations, and assist that individual to understand more clearly the role and function of anxiety and anxiety reduction methodologies in adjusting to pain and its impact on life.

The cognitive–behavioral approach to the treatment of pain focuses on the elements involved in helping the patient to cope with the pain being experienced by altering the patient's interpretation of the sensation of pain. There are various interpersonal and intrapersonal methods that can be used to divert attention in order to avoid or reduce the sensation of pain. A tailormade approach using the individual's own skills and resources is probably the most beneficial method.

The use of cognitive imagery in diverting attention from an unpleasant stimulus in pain sensation can frequently be an effective alternative. Focusing on a preoccupied topic of interest, as can often be experienced in the daydreaming process, can provide a favorable modality and encourage activity in the patient's attempt to cope with pain. The nurse may ask the patient to describe an absorbing article, book, or movie and then attend to the specific interests and preoccupations that the patient discusses. When this approach is combined with muscle relaxation exercises, the patient will benefit by a reduced level of pain sensation and thereby realize the altering effect of this sensation experience. Turk has discussed cognitive imagery in detail and provides steps in using cognitive-oriented imagery as a way of altering sensations. There are other treatment strategies that focus on sensations of the body, comparing sensations of pain in one part of the body with those in another part, allow chronic pain patients to address the discomfort they expressed, and use this discomforting experience as a way of preparing for the onset of future pain experiences as well as confronting and managing the current sensations of pain. In addition, it provides the individual an ability to cope with the feeling and sensations of critical moments when the pain can be most excruciating, and then contemplating how the present and future situations can be handled in gaining a mastery and confidence to be able to manage and control pain experience rather than be dependent on external forces, including medication to relieve or control the pain-related problem.

The health care professional should be aware that social support systems are very important in influencing adaptive coping processes, and should encourage those support systems to be an active ingredient in the treatment of the chronic pain patient. Each pain patient has a variable and unique requirement for different levels of support, and therefore the health care professional should attempt to tailor the level of spousal or significant others involvement in dealing with pain-related and maladaptive types of behavior.

There are a number of areas in which support individuals, including spouse or significant others, can be actively involved. One of these areas is exercise. Exercise activities play a significant role, both psychologically and physiologically, in the management of chronic pain. The initial efforts should be to establish tolerance levels as uniquely defined by the patient's level of tolerance for pain with exercise. Once the initial measurement baselines for tolerance levels are recognized, the establishment of a daily regime and exercise schedule can be initiated. Having a significant other involved in the program greatly affects the positive involvement of the pain patient in such activities.

Homework activities provide a key ingredient between therapy sessions for the pain patient and significant others. The assignment of out-of-therapy activities can serve a diagnostic purpose by helping the patient and significant others identify various maladaptive pain-related responses and thus make them more aware of factors that exacerbate or alleviate the pain condition. Homework activities show support and encourage confidence that coping procedures do exist and that the pain patient is not alone in coping with or resolving the ability to manage the pain-related disorder. The use of homework assignments also demonstrates to the patient and to the significant others that the pain condition will continue but that progress can be made in appropriately coping with the pain conditions. Finally, these activities can offer reinforcement and reward, with specific emphasis on self-reinforcement and self-reward as the pain patient achieves certain designated and expected goals that have previously been set through conjoint sessions during the regular therapy program.

The psychological approach to chronic pain conditions is a rapidly growing area of clinical research and discovery. Psychological approaches hold a great deal of promise in the regulation, management, and altering of sensations of pain. The literature tends to suggest the importance of cognitive and affective factors in pain perception and in the pain patient's expected response to nociceptive stimuli. As Melzack (1980) and others have emphasized, the psychological variables may modulate the pain perception directly by "closing the gate" through which the pain enters (Hendler, 1982). This will result in reduced pain and block the abnormal reverberatory neural activity that has been hypothesized as the critical underlying agent related to chronic pain disorders. Psychopharmacology has been an important key in bridging fundamental molecular biology to behavior. As a pragmatic psychobiological procedure, biofeedback has heightened awareness of the many contributions from behavioral therapy. These contributions include learning theory, contracting, desensitization, flooding, reciprocal inhibition, assertiveness training, approach-avoidance gradients, cognitive restructuring, and the crucial issues of adherence and compliance. All these techniques deserve more widespread application in treatment than they have received to date.

Physicians are in a unique position to recognize genetic, organic, and learned factors that underlie behaviors related to pain. Clinicians who attend to one factor without attending to the others can ignore critically important ingredients in understanding chronic pain patients.

Family Role in Chronic Pain. There is a growing literature (Cohler, 1983; Hulka, Kupper, and Cassel, 1972) supporting the hypothesis that family and significant others play critical roles in both adaptation to and maintenance of chronic pain. Furthermore, how a person defines symptomatology is based on consultation with significant others (Litman, 1974). And finally, family attitudes have been attributed to the response of patients and their subsequent recovery (Reiss, 1982).

Chronic pain impacts every dimension of life, and, by its very nature, it has major consequences for the family of the identified patient, especially in the areas of social, vocational, and recreational activities. The manner in which the family chooses to cope with the pain condition is significant in understanding the responsivity of the chronic pain patient to the pain condition. Engel (1977) and others (Payne and Norfleet, 1986; Turk and Holzman, 1986) have suggested a biopsychosocial perspective that emphasizes the importance of considering sociocultural and environmental aspects in addressing disease entities. This is particularly relevant to the chronic pain condition. Merskey and Spear (1965) and Merskey (1965) studied psychiatric patients who suffered from chronic pain complaints, as well as a sample of psychiatric patients without chronic pain. Gentry, Shows, and Thomas (1974) suggest close to 60 percent of low back pain patients had close family members with chronic low back pain or other debilitating disorders, and Turkat, Kuczmierczyk, and Adams (1984) noted that headache patients have more family members who suffer from headaches than healthy controls.

Studies assessing spousal relationships also demonstrate increased rates of pain complaints in spouses of chronic pain patients (Floyd, 1983; Flor, Turk, and Scholz, in press). While the incidence of chronic pain problems within families may be open to broad interpretation, they should nonetheless be viewed as etiologically relevant in significant factors in the maintenance of chronic pain conditions.

In an effort to address etiological factors, there is a broad range of support for hypotheses ranging from genetic (Devor, Inbal, and Govrin-Lippman, 1982) to psychodynamic (Violon, 1985) to learning theory. Perhaps the most prominent of these hypotheses rests with the learning theory approach. Whitehead, Federovicius, Blackwell, and Wooley (1979) and Wooly, Blackwell, Winget (1978) developed a model of learned illness behavior that addresses the role of instrumental conditioning of symptoms in the chronic pain patient. These researchers suggest that pain tolerance can be influenced by positive reinforcement of pain-related behaviors by significant others in the environment. Others have argued that a behavioral model of vicarious observational learning and subsequent reinforcement may best explain the high incidence of pain experienced by family members (Linton and Gotestam, 1985). One research study suggests that experimental subjects who were exposed to tolerant vs. intolerant models reported lower levels of pain and displayed higher pain tolerance in experimental pain induction studies (Miller and Kratchowill, 1979). Research on ethnocultural differences in illness behavior, pain perception and level of tolerance for pain clearly showed differences among ethnic groups, and this has been discussed in chapter 4 by Reid and Bush.

Family systems theorists have generated research in support of the family's role in the maintenance of pain symptomatology. (Meissner, 1974; Minuchin, Rosman, and Baker, 1978; Epstein, Bishop and Baldwin, 1981). This is usually realized through the extent to which marital satisfaction and expressed emotionality occur as a result of the pain condition and how the pain patient accommodates the pain experience. Chronic pain patients and their spouses often demonstrate considerable distress and marital dissatisfaction, as well as a statistically significant relationship between conflicts and pain levels in the marital and family setting.

Chronic pain as chronic illness must be viewed as a significant factor affecting family life. The extent to which attitudes and values of family members affected is influenced by an educational process that promotes autonomy and independence of the chronic patient is the extent to which the family can successfully accommodate a chronic pain patient in the family system. Research is needed to establish the relative determinants and coping resources and strategies that can help us to understand the most effective means of accommodating and assimilating chronic pain in the family network.

CONCLUSION

Health care professionals have for some time attempted to conceptualize, diagnose, and treat the complexity of chronic pain. Conceptually, three major models have involved a psychophysiological perspective on chronic pain syndromes. These include the neuromuscular pain model, the pain-spasm-pain cycle model, and the stress pain model. Each is based on the assumption that physiological changes interact closely with psychological variables produced or exacerbate a chronic pain condition. The neuromuscular model of pain stresses the contribution that abnormal patterns of muscle activity contribute to the development and maintenance of chronic pain. The pain muscles, pain spasms cycle argues that a specific event triggers reflex muscle spasms, which are often accompanied by vasoconstriction and the subsequent relief of pain-producing substances which achieve a chronic state for the individual. Finally, the stress pain model suggests that stressful life events can elicit physiological and psychological responses resulting in a chronic pain experience. Such stressful life events induce autonomic arousal and heighten muscle activity that leads to nociceptive stimulation resulting in anxiety, depression, and somatization associated with the pain condition. These emotional reactions to pain ultimately increase the pain condition and cause a cyclical pattern of stress, subsequent anxiety, depression, somatization, and chronic pain. Irrespective of the model, the nature of chronic pain will continue to be most meaningfully examined within the context of the unique quality of the person, the complexity of the environment, and the pathogenesis of the disorder causing the pain experience. Only be expanding our knowledge of the interaction of these critically important factors will we begin to understand the exact pathways of the disorder, the exogenous factors affecting a patient's response to pain and the endogenous characteristics that permit the pain patient the ability to achieve their level of coping sufficient to experience an acceptable quality of life.

REFERENCES

Andrasik, F., Blanchard, E.B., Arena, J.G., Saunders, N.L., and Barron, K.D. (1982), Psychophysiology of recurrent headache: Methodological issues and new empirical findings. *Behav. Ther.*, 13:407–429.

Arthritis Foundation (1985), *National Report.* Washington, DC: Arthritis foundation.

Basmajian, J.V., ed. (1983), *Biofeedback: Principles and Practice for Clinicians.* Baltimore: Williams & Wilkins.

Blanchard, E.B., Andrasik, F., Arena, J.G., Neff, D.F., Saunders, N.L., Jurish, S.E., Teders, S.J., & Rodichok, L.D. (1983), Psychophysiological responses and predictors of response to behavioral treatment of chronic headache. *Behav. Ther.*, 14:257–374.

Brena, S.F. (1983), Drugs and Pain: Use and misuse. In: *Management of Patients with Chronic Pain,* eds. S. F. Brena and S.L. Chapman. New York: Spectrum, pp. 121–130.

Butler, F. (1978), *Biofeedback, A Survey of the Literature.* New York: Plenum.

Cohler, B.J. (1983), Autonomy and interdependence in the family of adulthood: A psychological perspective. *Gerontol.*, 23:33–39.

Devor, M., Inbal, R., & Govrin-Lippman, R. (1982), Genetic factors in the development of chronic pain. In: *Genetics of the Brain,* ed. M. Lieblich Amsterdam: Elsevier Biomedical.

Dolce, J.J., & Raczynski, J.M. (1985), Neuromuscular activity and electromyography in painful backs: Psychological and biomechanical models in assessment and treatment. *Psychol. Bull.*, 97:502–520.

Engel, G.L. (1977), The need for a new medical model: A challenge for biomedicine. *Science*, 196:129–136.

Epstein, N.B., Bishop, D.S., & Baldwin, L.M. (1981), McMaster model of family functioning: A view of the normal family. In: *Normal Family Processes*, ed. F. Walsh. Guilford, New York.

Flor, H., Turk, D.C., & Scholz, O.B. (in press), Impact of chronic pain on the spouse: Marital, emotional, and physical consequence. *J. Psychosom. Res.*.

Floyd, F.J. (1983), Spouse observation and objective behavioral assessment of marital interaction. Paper presented at the annual meeting of the Association for the Advancement of Behavior Therapy, Washington, D.C.

Fordyce, W.E., & Roberts, A.H., Sternbach, R.A. (1985), The behavioral management of chronic pain: A response to critics. *Pain*, 22:113–125.

Gaarder, K.R., & Montgomery, S. (1981), *Clinical Biofeedback: A Procedural Manual for Behavioral Medicine.* Baltimore: Williams & Wilkins.

Gentry, W.D., Shows, W.D., & Thomas, M. (1974), Chronic low back pain: A psychological profile. *Psychosomat.*, 15:174–177.

Gottlieb, H., Strite, L., Koller, R., Madorsky, A., Hockersmith, V., Kleeman, M., & Wagner, J. (1977), Comprehensive rehabilitation of patients having chronic low back pain. *Arch. Phys. Med. & Rehab.*, 58:101–108.

Hendler, N. (1982), The anatomy and psychopharmacology of chronic pain. *J. Clin. Psychiat.*, 43:15–20.

Hulka, B.S., Kupper, L.L., & Cassel, J.C. (1972), Determinants of physician utilization. *Med. Care*, 10:300–309.

Kantor, T.G. (1984), Perpherally acting analgesics. In: *Analgesics: Neurochemical, Behavioral and Clinical Perspectives*, eds. M.J. Kuhar & G.W. Pasternak. New York: Raven Press, pp. 289–312.

Katon, W. (1984), Depression: Relationship to somatization and chronic medical illness. *J. Clin. Psychiat.*, 45:4–11.

Linton, S.J., & Gotestam, K.G. (1985), Controlling pain reports through operant conditioning: A laboratory demonstration. *Perceptual Motor Skills*, 60:427–437.

Litman, T.J. (1974), The family as the basic unit in health and medical care: A social and behavioral overview. *Soc. Sci. Med.*, 8:495–499.

Luce, J.M., Thompson, T.L., II, Getto, C.J., & Bynny, R.L. (1979), New concepts of chronic pain and their implications. *Hosp. Pract.*, 14:113.

Meissner, W.W. (1974), Family process and psychosomatic disease. *Internat. J. Psychiat. Med.*, 5:422–430.

Melzack, R. (1980), Psychological aspects of pain. *Pain*, 9:143–154.

Merskey, H. (1965), Psychiatric patients with persistent pain. *J. Psychosom. Res.*, 9:299–309.

———& Spear, F.G. (1965), *Pain: Psychological and Psychiatric Aspects*. London: Balliere.

Miller, N.E. (1980), Applications of learning and biofeedback to psychiatry and medicine. In: *Comprehensive Textbook of Psychiatry*, Vol. 1, 3rd ed., eds. H.I. Kaplan, A.M. Freedman, & B.J. Sadock. Williams & Wilkins, Baltimore, p. 468.

Miller, A.J., & Kratchowill, T.R. (1979), Reduction of frequent stomachache complaints by time-out. *Behav. Ther.*, 10:211–218.

Minuchin, S., Rosman, B., & Baker, L. (1978), *Psychosomatic Families*. Cambridge, MA: Harvard University Press.

Olton, D.S., & Noonberg, A.R. (1980), *Biofeedback: Clinical Applications in Behavioral Medicine*. Englewood Cliffs, NJ: Prentice-Hall.

Orne, M.T., (1980) ed. *Task Force Report, No. 19: Biofeedback*. Washington, DC: American Psychiatric Association.

Payne, B., & Norfleet, M.A. (1986), Chronic pain and the family: A review. *Pain*, 26:1–22.

Peper, E., Ancoli, S., & Quinn, M., eds. (1979), *Mind/body Integration: Essential Readings in Biofeedback*. New York: Plenum.

Reiss, D. (1982), The working family: A researcher's view of health in the household. *Am. J. Psychiat.*, 139:1412–1420.

Skevington, S.M. (1983), Social cognitions, personality and chronic pain. *J. Psychosom. Res.*, 27:421–428.

Turk, D.C., & Genest, M. (1979), Regulation of pain: The application of cognitive and behavioral techniques for prevention and remediation. In: *Cognitive-Behavioral Intervention: Theory, Research and Procedures*, eds. P.C. Kendall & S.D. Hollon. New York: Academic Press.

———Meichenbaum, D., & Genest, M. (1983), *Pain and Behavioral Medicine: A Cognitive-Behavioral Perspective*. New York: Guilford Press.

———Holzman, A.D. (1986), Chronic pain: Interfaces among physical, psychological, and social parameters. In: *Chronic Pain: A Handbook of Psychological Treatment Approaches*, eds. A.D. Holzman & D.C. Turk. Elmsford, NY: Pergamon, pp. 1–9.

Turkat, I.D., Kuczmierczyk, A.R., & Adams, H.E. (1984), An investigation of the etiology of chronic headache. The role of headache models, *Brit. J. Psychiat.*, 145:665–666.

Violon, A. (1985), Family etiology of chronic pain. *Internat. J. Fam. Ther.*, 7:235–246.

Whitehead, W.E., Federovicius, A.S., Blackwell, B., & Wooley, S. (1979), A behavioral conceptualization of psychosomatic illness: Psychosomatic symptoms as learned responses. In: *Behavioral Approaches to Medicine: Applications and Analysis*, ed. J.R. McNamara. New York: Plenum pp. 65-99.

Wooley, S.C., Blackwell, B., & Winget, C. (1978), A learning theory model of chronic illness behavior: Theory, treatment and research. *Psychosom. Med.*, 40:379–401.

18

Chronic Pain: The Family in Treatment

GENE W. BROCKOPP, PH.D
DOROTHY Y. BROCKOPP PH.D., R.N.

INTRODUCTION

Perceptions of the etiology and treatment of chronic pain have become increasingly complex, moving from simple cause and effect models to those in which multiple factors are considered. Simplistic views of both the treatment and etiology of chronic pain have generally accepted a physiologically based stimulus as the cause of the condition and have used a variety of medically oriented interventions as appropriate treatment. Unfortunately, this biomedical approach to conceptualizing and treating pain has met with little success for a large number of chronic pain patients. (Fordyce, Fowler, Lehmann, and DeLateur, 1968; Melzack, 1973; Payne and Norflett, 1986).

Approaches to chronic pain that have considered multiple factors relative to both etiology and treatment have taken psychosocial factors as well as physiological concerns into consideration. While the stimulus responsible for the individual's pain sensation may be physiologically based, the experience of pain is thought to be influenced (increased or decreased) by social and psychological variables. (Bonica, 1973; Crowley, 1975).

This more complex or holistic approach to conceptualizing chronic pain requires professionals working in the area to consider all facets of the individual's life when designing a plan of care. Thoughts, attitudes, behaviors, and relationships are believed to have the potential to exacerbate or diminish the discomfort experienced. Individual's expectations in relation to their plan, the social environment in which the pain occurs, and the experience of the sensation itself often combine to create new patterns of behavior. (Bellissimo and Tunks, 1984). Examples of such behaviors include overuse of analgesics, spending increasing amounts of time in bed, and withdrawing from interpersonal contacts. (Sternbach, 1984). These behaviors can be destructive to individuals and their relationships.

While there are approaches to the treatment of chronic pain that include the family (Bellissimo and Tunks, 1984; Roy, 1986), the purpose for such inclusion is usually to enable family members to assist patients to improve their condition. The family, or social environment in which the patient resides is seen as a tool that can help the patient to modify destructive behaviors and facilitate a pain-free or diminished pain state. If the behaviors of family members are thought to perpetuate or exacerbate the patient's pain, treatment is focused on erasing or diminishing the destructive behaviors (Waring, 1977; Block, 1981; Maruta, Osborne, Sanson, and Halling 1981).

Jeans and Rowat (1984), have suggested that a family may suffer from having a member experience chronic pain to such an extent that the family itself needs assistance. In such a case, the debilitated family would need to receive treatment before enlisting members' help on behalf of the patient. How to determine the appropriate level of involvement with the family of the chronic pain patient, however, is not clear. While the importance of including the patient's family to some extent in the treatment plan has been substantiated, clear directions for intervening have not been empirically validated (Flor, Turk, and Rudy, 1987).

Under these circumstances, it would seem advantageous to perform a comprehensive assessment on patients and their families—one that would be most likely to provide information that could give direction for treatment. Data regarding developmental issues that are routinely gathered when working with families, as well as information regarding the impact and characteristics of the patient's condition, are desirable when working in the domain of chronic pain. In the absence of clear, empirically based directives for providing care for the patient and the family, conducting a thorough assessment of the family's role in helping the patient to diminish, maintain, or exacerbate the pain experienced is probably worthwhile. Interventions can then be developed from the data collected and evaluative measures can be designed to assess their effectiveness in the treatment of chronic pain.

The family is conceptualized in this chapter as an open system of interrelated, interdependent parts. In this definition, the concept of family includes not only individual family members, it also includes their relationships, communication patterns, and interactions with the external environment. The role of the family in the treatment of pain then emphasizes the importance of understanding the impact of the patient's chronic pain condition on usual family functioning, the family's ability to perform its developmental tasks, and the family's strengths in terms of dealing with the various phases of a chronic illness.

As one member or pattern of internal–external interaction changes, the unit is affected. In response to change, the desire to maintain the family structure as experienced by its members becomes a powerful motivating force underlying both positive and negative behaviors. (Jackson, 1965). The challenge for individuals working with the families of chronic pain patients is to understand their traditional mode of functioning, strengths and weaknesses, and response to the patient's condition. With this information, an interdisciplinary team or a designate can then facilitate change that will enhance the lives of both patient and family members by working with the family's communication patterns and contracting with individual members as well as the unit as a whole to modify their behavior patterns.

The treatment of the patient with pain is limited in this chapter to the effects of the interaction between the patient and the family that occur as a result of the chronic pain condition. The authors recognize the need for a thorough physical and psychobehavioral evaluation of the patient in the development of an appropriate treatment plan. The addition of a family perspective to the treatment program is effective because patients are treated within the context in which they live. Given the complexity of the task, the use of an interdisciplinary team consisting of individuals who represent various areas of expertise and who are willing to both share information and learn from each other is strongly recommended.

THE FAMILY LIFE CYCLE

Human beings are thought to progress through a number of developmental stages. Depending on the stage in question, life events may be perceived and experienced in different ways. Discovering the existence of a chronic illness in adolescence for example, alters the lives of patients in a fashion that is somewhat different than if chronic illness was diagnosed during middle adulthood. The adolescent has expectations of the coming years as well as tasks to perform that are different from those of the middle-aged adult. Similarly individuals in other stages differ in their experience of life events. Because the individual's developmental stage is generally acknowledged as an important variable, it is usually considered in assessing and treating patients diagnosed with a chronic illness.

Families, not unlike individuals, undergo different phases of growth and can be expected to perform different tasks as they progress from their initial formation to eventual dissolution. Levinson (1978) described the family as experiencing building and maintenance periods as well as structure-changing phases. As families attempt to build or maintain their structure certain tasks are performed.

Families have traditionally been considered responsible for maintaining their members' physical well-being, allocating available resources, directing the division of labor, socializing its members, maintaining order within the unit, incorporating new members into the structure, releasing members as their developmental needs require them to leave, placing members in the larger society, and maintaining motivation and morale

(Duval, 1971). The pressure felt as a result of the developmental tasks expected of a family at a given point in time, can have an important influence on its ability to maintain itself and also support the chronic pain patient. For example, if the patient previously represented a major source of the family's financial support, or took a major role in assisting with household chores, the physical maintenance of the family may be in question as a result of the patient's condition.

Dealing with problems of physical maintenance, redirecting the division of labor, and reallocating resources are activities that can cause negative emotional responses toward the patient and the condition responsible for the changes in family functioning. Interventions can be designed to enable families to resolve destructive emotional responses to the situation and adopt new patterns of behavior. An understanding of a family's particular developmental tasks at the time of diagnosis and the unit's ability to redefine those tasks, given the impact of the patient's condition, permits the treatment team to design an effective plan of care in terms of the family's involvement.

Phases of a Chronic Illness

Rolland's (1987) model of a chronic illness identifies phases of a chronic condition that influences the choice of intervention at any given time. These phases, crisis, chronicity, and terminal, are linked by transition periods. Transition periods occur when families must reevaluate their functioning in view of new, illness-related, developmental demands. Successful transition depends on the way in which the family has completed the tasks of the previous phase. For example, if a family has been unable to resolve issues relating to the crisis period, they will have difficulty moving successfully into and through the chronic phase.

The three major threads of the model are the illness, the family, and the individual. Each of these threads responds over time to various external stimuli as well as to the interaction among these three variables. Illness-related events can influence family and patient. Developmental concerns of family members and patient can influence responses to the illness.

Illness within this model is described in terms of its onset, course, outcome, and incapacitation. Each of these variables can affect the choice of intervention as well as the patient and family's response to the condition. The onset may be acute or gradual. In the case of chronic pain, individuals may become suddenly aware of intense discomfort or the awareness of discomfort may be a gradual process with the awareness of the pain heightened as the intensity increases.

The course of the chronic illness may be progressive, constant, or episodic. An example of progressive chronic pain would be the pain of the cancer patient who may feel minimal discomfort until there is evidence of metastases to the bone. As the disease metastasizes to the bone the pain increases and in some instances is intractable (Baines and Kirkham, 1984). Constant pain is experienced by some individuals who have tumor-related headaches (Dalessio, 1984), and episodic pain is a common experience among patients with gastric ulcers (Blendis, 1984).

The outcome of the illness refers to the likelihood that the condition will shorten the patient's life span. According to Rolland (1987) an important factor in determining the effect of the outcome of the illness is the patient's and family's expectation regarding the patient's life span. Objective data regarding the outcome may not be as important as the patient's and family's perceptions. For example, although death may not be a likely outcome, if the patient and family believe that death is probable, their behavior will be based on that assumption.

Incapacitation is a factor that can have a devastating effect on both patient and family. How severely the patient is restricted, the kind of handicap experienced, and when the incapacitation occurs make a difference in the family's response to the patient's condition. If patient and family have a period of time to accustom themselves to the handicap, as in those diseases that are characterized by a progressive deterioration of the body, the individuals involved may cope more effectively (Rolland, 1987).

The crisis phase of Rolland's model is that period when the

patient and family are attempting to cope with the initial diagnosis and the accompanying symptoms. For the chronic pain patient the crisis phase may be that moment when the label "chronic pain" is applied for the first time. After a prolonged period of discomfort, the patient may be told that the condition appears to be chronic. At this time former hopes for a quick and simple solution to the problem may be erased.

There are illness-related tasks that need to be addressed by both patient and family in this phase. These tasks include learning to deal with the incapacitation suggested by the condition, various symptoms, and new environments such as hospitals and clinics. In this phase families need to ascribe a meaning to the patient's condition that can allow them to continue to live in a productive manner. They may also need to grieve for their former manner of functioning that is no longer possible (Moos, 1984).

The terminal phase is characterized by concerns related to separation, death, loss, and grief. For the chronic pain patient the terminal phase probably applies to those individuals whose pain is related to the diagnosis of a life-threatening illness. For example, it is estimated that 60 percent of cancer patients experience pain during the course of their disease and much of that pain is poorly controlled (Bonica, 1979).

Describing the chronic pain patient's condition in terms of Rolland's model provides a framework against which the information gathered in relation to the family's developmental life cycle can be plotted. Judgments regarding the intensity of the difficulties facing both patient and family can be made on the basis of the objective data obtained. Subjective responses of the individuals involved can complete the picture and appropriate interventions can then be designed.

The Family and the Assessment of the Chronic Pain Patient

Setting the stage for the assessment of the chronic pain patient in terms of the family's role is an important prelude to later treatment. If family members are included in the initial assessment a clear message is automatically given regarding their importance to the success of therapy. (Bellissimo and Tunks, 1984). If concern is expressed relative to the impact the patient's condition has had on family member's lives, a sense of empathy or caring can be conveyed.

Another valuable message that can be conveyed to families of chronic pain patients concerns the reason for including them in the treatment plan. Families should be told that their inclusion is based on a belief that families are always involved in their members' problems. Because families are involved in their members' problems, they can be of considerable help in assisting members to deal with a variety of concerns. The purpose of including family members in the treatment of the pain patient is not simply to identify possible pathology but to elicit their assistance in designing the best possible interventions for the patient (Bellissimo and Tunks, 1984). Even behaviors that may be viewed as destructive can be reframed as attempts on the part of family members to maintain their family structure in the face of a threatening event (Jackson, 1965).

Data pertaining to chronic pain patients and their families can be gathered using a paper and pencil test, face-to-face interviews, and/or observations of family members' interactions. Information regarding the family's position in the family life cycle and related developmental tasks can be readily accessed through questioning family members. The following list of developmental tasks identified by Duvall (1971) provides guidelines for assessing the tasks expected of most families.

Physical Maintenance—the provision of basic necessities such as food and shelter

Resource Allocation—the allocation of material goods, and emotional attention

Division of Labor—assigning chores in order to manage the household

Socializing Family Members—assisting family members to grow in a valued direction

The Inclusion and Release of Family Members—rearing children so that they are comfortable to leave at maturity

Maintaining Order—assigning sanctions in keeping with family norms

Placing Family Members in the Larger Society—schools, religious organization, and so on

Maintaining Motivation and Morale—developing a sense of family togetherness

During the process of collecting data relative to the performance of developmental tasks, the treatment team can assess the family's ability to solve problems. If former problem-solving skills are not effective in dealing with the difficulties caused by the patient's condition, the teaching of new skills can be incorporated into the treatment plan. Additional information regarding family members' emotional responses to their situation, patterns of communication, and interpersonal relationships can also be observed as data relative to developmental tasks are collected.

Describing the patient, the patient's illness, and the family in terms of Rolland's model can also be achieved during an assessment interview. Information regarding the phase of the illness, crisis, chronic, or terminal, as well as the other characteristics of a chronic illness identified by Rolland—onset, course, outcome, and incapacitation—can be of assistance in designing a plan of care. Given the objective data collected regarding tasks and developmental issues, the observations of the family as its members interact, and the subjective concerns and expectations of each family member, a picture of the general status of the family should emerge.

Specific difficulties identified in the assessment interview(s) can provide direction for working with the family. The overall picture of the family obtained from all data collected can provide a basis for judgments as to the degree to which the family needs to be involved in treatment.

Interventions and Their Evaluation

Possible family-related interventions based on the suggested data collection include intensive family therapy for those families in which serious pathology is found and a series of working sessions for those families whose problems are related to the patient's condition. Working sessions can involve the provision of support and reassurance for families in need, the modification of nonproductive patterns of communication within the family, and the formation of contracts with individual family members and the family as a whole, designed to introduce new behaviors or modify existing ones.

Support can be offered for those families whose suffering in relation to the patient's condition has depleted their energies. In addition to the support of the treatment team, methods for the family to care for themselves can be suggested. Problem-solving skills can be taught to families who have difficulty modifying their former roles or behaviors in order to meet their obligations.

For some families, the diagnosis of a chronic illness does not disrupt their functioning and they can of their own accord respond positively to the patient's needs. The assumption that all families should share an intense involvement in the treatment of the chronic pain patient is probably erroneous (Flor, Turk, and Rudy, 1987). A comprehensive assessment of the family and patient should provide direction for the treatment team as to the kind involvement that is most appropriate.

An evaluation of family-related interventions used in the treatment of the chronic pain patient can provide valuable clinical information related to the specific patient and can also contribute to a general framework for understanding the role of the family in treatment. A variety of measures are available for assessing family functioning that could be given before and after treatment in an attempt to evaluate those interventions aimed at improving the family's ability to work together. Interventions designed to improve the family's ability to communicate and problem solve can be tested within a single session. Feedback from family members in relation to their activities at home can also be used to evaluate the success of various treatment strategies.

Summary

An attempt has been made to describe the role of the family in the treatment of the chronic pain patient in terms of family need and developmental issues. The family is viewed as a possible patient, and the behaviors of family members are seen as largely directed toward the maintenance of the family structure. Developmental tasks expected of families are identified and a model defining the phases of chronic illness is presented.

An interdisciplinary team representing various areas of expertise assesses the patient and family and contracts with individual family members as well as the family as a whole to make the changes necessary to improve the patient's well-being. Systematic evaluation is suggested for all interventions in order to provide the best care possible and to begin to provide a framework for selecting appropriate family-oriented treatments.

References

Baines, M., & Kirkham, S. (1984), Carcinoma involving bone and soft tissue, In: *Textbook of Pain*, eds. P. Wall & R. Melzack. New York: Churchill Livingstone.

Bellissimo, A., & Tunks, E. (1984), *Chronic Pain: The Psychotherapeutic Spectrum.* New York: Praeger Publishers.

Blendis, L. (1984), Abdominal Pain. In: *Textbook of Pain.* eds. P. Wall & R. Melzack. New York: Churchill Livingstone.

Block, A. (1981), An investigation of the response of the spouse to chronic pain behavior. *Psychosom. Med.*, 43:415–422.

Bonica, J. (1973), Management of pain. *Postgrad. Med.*, 53:56–57.

———(1979), Importance of the problem. In: *Advances in Pain Research and Therapy*, eds. J. Bonica & V. Ventrafrida. New York: Raven Press.

Crowley, D. (1975), Chronic pain: Social aspects. In: *American Nurses Association Clinical Sessions.* New York: Appleton-Century-Crofts, pp. 257–266.

Dalessio, D. (1984) Headache. In: *Textbook of Pain*, eds. P. Wall & R. Melzack. New York: Churchill Livingstone.

Duvall, R. (1971), *Family Development.* Philadelphia: J.B. Lippincott.

Flor, H., Turk, D., & Rudy, T., (1987), Pain and families. II. Assessment and treatment. *Pain*, 30:20–45.

Fordyce, W., Fowler, R., Lehmann, J., & DeLateur, B. (1968), Some implications of learning in problems of chronic pain. *J. Chron. Dis.*, 21:179–190.

Jackson, D. (1965), Family rules: Marital quid pro quo. *Arch. Gen. Psychiat.*, 12:589–594.

Jeans, M., & Rowat, K. (1984), Counselling the patient and family In: *Textbook of Pain*, eds. P. Wall and R. Melzack. New York: Churchill Livingstone.

Levinson, D. (1978), *The Seasons of a Man's Life.* New York: Alfred A. Knopf.

Maruta, O., Osborne, D., Sanson, D., & Halling, J. (1981), Chronic pain patients and spouses. *Mayo Clinic Proced.*, Vol. 56:307–310.

Melzack, R. (1973) *The Puzzle of Pain.* New York: Basic Books.

Moos, R., ed. (1984) *Coping with Physical Illness, Vol. 2*, New Perspectives. New York: Plenum Press.

Payne, B., & Norflett, M. (1986), Chronic pain and the family: A review, *Pain*, 26:1–22.

Rolland, J. (1987), Chronic illness and the life cycle: A conceptual framework. *Fam. Proc.*, 26:203–221.

Roy, R. (1986), A problem-centered family systems approach in treating chronic pain. In: *Pain Management: A Handbook of Psychological Treatment Approaches*, eds. A. Holzman & D. Turk. New York: Pergamon Press.

Sternbach, R. (1984), Behavior therapy. In: *Textbook of Pain*. eds. P. Wall & R. Melzack. New York: Churchill Livingstone.

Waring, E. (1977), The role of the family in symptom selection and perpetuation in psychosomatic illness. *Psychother. Psychosom.* 28:253–259.

Part IV

PERSPECTIVES ON CHRONIC PAIN

Editorial Introduction

The complexity of chronic pain demands a cross-sectional approach that not only addresses theory, diagnosis, and treatment issues, but looks at innovative roles and concepts that may well be of benefit to the chronic pain patient. Dr. John Wilson of the Department of Behavioral Sciences, University of Kentucky College of Medicine provides such a cross-sectional approach when he addresses coping research in the study of chronic pain. Explored are current definitions of coping and a thorough review of selected research on the measurement of coping styles and the relationship of coping to the human response to pain. Suggestions are generated for the expansion of the conceptual framework of coping, and applying coping strategies to chronic pain management.

The role of the multidisciplinary chronic pain treatment team is addressed by clinical psychologist Dr. Nancy Moore of the V.A. Medical Center, Louisville, Kentucky. Specifically addressed are the disciplines constituting a multidisciplinary pain treatment team. Also explored are the problems encountered in interdisciplinary communication and potential conflicts among the disciplines represented. The composition of an ideal multidisciplinary team, free of the problems often encountered between disciplines, is also explored.

Pharmacotherapy in the treatment of pain and, more specifically, cancer pain, is addressed by Margaret Rankin, a nurse and faculty member at the University of Iowa College of Nursing. Specifically addressed are the categories and stages of cancer pain, the specifics of pain syndromes associated with cancer, and the multiplicity of medical approaches to the treatment and management of cancer pain.

The role of rehabilitation counseling in the management of chronic pain is explored by Dr. Richard J. Beck. As a rehabilitation counselor, he addresses the impact of Workman's Compensation claims and discusses counseling strategies which may be of benefit to returning a chronic pain patient to a productive life-style.

Pediatric pain is a unique area of study. Dr. Joseph Bush, Department of Psychology, Virginia Commonwealth University, addresses the prevalence and types of pain problems encountered in children. A broad developmental perspective on pain is presented which encompasses physical, cognitive, social, and behavioral factors. Dr. Bush also discusses the clinical significance of pain in children, including consideration of its importance relative to differential diagnosis, as well as to its impact on the developing child. Recommendations are made for assessing pain and factors relevant to its management in children, and a clinical summary of the literature on clinical pain management techniques associated with pediatrics are explored.

Dr. Rajan Roy, School of Professional Social Work at the University of Manitoba, Manitoba, Canada, explores the role of the clinical social worker in the treatment of chronic pain. Also addressed is the context of the patient–family relationship in the role of social work and, finally, a rationale for adopting this approach to maintain a systemic theme which attempts to understand the intrapsychic needs of the patient in the larger external system that incorporates both the medical and legal professions.

Finally, Chronic Pain and the Geriatric Patient explores issues in diagnosis and treatment from both a psychological and pharmaceutical perspective. Dr. Thomas W. Miller, professor, Departments of Psychiatry and Psychology, University of Kentucky, and Louis L. Jay, R.Ph., consulting pharmacist, University of Buffalo, Buffalo, New York examine the most prominent of pain syndromes facing the elderly, along with the analgesic medications frequently prescribed for pain management, as well as ancillary models frequently employed in the treatment of chronic pain. Summarized are approaches to behavioral assessment, cognitive appraisal, and education and selected management strategies in the treatment of chronic pain in the elderly.

"Concluding Thoughts on Chronic Pain" explores the major trends in understanding chronic pain and state-of-the-art management strategies. It becomes imperative that the health care provider recognize the value of multidisciplinary perspectives and interdisciplinary skills that will provide the best level of quality patient care for the chronic pain patient.

19

Applying Coping Research to the Study of Chronic Pain

JOHN F. WILSON, PH.D.

INTRODUCTION

The primary definition of coping is to struggle or encounter, and usually has connotations of a successful struggle. However, a sampling of definitions may help clarify the point. For some, coping is very narrowly defined as one's ability to reduce physiological activation (Rahe, 1974). Although this is certainly one function of coping, it is too narrow for the pain area. Others (Haan, 1963; Vaillant, 1977) view coping as a normal point along a continuum of adaptation on which "defense" or "defense mechanism" is the abnormal or pathological pole. One example of this would be the difference between sublimation and repression. Complex categorizations of ego mechanisms, such as Vaillant's (1977) hierarchy of psychotic, immature, neurotic, and healthy mechanisms, are typically most useful in conveying themes of adaptation across the life cycle. The difficulty of measuring this hierarchy makes application in the chronic pain setting difficult in any other than a case study format.

Models in a middle range of complexity have dominated the coping field in recent years. Stone and Neale (1984) defined coping as "those behaviors and thoughts which are consciously used by an individual to handle or control the effects of anticipating or experiencing a stressful situation" (p. 893). This definition excludes unconscious mechanisms and emphasizes anticipatory as well as reactive coping. For Lazarus and Folkman (1984), coping at the psychological level is "the process of managing external or internal demands that are appraised as taxing the resources of the person." This approach emphasizes process, management, and effort rather than trait, mastery, and automatic or effortless adaptation. Cronkite and Moos (1984) view coping responses as either "individual stylistic tendencies toward handling any difficulty, or as situation-specific coping efforts." The decision as to whether generic coping style or situation-specific coping process is more important remains a largely unanswered, empirical question. A revitalized trait approach is manifest in their distinction between coping responses and coping resources. Coping resources include psychological resources such as generalized attitudes about oneself or the world that influence coping responses or appraisal of threat. Self-esteem would be one example of a coping resource. The Moos formulation also emphasizes extraindividual resources, and often includes social support as a coping resource for an individual.

Pearlin and Schooler (1978) approach the problem from a more sociological level, and differentiate between social resources, psychological resources, and coping responses. Social resources consist of the interpersonal networks of family, friends, and workers. Psychological resources are considered to be personality characteristics such as self-esteem that help withstand threat. Coping responses are "specific behaviors, cognitions, and perceptions in which people engage when actually contending with life problems." Pearlin and Schooler (1978) emphasize that coping responses depend on the role within which the person is functioning. For example, ways of coping with work stress would be considerably different from ways of coping with marital stress, and would not even be measured with the same set of concepts.

Although the authors listed above differ in what each emphasizes on a conceptual level, there is considerable overlap in their operationalization of coping. In order to adequately address questions of conceptual clarity, I have elected to discuss in detail four measures of the ways people cope. Three measures are of generic ways of coping, and one was specifically designed to address issues of how people cope with chronic pain. The discussion of each will focus on the actual items to which people are asked to respond and on the conceptual organization of coping that each approach emphasizes. Tables 19.1 through 19.5 depict the labels and sample items of the ways of coping instruments used by Pearlin and Schooler (1978); Folkman and Lazarus (1980); Moos, Cronkite, Billings, and Finney (1983); Rosenstiel and Keefe (1983). I have chosen to review each scale by selecting one or two research reports generated by each set of researchers and reviewing them in detail rather than by surveying the much larger literature that has used these coping scales. I believe use of this reviewing strategy will facilitate identification of critical problems and conceptual dilemmas in the field of coping. When possible, research on coping by chronic pain patients will be emphasized.

The Problems of Everyday Living Scale

Pearlin and Schooler (1978) interviewed 2300 adults from the Chicago area. Respondents were asked about life strains, emotional stress, coping behaviors, and aspects of personality. Strain was defined as enduring problems that have the potential for arousing threat within four different life areas: marital, parental, household economic, and occupational roles. For example, strain within the marital role was measured by items assessing how accepted you felt by your spouse, items suggesting there was an equal amount of give and take in the relationship, and items explicitly rating your spouse on performance in the roles of sexual partner, breadwinner, and housekeeper. Stress was operationalized in terms of how well negative moods (upset, frustrated, worried) described your daily married life. It is important to note that this definition of strain corresponds closely to the concept of stressor in most psychological frameworks, and this notion of stress corresponds closely to the concept of strain or distress in the psychological literature. Although the labels are applied differently, the conceptual distinction between stressor as stimulus and distress as the response to that stimulus is maintained.

Coping responses were organized into seventeen coping behaviors with factor-analytic techniques. These coping behaviors were defined somewhat differently for each of the four role areas, but within each role, coping behaviors were organized according to three functions: attempts to modify the situation, attempts to control the meaning of the situation, and attempts to manage the stress of the situation. This conceptual framework, along with subscale labels and sample items from the scales, can be found in Table 19.1.

If coping responses are considered to be the things people do to reduce distress, psychological resources or personality variables represent some of the things people are in terms of enduring traits. Pearlin and Schooler (1978) considered such variables to represent the personal context within which coping occurs. They measured three personality variables: self-esteem, self-denigration, and mastery. Self-esteem and self-denigration refer to positive and negative attitudes about the self. Mastery refers to the extent to which one's life is considered to be under one's own control. Sample items from the mastery scale can be found in Table 19.1.

Pearlin and Schooler (1978) asked three basic questions about this relatively sophisticated model of stress, strain, coping, and personality. First, how effective are coping behaviors? Effectiveness is defined as how well a behavior reduces the relationship between strain and stress. Before taking coping into account, the regression coefficient between stress and strain is 0.62. As each of the six coping scales reported in Table 19.1 is introduced into the regression equation, the relationship between stress and strain is reduced, with the final coefficient being 0.30. Significant moderation of the stress–strain relationship by coping was also found for parenting and household economic role areas, but not for the occupational role area. Coping is considered to be effective, therefore, if you do not feel distressed when faced with a stressor. This essentially

TABLE 19.1

CONCEPTUAL FRAMEWORK, SUBSCALE LABELS AND SAMPLE ITEMS FROM THE PROBLEMS OF EVERYDAY LIVING SCALE (PEARLIN AND SCHOOLER, 1978)

Marital Role Area

A. Attempts to modify the situation
   1. Self-reliance vs. advice seeking
      a. asked the advice of relatives about getting along in marriage
      b. went to a doctor, counselor, or other professional person for marriage advice
   2. Negotiation
      a. tried to find a fair compromise in marriage problems
      b. sat down and talked things out

B. Attempts to control the meaning of the situation
   1. Selective ignoring
      a. told myself that marital difficulties are not important
      b. tried to overlook my spouse's faults and paid attention only to good points
   2. Positive comparisons
      a. with time, did my marriage get better
      b. how often did I appreciate my own marriage more after seeing what other marriages were like

C. Attempts to manage stress
   1. Controlled reflectiveness
      a. found myself thinking over marital problems
      b. yelled or shouted to let off steam (negative scored)
   2. Passive forbearance
      a. kept out of my spouse's way for a while when we had differences
      b. gave in more than halfway

D. Mastery as a personality trait
   1. had little control over the things that happen to me
   2. Often felt helpless in dealing with the problems of life

defines a buffer model of coping in which coping is viewed as a moderator of the relationship between stressors and distress (Baron and Kenny, 1986).

This approach is in contrast to measurement of more direct effects of coping in reducing absolute levels of distress, or the direct effects of coping in reducing the occurrence or intensity of stressors. In the Pearlin and Schooler example, direct effects would have been manifest in copers having either less marital role strain, or in copers having lower levels of distress. The preventive or proactive benefits of coping in reducing marital strain are not addressed, and thus coping in this model remains a reactive process.

Some direct effects of coping on distress were reported in Pearlin and Schooler's discussion of the differential effectiveness of individual coping behaviors. Although use of all six coping behaviors were independent predictors of reduced distress in the marital role area, differences in effectiveness were not large, and the pattern of differences was not consistent across the different role areas. Of particular interest was the finding that selective ignoring was associated with high levels of distress in the marital and parenting role areas, and low levels of distress in household economic and occupational role areas. This supports an interpretation of coping effectiveness as dependent on a fit between type of stressor and type of coping.

Although all six coping scales were associated with distress in the marital role area, Pearlin and Schooler raise an additional question about the extent to which use of a varied repertoire of coping might be more effective than use of one way of coping. Use of an extended repertoire, as defined by use of four or more behaviors was more effective at moderating the stress–strain relationship than use of only one behavior. This relationship, however, occurs primarily for marriage and parenting role areas and not for the occupational role area. This represents one attempt at viewing coping as a pattern of responses rather than as unidimensional phenomena.

The question of individual differences in use of coping mechanisms, and in how personality variables affect coping, is addressed in two ways. First, gender differences in use of coping were examined. Although the magnitude of the differences in coping behaviors for males and females is not great, females were more likely than males to use the selective ignoring coping behaviors that resulted in more distress in the marriage and parental role areas. The authors discuss a socialization and sex role learning interpretation of these findings, but it is possible that choice of coping behavior may not only be different for men and women but also that the same behavior may have different meaning for men and women. It does suggest that gender difference cannot be ignored.

Personality traits, the second aspect of individual differences, were assessed in the same manner as coping behaviors. Low self-denigration, high mastery, and high self-esteem were all associated with decreased distress and decreased correlation between stressors and distress for all of the role areas. When effects of coping behaviors and personality variables were assessed simultaneously, coping behaviors were reported to be more important than personality variables for the marital role area, equally important in the parenting and household economics areas, and less important than personality variables in the occupational role area. These analyses do not, however, discuss interactive questions; that is, they do not ask whether nonadditive effects of personality and coping may be occurring. Critical comparisons between individuals who have poor psychological resources (personality traits) but use effective coping behaviors, and individuals who have good psychological resources but do not use effective coping behaviors are not examined.

In summary, Pearlin and Schooler's complex structure of coping includes important distinctions between psychological resources or traits and actual coping behaviors; distinctions between stressor situations or role areas, and broader characteristics of the use of coping behaviors, such as whether a repertoire of coping is varied or constricted. Their structure of coping, however, does not address the direct or proactive effects of coping on the occurrence of intensity of stressors, the question of how chronicity of stressors may affect coping, and the interactive as well as additive effects of personality traits on coping. The pattern of their findings, though, both in the original report and in subsequent projects (Pearlin, Lieberman, Menaghan, and Mullan, 1981; Fleishman, 1984) represent a strong argument for more complex models of coping.

Concepts from the Pearlin and Schooler model of coping have recently been applied to chronic pain patients (Elliot, Trief, and Stein, 1986). The Problems of Everyday Living Scale was administered to fifty-five married chronic pain patients. The subjects for this study were obtained from inpatient and outpatient clinics, as well as from doctor's offices. Eighty-four percent of the sample reported the back as the primary site of pain, and the mean duration of their pain problem was 6.5 years. Seventy percent of the sample was unemployed and receiving compensation or disability income.

The focus of the study was on the marital role area. Elliot and her colleagues divided subjects into low, moderate, or high mastery groups according to scores on the mastery scale described in Table 19.1. Marital strain and personal distress were assessed in a way similar to that of Pearlin and Schooler's (1978) study. Coping behavior was assessed using five of the six coping dimensions reported in Table 19.1. The dimension of positive comparison was not reported. In comparison to subjects with low levels of mastery, high mastery levels were associated with lower levels of marital strain, lower levels of personal distress, greater use of negotiation, and less frequent use of selective ignoring, controlled reflectiveness, and passive forbearance.

It is particularly interesting to compare this study with the earlier Pearlin and Schooler (1978) data. Elliot and her colleagues essentially report a direct effect of mastery, a personality variable, on the intensity of marital stress, on the intensity of personal distress, and on the pattern of coping behaviors. The direct and indirect effects of coping behavior on distress are not discussed. Although direct relationships between negotiation, advice seeking, selective ignoring, or manage stress coping and either stressor level or distress are not reported, it is suggested that effective coping is characterized by greater use of negotiation and less use of selective ignoring and manage stress behaviors.

These results are consistent in showing the ineffectiveness of selective ignoring and the effectiveness of negotiation and controlled reflectiveness, but differ from earlier findings in that advice-seeking was related to decreased distress in the sample of 2300 adults and is not associated with mastery in the chronic pain sample. It also appears that the direction of effect in the use of passive forbearance differs in the two samples, with passive forbearance having a positive effect in the Pearlin and Schooler study, and being associated with poorer mastery levels in the chronic pain study. It is difficult to make more definitive statements about the results because these two studies reflect a basic problem in research on coping and stress: no two studies operationalize the coping process in the same way. Even when the same questionnaires are used, comparability is made difficult due to use of different subscales, omission of some variables, and differences in analysis techniques. Differences in style of analysis may be due to differences in the disciplinary backgrounds of the researchers. In the above study with chronic pain patients, the researchers assumed that a personality variable, mastery, was the crucial organizing variable within the coping process. This determined not only what was examined, but more importantly what was not reported. Pearlin and Schooler's analysis used methods more commonly used in sociology, where correlational data is not seen as an absolute barrier to establishing some degree of causal sequence. Elliot and her colleagues approach the topic with the assumption that personality variables are more central to adaptation than are coping behaviors, and in fact determine coping behaviors. With the opposite assumption, subjects would have been categorized according to use of coping behaviors, and mastery scores would have been the dependent variable. Perhaps most importantly, coping effectiveness in the original Pearlin and Schooler model is based on coping as a buffer, whereas in the approach of Elliot and her colleagues, the emphasis is on assessment of direct effects of coping on stress and strain.

This should not be taken as a criticism of either group of researchers, but as an ongoing problem in making sense of literature in the area of stress and coping. These implicit assumptions and analysis decisions have practical significance in that they focus attention on one part of a complex system, and suggest that intervention at that point may be effective in reducing distress. Elliot and her colleagues suggest their results support programs for treating pain patients by increasing their sense of mastery. Although this may be true, the attempt to simplify data analysis by adopting a less complex model may be limiting our understanding of the effects of interventions to assist chronic pain patients. Multidisciplinary approaches to analysis would yield a more complete picture of coping processes.

Pearlin and Schooler's (1978) structure of coping is the most complex of the four models selected for discussion in this chapter in its use of multiple role areas of strain. Discussion of measures of coping derived by other researchers will focus more on conceptual developments in the area of responses and social resources.

Health and Daily Living Form

Cronkite and Moos present a model of the coping process that incorporates much of Pearlin and Schooler's approach with an added emphasis on concepts of social support and family environment variables. This formulation often includes perceptions of both spouses and measurement of family variables. One important difference between Pearlin and Schooler's approach and that used in the Health and Daily Living Form is the nature of the respondent's task. Whereas Pearlin and Schooler (1978) asked subjects to say how they typically responded to stress within a role area, Moos et al. (1983) asks subjects to report about their behavior and thoughts in response to stressful events which are important to them and which have occurred recently. Thoughts and behaviors are assessed with a checklist or with a Likert-type response format measuring frequency of use. Billings and Moos (1981) describe two conceptual frameworks for sorting out such coping data. One framework, referred to as the method of coping, divides the ways of coping identified by subjects into active cognitive attempts to resolve the stressor, active behavioral attempts to resolve the stressor, and cognitive and behavioral attempts to avoid the problem or reduce emotional tension. A second framework, which involves the same item pool sorted in a different way, refers to the focus of coping. Problem-focused coping includes attempts to modify the source of the stress. Emotion-focused coping includes attempts to manage the emotional effects of being under stress. Sample items from these frameworks can be found in Table 19.2.

TABLE 19.2

CONCEPTUAL FRAMEWORK, SUBSCALE LABELS AND SAMPLE ITEMS FROM THE HEALTH AND DAILY LIVING FORM (MOOS ET AL., 1983)

A. Method of coping scoring entered
   1. Active cognitive coping
      a. prayed for guidance
      b. considered several alternatives
      c. accepted it, nothing could be done
   2. Active behavioral coping
      a. tried to find out more about it
      b. talked with spouse or relative
      c. let my feelings out somehow
   3. Avoidance coping
      a. took it out on other people when I felt angry
      b. refused to believe it happened
      c. tried to reduce tension by eating, drinking, or smoking

B. Focus of coping scoring criteria
   1. Logical analysis
      a. considered several alternatives
      b. went over the situation in my mind to try and understand
      c. tried to step back and be more objective
   2. Information seeking
      a. tried to find out more about it
      b. talked with spouse or relative
      c. prayed for guidance
   3. Problem solving
      a. made a plan of action and followed it
      b. took things one day at a time
      c. tried not to act too hastily
   4. Affective regulation
      a. tried to see the positive side of the situation
      b. got away from things for a while
      c. tried to reduce tension by exercising more
   5. Emotional discharge
      a. took it out on other people when I felt angry or depressed
      b. let my feelings out somehow
      c. tried to reduce tension by eating, drinking, or smoking more

Results from two studies will be used to highlight conceptual problems in the measurement of coping. In the first study, Billings and Moos (1981) studied a random selection of families in the San Francisco area to determine how coping and social resources affected the relationship between life stress and functioning. The relationship between negative life events and outcome measure of depression, anxiety, and physical symptoms was reduced or "buffered" by both coping responses and social resources. Direct effects of coping on level of distress were puzzling. Avoidance coping was associated with higher levels of distress. Active cognitive coping was associated with lower levels of distress. Active behavioral coping, though largely unrelated to distress, was associated with higher levels of anxiety in males. The interrelationship of coping responses and social resources was also demonstrated by analyses showing that people using avoidance coping had fewer social resources.

A second study using this framework (Cronkite and Moos, 1984) was conducted as a prospective study of 249 families in the San Francisco area who were interviewed twice approximately twelve months apart. Coping data, however, was apparently gathered only during the second interview, and was categorized this time into only two categories of approach and avoidance coping. Approach coping was not related to measures of distress, whereas avoidance coping was associated with greater distress at both initial and follow-up measurements. Higher levels of stressful life events were associated with greater levels of both approach and avoidance coping. Personality variables such as self-esteem showed puzzling relationships with outcome variables. For males, high self-esteem was associated with greater use of approach and lesser use of avoidance coping, whereas for females, self-esteem was associated with more frequent life events. Interactive effects of your spouse's coping on your adaptation were examined, but only two of seventy-two interaction terms were significant. There did, however, appear to be evidence for a stress-amplifying effect when both partners used avoidance strategies. The results of these two studies provide only weak support for the hypothesis that approach coping is beneficial, and somewhat stronger support that avoidance coping is related to higher levels of distress. There is also support for the hypothesis that your spouse's functioning and style of coping are important for your adaptation, but are unclear determinants of distress.

It is interesting to note that earlier conceptual distinctions about the problem or emotion or "focus" of coping are not reported or are stated as being similar to results reported for approach and avoidance coping. Conceptual frameworks have typically not been consistently applied from study to study in the coping literature. Once again, interpretation is complicated by the fact that different formulations of the same questionnaire items are used in each study. The situation becomes even more complex when one tries to determine the meaning of a particular coping scale. For example, in the Billings and Moos (1981) study, the item "prepared for the worst" is classified as an avoidant response, whereas "prayed for guidance and strength" is classified as an active cognitive response. "Exercised more" is classified as an active behavioral response, whereas "tried to reduce tension by smoking or eating more" is classified as a avoidance response. If the concept of avoidance is to be more than just a label for a factorially defined cluster, the meaning of individual items must be more clearly specified. Preparing for the worst could be an avoidant response, but it also could be a very active cognitive or behavioral sequence of events directly focused on altering a stressor. Praying for guidance could be a very direct attempt to seek advice and develop a plan, but it also could be a means of avoiding any further coping or at least postponing further efforts.

A second problem within the meaning dimension of items is the shift in meaning and perhaps factorial structure of the scales in different projects. The Billings and Moos (1981) study described a nineteen-item scale; the Cronkite and Moos (1984) scale consisted of seventeen items. The manual for the Health and Daily Living Form (Moos et al., 1983) lists more than twenty-eight items, and places "prepared for the worst" in the category of active cognitive coping rather than avoidance coping. Differences in the pool of items should certainly be expected as concepts of coping evolve, but when "items" switch from concept to concept, comparison of results across studies becomes almost impossible. Thus, although the coping formulations derived from the Health and Daily Living Form have produced important empirical findings, the meaning of those findings may only be peripherally related to the stated concepts of approach and avoidance coping. The desire to simplify coping categories has produced a conceptual framework of approach and avoidance coping that does not necessarily reflect the complexity of the coping process or the reality of the behaviors being measured as "approach" or "avoidance" behavior.

The Ways of Coping Checklist

The ways of coping checklist (WCC) was developed by Folkman and Lazarus (1980) in an attempt to more adequately study the process of coping. The study of enduring personality traits was considered to be a relatively poor predictor of outcomes in stress studies and to be a relatively poor descriptor of how people actually cope with both major and minor problems. Through open-ended questionnaires, a sixty-eight-item checklist of behaviors and thoughts was constructed through subjects' responses as to how they had coped in a stressful situation. The WCC was explicitly formulated to not be a trait measure, and it was anticipated that coping behaviors would change as a function of the type of stressful situation and of the temporal stage of adaptation to that stressor.

The major conceptual framework shaping the clustering of items within this checklist was the distinction between problem-focused and emotion-focused coping (Folkman and Lazarus, 1980; Lazarus and Folkman, 1984). Problem-focused coping reflects attempts to modify the problem that has caused an appraisal of threat. Emotion-focused coping reflects attempts to modify the emotional consequences of an appraisal of threat. More recent formulations have also operationalized two concepts from Lazarus and Folkman's (1984) larger model of stress, appraisal, and coping. Primary appraisal is the cognitive process through which a person judges a stimulus to be negative, positive, or irrelevant. Secondary appraisal is the cognitive process through which a person evaluates his options for coping.

Folkman, Lazarus, Gruen, and DeLongis (1986) operationalized primary and secondary appraisal and used a revised form of the Ways of Coping checklist to study relationships between coping and physical and psychological symptoms of distress in eighty-five married couples living in northern California. Subjects were interviewed once a month in their homes for five months, and were asked to respond to questions about the most stressful event experienced during the previous week. Results of the five interviews were aggregated to form indices of coping and adaptation. Examples of the subscales and items used to assess appraisal variables and problem- and emotion-focused coping can be found in Table 19.3.

TABLE 19.3

CONCEPTUAL FRAMEWORK, SUBSCALE LABELS AND SAMPLE ITEMS FROM THE REVISED WAYS OF COPING CHECKLIST (FOLKMAN AND LAZARUS, 1985)

A. Problem Focused Coping
   1. Confrontive coping
      a. stood my ground and fought for what I wanted
      b. expressed anger to the person causing the problem
   2. Planful problem solving
      a. knew what had to be done so I doubled my efforts to make things work
      b. made a plan of action and followed it

B. Emotion Focused Coping
   1. Distancing
      a. went on as if nothing had happened
      b. tried to forget the whole thing
   2. Self-control
      a. tried to keep my feelings to myself
      b. kept others from knowing how I felt
   3. Seeking social support
      a. talked to someone who could do something concrete about the problem
      b. accepted sympathy or understanding from someone else
   4. Accepting responsibility
      a. criticized or lectured myself
      b. realized I brought the problem on myself
   5. Escape-avoidance
      a. wished the situation would go away
      b. tried to make myself feel better by eating, drinking, smoking, using medications
   6. Positive reappraisal
      a. changed or grew as a person in a good way
      b. found new faith, prayed

In addition to these variables, measures of mastery (Pearlin and Schooler (1978) and of interpersonal trust were administered. Adaptational status was assessed using a checklist of psychological symptoms and health status. Personality, appraisal, and coping variables were found to be related to both psychological symptoms and health status. Seventeen of twenty correlations between predictor variables and psychological symptoms of distress were statistically significant. The personality variables of mastery and interpersonal trust were negatively correlated with distress, and primary appraisal and coping subscales were positively correlated with distress as measured by psychological symptoms. Ten of the correlations were larger than 0.30. Relationships to health status were less impressive. Eleven of twenty correlations were significant, none larger than 0.30. Although the magnitude of the relationships with health status were not large, coping variables were negatively correlated with health status.

When analyzed in a multiple regression format, problems of multiple collinearity limit the power of the analysis. Correlations between the eight coping subscales ranged from 0.00 to 0.52, with a mean of 0.37. Analysis of individual coping scale effects, therefore, lacked statistical power. When considered as a single regression equation, predictor variables accounted for 16 percent of the variance in somatic health; but the adjusted *R* squared was not significant. A regression equation explained 43 percent of the variance in psychological symptoms, with an adjusted *R*-squared of 36 percent. It perhaps should not be surprising that coping and appraisal variables were not strongly related to health status, because, as Folkman and her colleagues point out, only 6 percent of the 750 stressful encounters reported by the subjects were health related phenomena. Overall, however, the results do not provide a greater understanding of what constitutes effective or healthy coping in a health related situation.

I believe this study illustrates three major issues that have yet to be confronted in the study of coping and stress. First, many studies use population sampling that produces a wide range of "stressors." There is little theoretical reason to suppose that widely differing stressors should be characterized by similar patterns of coping. Aggregating data in this manner may tend to obscure situation-specific coping patterns. Aggregating across stressors may also tend to emphasize the effects of stress on coping; that is, increasing stress should increase the number of coping responses. This may account for the positive correlations between stress and coping that are found in population studies looking for direct coping and stress relationships. It is much more likely that coping benefits will be evident when measured in the context of specific stressor–coping–distress relationships, as in the "buffer" models of Pearlin and Schooler (1978) and Billings and Moos (1981).

Second, different patterns of findings reflect a recurring problem of just how to lump or split coping processes. The need to go beyond single categories of problem- and emotion-focused coping and split the item pool into a larger number of more conceptually specific coping styles produces analytic problems because of the natural intercorrelation of coping behaviors. As Folkman and Lazarus (1980) have pointed out, 98 percent of subjects use both problem- and emotion-focused coping in any stressful encounter. But the use of eight intercorrelated coping subscales presents enormous difficulties in analyzing even simple regression main effects, and allows no opportunity to look at interactions or combinations of coping behaviors. Thus, if we lump coping behaviors into one or two categories, we can obtain significant results, but at the cost of being unable to interpret our findings. If they are split into interpretable subscales, the power of the analysis evaporates.

Third, although ways of coping checklists were developed in order to more adequately assess "process" aspects of coping, none of the studies reviewed here have actually looked at the process of coping with a particular stressor. Subjects are asked to say retrospectively how they coped with a stressor; and even when outcome measures are longitudinally gathered, none of the studies reviewed here address the question of how coping behaviors in response to threat are sequenced. This may be a third reason why answers to the question of what constitutes effective coping have been elusive.

A study by Folkman and Lazarus (1985), however, does provide a view of coping process that may provide a model for further studies. They posited three criteria for adequately studying coping as a process. Coping must be examined in response to a specific stressor. Coping must be measured by what the individual actually does in response to the stress. Coping and distress must be measured at multiple times in the coping process. Coping and distress measures were assessed at three points in the lives of college students preparing for, taking, and responding to the results of a college examination.

Coping was assessed using a further revision of the Ways of Coping Checklist. The three-step procedure used by Folkman and Lazarus in producing the scales is important to note in some detail. They eliminated nine items from the sixty-six item pool due to high skewedness and restricted variance. Factor analysis produced a six-factor solution, which with an oblique rotation produced a conceptually interpretable set of factors. Fifteen items that failed to load clearly on any one factor were then eliminated. As a final step in the process, one emotion-focused factor was divided into three factors on theoretical grounds. This process yielded eight subscales; sample items from these scales can be found in Table 19.4. Coefficient alpha for these subscales ranged from 0.56 to 0.85. This process of scale construction eliminated items with restricted variance and items with multiple loadings on different factors. Although such procedures are valid statistically, items with restricted variance reflect coping behaviors used by nearly everybody or by almost nobody. Knowledge about such universal or absolute coping items may be important in terms of conceptual development, even if they cannot be effective predictors within a particular study. Exclusion of items loading on many factors is also statistically and conceptually valid, but once again, if "sense" is to be made of a complex literature, the extent to which such items reflect poor item wording or reflect behaviors that do represent multiple concepts cannot be determined if one does not know how they vary across populations and types of stressful situations. Also important was the authors' conceptual decision to split a factorially derived cluster of items into three more conceptually interpretable subscales. This use of factor analytic techniques in a manner balanced by demands of theory and conceptual development is far preferable to more simple data-reduction use of factor analysis.

Folkman and Lazarus (1985) noted significant changes in coping from an anticipatory stage before the examination to a waiting stage after the examination, but before grades were announced. Problem-focused coping and seeking social support declined dramatically, whereas distancing increased.

TABLE 19.4

CONCEPTUAL FRAMEWORK, SUBSCALE LABELS AND SAMPLE ITEMS FROM THE REVISED WAYS OF COPING CHECKLIST (FOLKMAN AND LAZARUS, 1985)

1. Problem focused coping (11 items)
   a. I try to analyze the problem in order to understand it better
   b. I'm making a plan of action and following it

2. Emotion-focused coping
   a. Wishful thinking (5 items)
      (1) Wish that I can change what is happening or how I feel
      (2) Wish that the situation should go away or somehow be over with
   b. Distancing (6 items)
      (1) Try to forget the whole thing
      (2) I'm waiting to see what will happen before doing anything
   c. Emphasizing the positive (4 items)
      (1) Look for the silver lining, so to speak; try to look on the bright side of things.
      (2) I'm changing or growing as a person in a good way
   d. Self-blame (3 items)
      (1) Criticize or lecture myself
      (2) Realize I brought the problem on myself
   e. Tension-reduction (3 items)
      (1) Try to make myself feel better by eating, drinking, smoking or using drugs or medications, etc.
      (2) I jog or exercise
   f. Self-isolation (3 items)
      (1) Avoid being with people in general
      (2) Talk to someone to find out more about the situation.

3. Mixed problem- and emotional-focused coping
   a. Seeking social support (7 items)
      (1) Talk to someone to find out more about the situation.
      (2) Accept sympathy and understanding from someone.

Changes in coping were also noted as the process moved from the waiting stage to the outcome stage, when results of the exam were announced. Wishful thinking and distancing decreased. Coping patterns at the outcome stage were also influenced by the performance measure of grade on the examination. Students receiving poor grades used more emotion-focused forms of coping. These findings provide support for the hypothesis that the timing as well as the use of a coping behavior may be an important predictor of outcome in a stressful encounter. One could hypothesize, for example, that use of distancing would be adaptive during the waiting phase and maladaptive during the anticipatory stage. One could also hypothesize that in a different stressor, for which preparation may be less crucial than an examination, distancing might well be most adaptive during the anticipatory phase.

Folkman and Lazarus' outcome measures consisted of adjective scales measuring emotional state. During the anticipatory stage outcome was assessed with "threat" emotions (worried, fearful, anxious) and by "challenge" emotions (confident, hopeful, and eager). Adaptation during the outcome stage was assessed as "harm" emotions (angry, disappointed, sad, guilty) and "benefit" emotions (pleased, happy, exhilarated, relieved). Primary appraisal or "stakes" factors were assessed in regard to how important the exam was perceived to be and in how difficult the exam was anticipated to be. A "secondary appraisal" or control factor was also measured in terms of how much in control the subject felt about the examination.

Multiple regression analyses were used to analyze how well coping and appraisal variables predicted threat challenge, harm, and benefit. During the anticipatory stage, threat was associated with the two appraisal variables of exam difficulty and importance and with use of the coping behaviors of wishful thinking and seeking social support. Challenge emotions during the anticipatory stage were related to exam difficulty and exam importance, to sense of control, to problem-focused coping, and inversely to self-isolation coping. Harm emotions during the outcome stage were related to poor exam performance and to use of self-blame and wishful thinking coping behaviors. Benefit emotions during the outcome stage were related to exam performance, to feelings of control, and to use of seeking social support and tension-reduction coping behaviors. Total variance explained in threat, challenge, harm, and benefit ranged from 48 to 61 percent. Outcome measures during the waiting stage were not discussed.

Three conclusions can be drawn from this study of coping processes during a college examination. First, important changes in coping behavior occurred as the process of coping with the exam unfolded. Second, in terms of analytic strategy, significant findings emerged even though multicollinearity among the eight coping scales (mean intercorrelation=0.39) was greater than the Folkman, Lazarus, Dunkel-Schetter, DeLongis, and Gruen (1986) community study. The use of a specific stressor and repeated measurements may be a key way to increase the chance of finding significant relationships with multiple coping variables. Third, measures of primary and secondary appraisal and measures of positive and negative outcomes appear to be useful conceptual advances that increase understanding of the process of coping without unduly increasing the complexity of the analysis task (Folkman et al., 1986).

Summary of Themes from Ways of Coping Approaches

A summary of themes derived from the brief reviews of the three research groups discussed above may be useful prior to discussing the specific application of coping behavior research to the topic of chronic pain. Three themes can be abstracted from research using the structure of coping model developed by Pearlin and Schooler (1978). First, coping effectiveness was primarily assessed in terms of how well one's coping behavior reduced the relationship between stress and distress, rather than how well it prevented stress. This distinction between coping as a buffer between stress and distress and coping as a preventor of stress, is often overlooked in the analysis of coping effects. Second, the effectiveness of coping clearly depended on specific aspects of the situation or role area in which coping took place, such that effective coping behaviors in one role area would be harmful in another role area. Third, concepts of personality, such as self-esteem and mastery were important predictors of distress, but relationships between personality and coping behaviors and especially interactive or nonadditive effects of personality and coping variables on stress or distress measures were not assessed or reported.

Concepts derived from the Health and Daily Living Form (Cronkite and Moos, 1984) also emphasized personality variables and the buffering effects of coping. These authors, however, more explicitly included concepts of social support or social resources within their model of coping, demonstrating important relationships between type of coping and level of social resources. Moos and his colleagues have also broadened the focus of coping to include family environment variables and more specifically, the coping styles of one's spouse as important predictors of your own coping effectiveness.

The Ways of Coping Checklist format adopted by Lazarus and Folkman has evolved into a complex model using personality concepts, and measures of primary and secondary appraisal processes as well as specific coping thoughts and behaviors. Typical measures of distress have been expanded to include positive adaptive modes such as challenge and benefit as well as threat and harm, and for the first time, actual coping processes have been effectively operationalized as a longitudinal process. The inclusion of positive and negative outcome measures is especially important. Folkman and Lazarus (1985) noted that correlations between positive and negative emotions were not significant in the anticipatory and waiting phases of coping and only become significant during the outcome phase of a stressful situation. Coping may differentially affect positive and negative outcomes. This broadened notion of outcome or adaptation mirrors the word of Bryant and Veroff (1982) who demonstrated that the structure of psychological well-being includes two types of personal competence: the ability to enact positive affect and the ability to cope with stress or reduce negative affect.

Significant theoretical and methodological problems still plague all of the approaches reviewed in this section. Measurement of how an individual copes in a specific stressful situation produces problems in disentangling the effects of stress as a stimulus for increased coping from the effects of coping as a reducer of distress. Measurement in terms of how an individual typically copes with a stressor risks overlooking specific matches between coping and stressor characteristics in determining effectiveness. All of the approaches described above face the problem of shifting factorial structures of their coping instruments and have not yet evolved an analysis strategy that avoids the problem of lumping coping behaviors into limited numbers of categories and having uninterpretable coping styles, or splitting coping behaviors into numerous subscales and facing problems of multicollinearity and diminished statistical power. None of the approaches have yet addressed the larger questions of how interactive patterns of coping behaviors may have different effects on distress than coping behaviors assessed in a "main effects" multiple regression model. All of these issues should serve as background for the following discussion of a measure of coping behaviors specific to the chronic pain setting.

Coping with Chronic Pain—Coping Strategies Questionnaire (CSQ)

The Coping Strategies Questionnaire was developed by Rosenstiel and Keefe (1983) to quantitatively assess the efforts made by chronic pain patients to control their pain. The instrument was originally designed to assess six cognitive and two behavioral coping strategies patients used when they felt pain. Subscales and sample items of the Coping Strategies Questionnaire can be found in Table 19.5. In addition, respondents are typically asked to rate their overall ability to control pain and to decrease pain.

Rosenstiel and Keefe (1983) studied the relationship between pain strategies, patient characteristics and adjustment in sixty-one chronic low back pain patients. One coping strategy, increasing pain behavior, was dropped due to lack of internal consistency. Factor analysis reduced the remaining pain strategies to three factors. Cognitive coping and suppression included reinterpretation, coping self-statements, and ignoring items. Helplessness included the catastrophizing and increasing activity subscales as well as the assessments of ability to control and decrease pain. The third factor, diverting attention, included the praying and diverting attention subscales.

These derived factors were unrelated to either duration of chronic pain, presence of disability payments, or number of surgeries. Coping strategies were related to measures of pain and functioning. Patients with high scores on cognitive coping

TABLE 19.5

CONCEPTUAL FRAMEWORK, SUBSCALE LABELS AND SAMPLE ITEMS OF THE PAIN STRATEGIES QUESTIONNAIRE (ROSENSTIEL AND KEEFE, 1983)

1. Diverting attention (6 items)
   a. I count numbers in my head or run a song through my mind
   b. I try to think of something pleasant
   c. I think of things I enjoy doing

2. Reinterpreting pain sensations (6 items)
   a. I try to feel distant from the pain, almost as if the pain was in someone else's body
   b. I just think of it as some other sensation, such as numbness
   c. I pretend it is not a part of me

3. Catastrophizing (6 items)
   a. It is terrible and I feel it is never going to get any better
   b. It is awful and I feel that it overwhelms me
   c. I feel I can't stand it anymore

4. Ignoring sensations (6 items)
   a. I don't think about the pain
   b. I tell myself it doesn't hurt
   c. I ignore it

5. Praying or hoping (6 items)
   a. I pray to God it won't last long
   b. I have faith in the doctors that someday there will be a cure for my pain
   c. I rely on my faith in God

6. Coping self-statements (6 items)
   a. I tell myself to be brave and carry on despite the pain
   b. I tell myself that I can overcome the pain
   c. I see it as a challenge and don't let it bother me

7. Increased behavioral activities (6 items)
   a. I try to be around other people
   b. I do something I enjoy, such as watching TV or listening to music
   c. I do something active, like household chores or projects

and suppression were more likely to report functional impairments. Patients with high scores on the helplessness factor were more likely to be high on measures of depression and anxiety. Patients with high scores on the factor of diverting attention and praying reported higher levels of pain and more functional impairment.

The authors suggest that previous reports of the benefits of use of similar strategies (Spanos, Horton, and Chaves, 1975;

Rybstein-Blinchik, 1979) were due to differences between chronic and acute pain settings. They suggest that use of self-control strategies may not be effective over prolonged periods of time. They do suggest, however, that measurement of coping strategies should occur on repeated occasions to more adequately test the hypothesis that use of such strategies is related to poor adaptation.

The suggestion that chronic pain patients with different sites of pain may also differ in use of pain strategies, was explored by Keefe and Dolan (1986). Pain behavior and pain coping strategies were assessed in thirty-two low back pain and thirty-two myofascial pain dynsfunction patients. Although the factors derived from the pain strategy items had identical labels, it was unclear whether the two effectiveness ratings were included in the helplessness factor. In any event, patients with low back pain used significantly more attention diversion and praying and hoping, and significantly more total strategies than the myofascial pain dysfunction patients. Differences on one other factor, cognitive coping and suppression, also showed a large mean difference between back and myofascial pain patients, but enormous variability in the scores of the back pain patients prevented statistical significance. This suggests that differences in variability as well as differences in mean level of coping might be important characteristics to evaluate in future studies. Pain behaviors were also assessed, and the low back pain patients exhibited more guarding, bracing, and rubbing then the myofascial pain patients. The two groups of patients did not differ in their self-assessment of their ability to decrease pain or in their level of control over pain. The authors suggest that these data underscore the discrepancy between what chronic pain patients say and what they actually do, although no evidence is presented to suggest that low back pain patients are reporting use of coping strategies that they are not using.

Turner and Clancy (1986) studied relationships between pain coping strategies and outcome of cognitive–behavioral and operant treatment approaches for seventy-four chronic low back pain patients. The factor structure of the pain strategy items was similar to that derived by Rosenstiel and Keefe (1983) in that the labels of two factors were identical, but Turner and Clancy's analysis switched the coping self-statements subscale from the previous cognitive coping and suppression factor to the helplessness factor. In addition, increasing activity level was switched from the old helplessness factor to a new diverting attention and praying factor. Thus, none of the originally derived factors are identical to the new factors and one, helplessness, had two subscales deleted from it and one subscale added to it. It is clear, therefore, that although factor labels may remain relatively consistent, the factorial structure of the CSQ is far from fixed.

Analysis of the relationship between use of pain strategies and measures of distress and functional impairment suggested results similar to the original Rosenstiel and Keefe (1983) findings. Depression, disability, and physical impairment were associated with high scores on the helplessness factor. Use of denial strategies was associated with low levels of activity. A different picture emerges, however, when differences in levels of pain strategies between cognitive, operant, and control groups are examined after completion of therapy. Differences were reported for four of the seven subscales. Both cognitive and operant groups reported lower catastrophizing scores and a higher coping self-statement score than did a waiting list control group. The operant treatment also reported higher scores on the ignoring sensations subscale than did the cognitive treatment group.

Within-group comparisons suggest that there were significant changes in use of pain coping strategies for each group. The cognitive treatment group increased in use of coping self-statements, diverting attention, and ignoring strategies, and decreased in catastrophizing. The operant treatment group increased in ignoring strategies and decreased in catastrophizing, and the waiting list control group registered a decrease in the use of coping self-statements. Further evidence of treatment-specific change can be found in correlations between change in coping behaviors and changes in pain intensity and functional disability. Decreased pain intensity was associated with increased use of praying and hoping and decreased catastrophizing.

Findings from this study are important because they emphasize the need to study patterns of change in coping strategies, and suggest that subtle but important differences exist within factors derived from the pain strategies questionnaire. For example, although attention diversion and praying and hoping are clustered in the same factor, only praying and hoping was associated with decreased pain. Praying and hoping may be correlated with attention diversion strategies, but have very different significance for chronic pain than does attention diversion. Perhaps most importantly, this illustrates the difference between longitudinal and cross-sectional analysis of relationships between pain strategies and measures of distress and functioning. Cross-sectional analyses show positive relationships between pain and coping strategies. The longitudinal analysis of Turner and Clancy (1986) demonstrates positive effects of changes in coping strategies.

A partial look at the relationship between scores on the CSQ and outcome of surgical rather than psychological treatment can be found in a report by Gross (1986), who studied back pain patients undergoing surgery for the first time. Average length of time between the most recent onset of back pain was 1.5 years, and thirteen of the fifty patients were receiving compensation or had a compensation decision pending at the time of the surgery. Gross interviewed subjects prior to surgery, prior to discharge from the hospital, and three to six weeks after discharge. The CSQ was administered only prior to surgery. Postsurgical interviews consisted of standard measures of pain and adjustment, anxiety, and depression.

Three factors were identified from the CSQ. Active coping and suppression consisted of coping self-statements, cognitive distraction, increased activities, and ignoring sensations subscales. A loss of control factor consisted of the catastrophizing subscale and the ability to control pain rating. A third factor, labeled self-reliance, consisted of the ability to decrease pain rating and a negatively loaded prayer and hoping subscale. It is unclear from the report whether factor-based or factor scoring was used in the construction of the scales.

Gross (1986) reports that high scores on self-reliance and on active coping and suppression factors and low scores on the loss of control factor were associated with high levels of presurgical adjustment. Medical status variables, such as type of disc and disability status, were not related to scores on the CSQ factors. Relationships between CSQ factors and postoperative adjustment were assessed using hierarchical regression techniques in which medical status, preoperative pain, and somaticization personality style were control variables that were entered into the analysis prior to CSQ factors. The three CSQ factors were not significantly associated with outcome measures prior to discharge from the hospital but were found to be associated with pain and subjective estimate of surgical outcome. Patients high on the self-reliance factor and high on the loss of control factor reported lower pain scores and rated surgical outcome more positively than did low scorers.

Loss of control scores are therefore positively related to pain prior to surgery and negatively related to pain after surgery. These findings are very difficult to interpret. The author notes that loss of control is uncorrelated with outcome when assessed as a simple correlation, but becomes significantly related only when analyzed in conjunction with the self-reliance factor, which is negatively correlated with loss of control. Gross suggests that there may be patterns of strategy use, in which specific combinations of strategies reflect subgroups of patients who differ significantly in outcome, but no subanalyses are reported to support such an interactive model. It is unfortunate that the longitudinal data gathered in this project was not examined in a manner that allows examination of changes in pain scores. The confusing pattern of results with the loss of control subscale strongly suggests use of study designs that allow assessment of interactive as well as direct main effects of coping strategy. Without subanalyses, the use of main effects regression approaches may be uninterpretable.

The CSQ has also been used with chronic pain patients that have not been as extensively analyzed as low back or myofascial pain dysfunction patients. Keefe and his colleagues (Keefe, Caldwell, Queen, Gil, Martinez, Crisson, Ogden, and Nunley, 1987) administered the CSQ to fifty-one patients with chronic osteoarthritis of the knee. Average age of the subjects was 63.8 years and average duration of pain complaints was 10.3 years. Only 17 percent were receiving disability and only 8 percent were using narcotic medications. Thus relationships between pain strategies and coping could be examined without as much concern for the complicating factors of secondary gain and medication use.

A factor analysis of the CSQ revealed two factors: One, labeled self-control and rational thinking, consisted of the catastrophizing subscale and the two ratings of ability to control and decrease pain. The other, labeled coping attempts, consisted of the other six subscales. The self-control and rational thinking factor was significantly related to measures of pain, psychological and physical disability, and psychological symptoms. No significant effects are reported for the coping attempts factor. These findings underscore the importance of the catastrophizing subscale and the effectiveness ratings, which comprised the self-control and rational thinking factor, and also raise the possibility that the factor structure of the CSQ may differ for different populations of chronic pain patients.

Summary of Research Using Coping Strategies Questionnaire

The CSQ represents a significant theoretical advance in the study of chronic pain. Coping Strategies Questionnaire items reflect an attempt to assess patients' actual cognitive and behavioral efforts to cope with pain, and offers a useful alternative to the more standard measures of personality traits, such as locus of control or MMPI scales. As such, its development mirrors attempts to assess ways of coping independently from trait concepts of personality that have recently characterized the study of stress and illness within personality and social psychology. Although the development of the CSQ has already produced new knowledge about coping processes of chronic pain patients, several significant conceptual and methodological problems remain.

First, the items of the CSQ differ markedly in degree of specificity. Most items relate a very specific cognitive and behavioral attempt to cope with pain: "I pretend it is not a part of me"; "I try to be around other people." Other items reflect an evaluation of the distress level of the pain as well as a self-statement: "It is awful and I feel that it overwhelms me." Still others reflect a rating of overall ability to control or reduce pain: "How much control do you have over pain." Significant relationships between CSQ factors and dependent measures of pain and distress have been much more frequently reported for factors based on distress level and overall ability items than for factors based on more specific cognitive and behavioral items. Catastrophizing, in particular, appears to be an important correlate of poor adjustment as well as a component that changes in response to psychological therapy. But conceptually, if ratings of a person's ability to control or reduce pain are not related to the remaining items on the CSQ, the construct validity of the scale must be questioned.

If a person's rating of his or her ability to control pain is not associated with most of the strategies measured in the CSQ, one must ask how that person does control pain. In its original form, the CSQ consisted of seven factors plus two effectiveness ratings. I believe the effectiveness ratings should have remained separate from analysis of CSQ subscales because they reflect not a coping behavior but an overall assessment of coping ability. In the ways of coping literature reviewed earlier in this chapter, the practice of combining effectiveness measures with discrete coping behavior would be equivalent to combining Pearlin and Schooler's mastery scale with actual coping behaviors, or in combining Folkman and Lazarus' secondary appraisal measures with their ways of coping scales. This mixing of conceptual levels may obscure important questions. For example, perceived sense of control ability may be a moderator variable determining whether or not a particular pain strategy is effective. Clustering effectiveness of coping ratings with ratings of actual behaviors will only complicate the task of understanding when coping behaviors are effective, how coping behaviors change over time, and how coping behaviors may relate to the effectiveness of both medical and psychological treatments.

Second, too little attention has been directed at absolute levels of use of coping behavior and absolute level of effectiveness. For example, mean ratings of ability to control pain (0–6 Likert type scale), range from 2.4 to 3.6 in the four studies in which mean ratings are reported (Rosenstiel and Keefe, 1983; Keefe and Dolan, 1986; Turner and Clancy, 1986; Keefe et al, 1987). Mean values of individual subscales have even greater ranges. Use of praying or hoping strategies ranged from 1.2 to 3.6. Use of coping self-statements ranged from 1.1 to 4.1. Others, such as reinterpretation strategies, ranged only from 0.9 to 1.1. Such differences make comparisons of results from regression analyses in different studies extremely difficult. A significant relationship between praying or hoping strategies and pain, for example, may have different meaning in a population in which mean use of the strategy is 1.1 than for a population in which mean use is 3.6. Mean levels of coping strategy use could be examined in a population of chronic pain patients who differ in the length of time in pain, as in the "ancient" pain patients described by Swanson, Maruta, and Wolff (1986).

Third, use of factor-analytic techniques as the primary tool for conceptual development unduly constricts the evolution of the coping concept. Early development of measures such as the ways of coping emphasized gathering as wide a pool of coping items as possible. It is important to note that early use of factor analysis with the ways of coping scale did not produce useful dimensions of coping, and more recent work has emphasized smaller clusters of items that are selected for conceptual validity as well as for factorial validity (Folkman and Lazarus, 1985; Vitaliano, Russo, Carr, Maiuro, and Becker, 1985; Vitaliano, Maiuro, Russo, and Becker, 1987). At this stage in the development of instruments to measure coping, the goal of lumping items into large dimensions may not be productive. Factor analysis should certainly remain a useful tool, but lack of consistent findings with "factors" such as the loss of control factor reported by Gross (1986) or the different relationships found between coping and pain for the diverting attention and praying or hoping components of a "factor" reported by Turner and Clancy (1986) should be a caution to researchers. I would argue that a useful approach might be to add more items to the CSQ before further attempts at establishing coherent factor clusters were made. Revisions of the Ways of Coping Checklist have added items relating to prayer and use of humor based on open-ended responses from subjects. Perhaps the item base of the CSQ could be broadened in the same manner. Early reports of the scale originally included "pain behavior" items. Perhaps these were prematurely deleted from the scale. Additional items specifically related to medication administration as a coping strategy might also be useful.

Finally, the study of coping processes has been evolving toward a model that includes traditional personality traits (e.g., mastery) that serve as a context in which coping occurs; measures of primary and secondary appraisal, measures of social support, and measures of actual cognitions and behaviors. Although interactive as well as direct effects of these levels have not been effectively analyzed, it is clear that the process of coping must be examined in longitudinal studies that make it possible to study changes in outcome measures as a function of changes in coping strategies. Only in this way can the effects of pain as a stimulus to increased coping be disentangled from the effects coping may have on reducing pain.

Applications and Potential of Coping Strategies and Chronic Pain

Research reviewed in the first section of this chapter suggests that concepts of coping are becoming increasingly important variables in understanding human response to stress. The study of chronic pain has tended to focus on concepts such as personality traits that may aid in the psychological assessment of chronic pain patients and help in making distinctions between organic and psychogenic pain and in identifying patterns of personality characteristics that may describe a pain-prone personality type. A recent review (Turk and Rudy, 1986) has questioned the utility of the organic–psychogenic distinction in the light of new psychobiological evidence and the extension of theories of pain far beyond the sensory-physiologic models of Cartesian dualism. Others have noted that use of updated norms for MMPI scales markedly reduces the number of chronic pain patients who might be classed as psychologically disturbed (Ahles, Yunus, Gaulier, Riley and Masi, 1986). I would suggest that concepts of coping which have traditionally reflected normal rather than psychopathologic defenses against stress may provide insights into the responses of chronic pain patients that personality traits would not provide. In this section, suggestions for further development of the coping concept will be combined with suggestions for new analysis strategies. Promising conceptual developments that may expand the concept of coping beyond the largely cognitively based CSQ items will be discussed. Finally, examples drawn from the use of coping concepts from the acute pain literature will be cited.

EXTENSIONS OF THE CONCEPT OF COPING: STRATEGY AND TACTICS

Throughout the coping literature, the terms *strategy* and *tactics* have typically been used interchangeably. I would suggest that it is important to distinguish between these two terms, particularly if coping is to be applied to a chronic rather than an acute stress situation. Distinctions between strategy and tactics are most clearly delineated in the military. Whereas the term *tactics* is used to describe the detailed conduct of military operations and the maneuver of troops on a small scale, *strategy* involves more macrocosmic decisions about when and where to fight, how to plan for unseen contingencies, and how to achieve one's objectives without fighting at all. In essence, tactics involve how to conduct a battle; strategy involves how to conduct a war (Clausewitz, 1896; Liddell Hart, 1967). Although coping with chronic pain is certainly a series of battles, in another sense it is a "war," and our concepts should include strategic level variables.

Three applications for further research in coping and pain can be developed from the military distinction between strategy and tactics. First, the effectiveness of a "defense" depends on an appropriate match between one's grand strategy and one's tactical capabilities. On one level, measures of personality traits may reflect strategic predispositions to view the world in a particular way, comparable to what one calls strategic policy in a military sense. Specific measures of coping behaviors such as "Diverting Attention" reflect tactics in response to a specific stressor. If one has a strategic predisposition or policy to view the world as outside of one's control, as is represented in trait measures of locus of control or mastery, not only will one's deployment of coping tactics be different, but the effectiveness of those tactics may depend on the fit between tactics and strategy. This suggests that personality variables that may reflect more general strategies must be evaluated both in terms of their direct effects on coping and in terms of their interactive effects with coping tactics on measures of outcome in a stressful situation. Evidence supporting this contention can be drawn from the work of Katharine Parkes (1984) who showed that locus of control scores interacted with the subject's appraisal of whether something could be done about the situation in determining scores on the Ways of Coping Checklist. Similar results were reported for another more "strategic" concept, the tendency to be optimistic or pessimistic (Scheir, Weintraub, and Carver, 1986). Interactions between strategic and tactical coping variables suggest that strategic considerations may influence choice of coping and outcome in stressful situations. On a analytic level, the process of "correcting" for personality variables by entering them first in a regression analysis becomes theoretically inappropriate when applied within a framework of strategy and tactics.

Second, strategic considerations are also involved in assessing when one fights or avoids fighting. Pearlin and Schooler (1978) showed that selective ignoring was beneficial in the occupational realm but destructive in the marital realm. The decision to use a tactic in one role but not in the other role is a strategic decision. Measures of how effectively one deploys coping tactics in terms of deciding when to use or when to stop using a particular coping tactic may be better measures of an effective defensive posture than are simple measures of coping tactics. This connotation of strategy as a concept at a higher level than coping tactics mirrors concepts of cognitive strategies in the field of developmental psychology (Paris and Lindauer, 1982) and metamemory strategies in the field of memory research (Zelinski, Gilewski, and Thompson, 1980). In the field of chronic pain, strategic considerations may play an important role in determining how well a patient functions not only in dealing with the immediacy of the pain but with the implications of that pain for other role areas of his or her life. Strategic considerations are also present in assessing the impact of a chosen coping style for pain on strain in other role areas of the person's life.

Finally, effective strategy evolves out of an understanding of one's tactical capabilities. Changes in strategy may be a result of changes in coping abilities. Cognitive and behavioral treatments for chronic pain may influence coping tactics in the short term but may also influence strategic variables in the long-run. In addition, strategic as well as tactical changes may be the focus of cognitive and behavioral treatment approaches. Biofeedback and relaxation treatments for chronic headache patients have been reported to produce changes in depression and trait anxiety level, even when changes in headache frequency did not occur (Blanchard, Andrasik, Appelbaum, Evans, Myers, and Barron, 1986). Such changes are often attributed to nonspecific effects of treatments, but may reflect changes in strategic outlook.

One essential difference between a tactical and a strategic orientation to coping effects is the hypothesis that knowing how tactics are used may be just as important as knowing which tactics are used. Analysis of data obtained from a study of elective surgery patients provides an illustrative example from the study of acute pain (Wilson, 1981). An overall measure of coping ability was constructed from patients' responses to a questionnaire designed to assess their ability to exert emotion-focused and problem-focused coping. An example of an item from the emotion-focused scale was: "I am able to be calm and controlled when faced with disturbing events." An example of an item from the problem-focused component was: "When I am going to leave on vacation, I always make sure that everything is arranged in advance, so that I don't have to do things at the last minute." The questionnaire attempts to assess the effectiveness of the subject's coping tactics rather than which tactics were used. This same questionnaire also asked subjects to describe how persistent they tended to be in their coping efforts. A sample item from the persistence subscale was: "I like to stick to what I am doing, no matter how long it takes me to finish." The persistence scale represents a strategic concept in that it depicts how an individual uses coping tactics rather than which tactics they use. Individuals who scored high on the coping effectiveness scale used less medications after surgery (Wilson, 1981). More interesting for purposes of example, however, coping effectiveness and persistence interacted in determining use of medications following surgery. Mean numbers of injections of morphine used following surgery for patients at low and high levels of coping ability and low and high levels of persistence can be found in Table 19.6.

TABLE 19.6

MEAN NUMBER OF INJECTIONS OF MORPHINE REQUIRED AFTER SURGERY FOR PATIENTS AT HIGH AND LOW LEVELS OF TACTICAL COPING ABILITY AND AT HIGH AND LOW LEVELS OF STRATEGIC PERSISTENCE.

Coping Ability	Persistence	n	Injections
Low	Low	27	14.5
Low	High	18	8.7
High	Low	11	9.3
High	High	18	9.1

The significant interaction between persistence and coping [F (1,69) = 5.06, $p<0.05$] indicates that lack of persistence in coping efforts only made a difference in medication use at low levels of coping ability. It should be noted that although persistence and coping ability are correlated [r (71) = 0.29, $p<0.05$], analysis of subjects who do not fit the modal pattern of being high on both coping and persistence or low on both coping and persistence reveals a relationship between strategy and tactics that would not be evident from analytic models that emphasize only main effects and not interactive effects.

EXTENSIONS OF THE CONCEPT OF COPING: MEASUREMENT AND ANALYSIS

Coping Assessment with Hypothetical Situations

Usefulness of coping research in the chronic pain area would be enhanced by broadening approaches to measurement and analysis. Research with the CSQ has focused on how patients typically respond to painful situations. Research with more general ways of coping has tended to ask about a specific stressor that is generated by the subject. Another approach in other areas of coping research provides all subjects the same set of hypothetical situations, the same set of hypothetical responses, and generates a specific score on one or many dimensions of coping. The advantage of this approach is that it allows one to provide a common stimulus to a diverse population and to tailor stimuli and response categories to areas of special interest. One example of such a coping instrument is the Monitor-Blunter scale (Miller, 1987). The scale was constructed to measure people's preferred style of dealing with threat-related cues (Miller and Mangan, 1983). Monitors respond to threat by seeking information. Blunters respond to threat by attempting to avoid information. This dimension is assessed by providing subjects with four hypothetical situations that involve stress. For example, subjects may be asked to imagine that they are afraid of the dentist and have to get some dental work done. They are then asked to indicate whether they would be likely to try any of ten monitoring and blunting responses to being in this situation. Examples of monitoring responses include the following: "I would ask the dentist exactly what he was going to do; I would watch the flow of water from my mouth to see if it contained blood." Examples of blunting responses include the following: "I would try to think about pleasant memories"; "I would do mental puzzles in my mind." Scores on dimensions of monitoring and blunting are generated from this approach. Although designed to assess one particular aspect of a person's style of coping with threat, the methodology used may be a useful way to provide common stressful stimuli. It is also possible to blend a common response format with an open-ended response format so that new coping patterns could be identified.

A more elaborated set of defense mechanisms produced by a similar methodological format is the Defense Mechanisms Inventory (Gleser and Ihilevich, 1969). Scores on dimensions derived from Freudian conceptions of defense mechanisms (e.g., turning against self, projection intellectualization) are generated by obtaining responses to hypothetical situations such as being splashed with mud by a passing car. A unique aspect of the Defense Mechanisms Inventory is a response format in which subjects are asked not only how they would respond to a situation, but how they would not respond. This generates additional information about an individual's repertoire of defenses and may be a useful measurement technique. In addition, this instrument has been found to be related to use of medications for pain and to level of epinephrine and norepinephrine output in patients facing an acute pain situation (Wilson, 1982). Thus, both the Defense Mechanisms Inventory and the Monitor-Blunter scale may be useful measurement approaches for extending coping concepts to chronic pain patients.

Coping Assessment Through Measures of Pain Behavior

In addition to development of new paper-and-pencil approaches to the measurement of coping, other aspects of the response to pain might be considered to be coping behaviors. For example, facial expressions of pain (LeResche and Dworkin, 1984; Craig and Patrick, 1985), as one aspect of pain behavior, may reflect a response to acute pain that becomes part of an integrated coping response pattern in chronic pain. Depression and medication use were found to be associated with measures of facial pain behavior in chronic patients (Keefe, Wilkins, Cook, Crisson, and Muhlbaier, 1986). Patrick, Craig, and Prkachin (1986) reported that self-reports of acute pain were affected by having a stoic model in the experimental setting, whereas observer judgments of facial pain were not altered. Experiments such as those of Ekman, Levenson, and Friesen (1983) have demonstrated that emotional states can be altered by altering facial expressions, suggesting that some aspects of pain behavior may augment pain rather than just being symptomatic of negative emotional states. The concept of "nocebo" response as a conditioned increase in pain due to the manner in which a patient focuses on pain (Schweiger and Parducci, 1981) may provide a model in which to examine complex relationships between pain and pain behavior. More comprehensive measures of pain tactics and strategy may therefore include nonverbal aspects of response to pain as well as traditional paper-and-pencil assessment of cognitive behaviors.

Coping Assessment Through Language

Questions of measurement of pain are also relevant to issues of coping. The response to chronic pain may include changes in coping processes at both strategic and tactical levels. However, the complexities of the pain experience suggest that pain itself, or at least the ability to express pain, may change as pain evolves from being an acute episode to being a chronic condition. Reading (1982) reported that chronic pain patients used more affective and reaction responses to the McGill Pain Questionnaire than did acute pain patients. Melzack (1984) has described enormous variation in adjective use on the McGill Pain Questionnaire among chronic pain patients with different sites of pain. The manner in which chronic pain patients express their pain and the extent to which this expression changes over time may be crucial to understanding the process of coping with chronic pain.

Recent philosophical (Scarry, 1985) and linguistic (Morris, 1986) analyses of the pain phenomena suggest that the inexpressibility of physical pain tends to defeat language. A corollary of their lyrical presentations of pain in history and literature is that coping or mastery may be associated with pain becoming expressible in language for individual patients. On the other hand, the chronic pain situation may alter expressive patterns as "staff and family learn to ignore complaining patients . . . and intensify a silence which already exists at the heart of pain" (Morris, 1986, p. 91). In any event, linguistic analysis of pain expression could be a key to understanding coping processes in chronic pain as being an indicator of adaptation as well as an index of pain intensity.

Further Applications in Chronic Pain

The use of concepts of coping in the study of chronic pain may be especially promising in assessing the importance of family functioning, and in clarifying recent work on psychobiological models of pain perception. Studies of family influences on chronic pain have generally focused on demographic variables such as birth order, social class, and family size, or on features of the family's role in maintaining pain (Payne and Norfleet, 1986). The work by Cronkite and Moos (1984) demonstrated that the spouse's coping patterns were influential in determining one's own distress in response to a stressor. Given the enormous impact of chronic pain on family functioning, analysis of family coping styles either as a unit or through key individuals such as a spouse, may be useful in understanding the adaptational patterns of chronic pain patients. A study of family functioning in adolescent chronic pain provides a developmental example of the potential usefulness of coping concepts in understanding family functioning (Dunn-Geier, McGrath, Rourke, Latter, and D'Astous, 1986). Dunn-Geier and her colleagues analyzed videotaped interaction patterns and reported that the adolescent who is not coping well with chronic pain is likely to have a mother who discourages active coping, and to become more overprotective in the pain situation. Characterization of family as well as individual coping styles may be a useful way to extend coping concepts into the chronic pain setting.

Enormous differences among individuals in pain threshold and tolerance have always been problematic for pain researchers. Jamner and Schwartz (1986), have reported differences in affective responses to laboratory-induced pain based on responses to the lie scale of the Eysenck Personality Inventory. Individuals who were characterized as being "self-deceptors" accepted much greater levels of pain than did low-deceptors.

Although interpretation of the meaning of responses to the Eysenck Personality Inventory are problematic, the authors suggest that significantly higher scores on this scale reported for chronic pain patients (Woodforde and Merskey, 1972) may be related to biologic variation in endogenous opioids related to the chronic pain experience. The dysregulation theory posited by these authors suggests that differences in coping style may be related to biologic differences in pain control systems. Although these hypotheses are clearly speculative, recent work examining variation in medication use in acute pain patients who have administered their own opiate medications through a technique called patient-controlled analgesia (Graves, Foster, Batenhorst, Bennet, Baumann, 1983), suggests that coping styles are correlated with amount of medication required after surgery (Wilson and Bennet, 1984). Other researchers (Tamsen, Sakurada, Wahlstrom, Terenius, and Hartvig, 1982) have related medication use after surgery to preoperative endorphin levels in cerebrospinal fluid. Still others (Johansson, Almay, Von Knorring, Terenius, and Astrom, 1979) have tried to relate personality traits to endorphin levels. Thus, although mediating mechanisms have not been specified, relationships between coping styles and biologic mechanisms of pain inhibition systems may be a promising area of inquiry.

Coping styles, therefore, might well assess physiological as well as psychological aspects of the pain process. An example of the usefulness of such an approach, even while staying on the level of questionnaire measurement of key variables, can be drawn from a research project assessing relationships between coping style and medication use in surgery patients using patient-controlled analgesia rather than conventional intramuscular injections (Wilson and Bennet, 1984). Measures of coping style similar to that described for the study of elective surgery patients (Wilson, 1981) reported earlier in this chapter were administered to a population of mixed elective surgery patients who were receiving patient-controlled analgesia as their postoperative dosing regimen. In addition to measures of subjects' emotion-focused control ability ("I am able to be calm and controlled when faced with disturbing things"; "Even if I feel nervous or frightened inside, people don't notice it because

I act calm on the outside"), a questionnaire measure interpreted as measuring their typical level of emotional arousal under stress was administered. Sample items from this scale include the following: "I have trouble sleeping when I am worried or nervous about something that is going to happen the next day"; "When something upsetting happens, I will have trouble relaxing and falling asleep that night." Table 19.7 depicts the amount of morphine used per day for surgery patients who were high or low on measure of emotional control and high or low on measures of emotional arousability.

TABLE 19.7

MEAN NUMBER OF MILLIGRAMS OF MORPHINE SELF-ADMINISTERED PER 24 HOURS BY SURGERY PATIENTS WITH HIGH AND LOW SCORES ON EMOTIONAL CONTROL AND EMOTIONAL AROUSABILITY SCALES

Arousability	Emotional Control	n	Mean	SD	Range
Low	Low	8	26.7	18.7	8–66
Low	High	9	27.1	16.5	6–56
High	Low	12	51.9	34.8	12–131
High	High	6	27.5	15.9	15–59

Both Arousability ($F\ (1,31) = 12.40$, $p<0.01$) and Emotional Control ($F(1,31) = 7.01$, $p < 0.05$) are independent predictors of medication use. The interaction between arousability and emotional control ability, however, is also statistically significant ($F(1,31) = 4.61$, $p < 0.05$). The shape of this interaction (see Table 19.7) suggests that low medication use is a function of either low arousability or high emotional control. The combination of high arousability and low emotional control ability is particularly volatile, as expressed in markedly greater medication use, greater variability, and greater range. Although the interpretation of the meaning of the "arousability" and emotional control scales is open to question, these results linking coping and medication use suggest that further exploration of questionnaire and physiological measures of coping processes and outcomes in painful situations would be conceptually important.

CONCLUSIONS

This chapter has attempted to describe the evolution of measures of coping style and process in the larger field of personality and social psychology, to discuss initial attempts to apply concepts of coping to the chronic pain setting with the Coping Strategies Questionnaire, and to suggest promising extensions of the concept of coping that may be especially useful in the study of chronic pain. The study of coping has evolved from a fixed, rather deterministic notion of personality trait into a fluid, much more process oriented approach that recognizes that coping variables function as both independent and dependent variables as one's time perspective varies. The studies reviewed in this chapter suggest several important directions for research on coping and chronic pain.

First, instruments to assess coping should be broadened to assess not only how individuals cope with "pain" but how those coping patterns interact with stress and strain in the chronic pain patient's major roles in life as a member of a family and as a member of a workplace. Attempts should be made to assess not only how an individual copes with pain, but also how effective each attempt is. Broader inclusion of the family both as an index of social resources or social support, but also in terms of family or spouse coping style will also be crucial in assessing coping effectiveness and in helping to predict treatment outcome.

Second, studies of coping in chronic pain patients should be more process-oriented. Failure to assess change in coping behaviors over time has made it difficult to disentangle the effects of pain on coping from the effects of coping on pain. A process approach could also be instrumental in better describing the manner in which acute pain episodes metamorphose into what is termed *chronic pain*.

Third, measures of outcome should differentiate between adaptation as a positive dimension versus adaptation as a reduction in distress. The phrase "mixed emotions" that emerged from the Folkman and Lazarus (1985) study of threat, challenge, benefit, and harm in college students facing an exam surely is more important in the complex network of emotions that represents responses to chronic pain.

Fourth, distinctions between coping as a tactical process and coping as a strategic process suggest that attempts should be made to develop concepts of people's strategies for coping with pain as well as the explicit tactics used in a pain episode. The strategic–tactical distinction also implies that analysis approaches must include assessment of buffering effects of coping as well as direct main effects of coping on outcome, and that interactive effects of coping tactics and coping strategies may more adequately represent the complexity of the coping process. Baron and Kenny (1986) suggest that choice of analytic techniques for assessing moderator and mediator variables depends on specific characteristics of the data, but include analysis of variance (Winer, 1971), complex multiple regression (Cohen and Cohen, 1983), and linear structural equations (LISREL) (Joreskog and Sorbom, 1984).

The importance of coping concepts for understanding chronic pain patients has been noted by outstanding pain researchers (Turk and Rudy, 1986; Keefe and Gil, 1986). But our understanding of the relationship between psychological variables hasn't recognized the extent of individual differences in how these variables relate to one another. Linton and Gotestam (1985) studied sixteen chronic pain patients over a period of six weeks. Measures of pain and mood were assessed daily. When analyzed as a group, pain and depression were positively correlated. But when analyzed as individuals, pain was significantly positively correlated with depression for eleven patients, uncorrelated with depression for two patients, and significantly negatively correlated with depression for three patients. Important differences in coping–pain relationships may only be discovered through time-series methods of study (Keeser and Bullinger, 1984).

The study of coping has oscillated between relatively rigid application of traitlike concepts and attempts to integrate qualitative life-history and case study data. Recent work by Taylor (1983) describing the complex manner in which breast cancer patients coped by maintaining and modifying illusions, certainly broadened the concept of denial, and illustrates the importance of understanding the contextual meaning of coping. The process of coping for chronic pain patients involves in some way making sense of pain. Research on coping must be broadened so that constructs of coping developed through traditional psychometric approaches can be enriched by qualitative and case-study data. Pain researchers still struggle constantly with how to measure pain. This inexpressibility is captured by an Emily Dickinson poem quoted by David Morris (1986).

> Pain—has an Element of Blank—
> It cannot recollect
> When it begun—or if there were
> A time when it was not—
>
> It has no Future—but itself—
> Its Infinite contain
> Its Past—enlightened to perceive
> New Periods—of Pain.

Although concepts of coping may also be ultimately inexpressible, attempts to describe the struggle of pain patients to cope with pain and its meaning for their lives should try to capture the meaning and process dimensions that are the goals of current models of coping.

REFERENCES

Ahles, T.A., Yunus, M.B., Gaulier, B., Riley, S. D., & Masi, A.T. (1986), The use of contemporary MMPI norms in the study of chronic pain patients. *Pain*, 24:159–163.

Baron, R.M., & Kenny, D.A. (1986), The moderator–mediator variable distinction in social psychological research: Conceptual, strategic, and statistical considerations. *J. Pers. & Soc. Psychol.*, 51/6:1173–1182.

Billings, A.G., & Moos, R.H. (1981), The role of coping responses and social resources in attenuating the stress of life events. *J. Behav. Med.* 4/2:139–157.

Blanchard, E.B., Andrasik, F., Appelbaum, K.A., Evans, D.D., Myers, P., & Barron, K.D. (1986), Three studies of the psychologic changes in chronic headache patients associated with biofeedback and relaxation therapies. *Psychosom. Med.*, 48/1, 2:73–83.

Bryant, F.B., & Veroff, J. (1982), The structure of psychological well-being: A sociohistorical analysis. *J. Pers. & Soc. Psychol.*, 43/4:653–673.

Clausewitz, K. von. (1896), *On War*, Vol. 1. New York: Barnes & Noble, 1966.

Cohen, J., & Cohen, P. (1983). *Applied Multiple Regression/Correlation Analysis for the Behavioral Sciences*, 2nd ed. Hillsdale, NJ: Erlbaum.

Craig, K.D., & Patrick, C.J. (1985), Facial expression during induced pain. *J. Pers. & Soc. Psychol.*, 48/4:1080–1091.

Cronkite, R.C., & Moos, R.H. (1984), The role of predisposing and moderating factors in the stress–illness relationship. *J. Health & Soc. Behav.*, 25:372–393.

Dunn-Geier, B.J., McGrath, P.J., Rourke, B.P., Latter, J., & D'Astous, J. (1986), Adolescent chronic pain: The ability to cope. *Pain*, 26:23–32.

Ekman, P., Levenson, R.W., & Friesen, W.V. (1983), Autonomic nervous system activity distinguishes among emotions. *Science*, 221:1208–1210.

Elliott, D.J., Trief, P.M., & Stein, N. (1986), Mastery, stress, and coping in marriage among chronic pain patients. *J. Behav. Med.*, 9/6:549–558.

Fleishman, J.A. (1984). Personality characteristics and coping patterns, *J. Health & Soc. Behav.*, 25:229–244.

Folkman, S. & Lazarus, R.S. (1980), An analysis of coping in a middle-aged community sample. *J. Health & Soc. Behav.*, 21:219–239.

—— ——(1985), If it changes, it must be a process: A study of emotion and coping during three stages of a college examination. *J. Pers. & Soc. Psychol.*, 48:150–170.

—— ——Dunkel-Schetter, C., DeLongis, A., & Gruen, R.J. (1986), Dynamics of a stressful encounter: Cognitive appraisal, coping, and encounter outcomes. *J. Pers. & Soc. Psychol.*, 50/5:992–1003.

—— ——Gruen, R.J., & Delongis, A. (1986), Appraisal, coping, health status, and psychological symptoms. *J. Pers. & Soc. Psychol.*, 50/3:571–579.

Gleser, G.C., & Ihilevich, D. (1969), An objective instrument for measuring defense mechanisms, *J. Consult. & Clin. Psychol.*, 33:51–60.

Graves, D.H., Foster, T.S., Batenhorst, R.L., Bennett, R.L., & Baumann, T.J. (1983), Patient-controlled analgesia. *Ann. Intern. Med.*, 99:360–366.

Gross, A.R. (1986), The effect of coping strategies on the relief of pain following surgical intervention for lower back pain. *Psychosom. Med.*, 48/3, 4:229–241.

Haan, N. (1963), Proposed model of ego functioning: Coping and defense mechanisms in relationship to IQ change. *Psycholog. Monogr.*, 77:1–23.

Hart, B.H. Liddell (1967). *Strategy: The Indirect Approach.* London: Faber & Faber.

Jamner, L.D., & Schwartz, G.E. (1986), Self-deception predicts self-report and endurance of pain. *Psychosom. Med.*, 48:211–223.

Johansson, F., Almay, B.G.L., Von Knorring, L., Terenius, L., & Astrom, M. (1979), Personality traits in chronic pain patients related to endorphin levels in cerebrospinal fluid. *Psychiat. Res.*, 1:231–240.

Joreskog, K.J., & Sorbom, D. (1984). *LISREL-VI—Estimation of Linear Structural Equations by Maximum Likelihood Methods*, 3rd ed. Mooresville, IN: Scientific Software.

Keefe, F.J., Caldwell, D.S., Queen, K.T., Gil, K.M., Martinez, S., Crisson, J.E., Ogden, W., & Nunley, J. (1987), Pain coping strategies in osteoarthritis patients. *J. Consult. & Clin. Psychol.*, 55:208–212.

——Dolan, E. (1986), Pain behavior and pain coping strategies in low back pain and myofascial pain dysfunction syndrome patients. *Pain*, 24:49–56.

——Gil, K.M. (1986), Behavioral concepts in the analysis of chronic pain syndromes. *J. Consult. & Clin. Psychol.*, 54:776–783.

——Wilkins, R.H., Cook, W.A., Jr., Crisson, J.E., & Muhlbaier, L.H. (1986), Depressing pain, and pain behavior. *J. Consult. & Clin. Psychol.*, 54:665–669.

Keeser, W., & Bullinger, M. (1984), Process-oriented evaluation of a cognitive behavioural treatment for clinical pain: A time-series approach. In: *Neurophysiological Correlates of Pain*, ed. B. Bromm. New York: Elsevier Science, pp. 417–428.

Lazarus, R.S., & Folkman, S. (1984). *Stress, Appraisal, and Coping*. New York: Springer.

LeResche, L., & Dworkin, S.F. (1984), Facial expression accompanying pain. *Soc. Sci. Med.*, 19/12:1325–1330.

Linton, S.J., & Gotestam, K. (1985), Relations between pain, anxiety, mood and muscle tension in chronic pain patients. A correlation study. *Psychother. Psychosom.*, 43/2:90–95.

Melzack, R. (1984), Measurement of the dimensions of pain experience. In: *Pain Measurement in Man. Neurophysiological Correlates of Pain*, ed. B. Bromm. New York: Elsevier Science, pp. 327–348.

Miller, S.M. (1987), Monitoring and blunting: Validation of a questionnaire to assess styles of information seeking under threat. *J. Pers. & Soc. Psychol.*, 52:345–353.

———Mangan, C.E. (1983), Interacting effects of information and coping style in adapting to gynecologic stress: Should the doctor tell all? *J. Pers. & Soc. Psychol.*, 45:223–236.

Moos, R.H., Cronkite, R.C., Billings, A.G., & Finney, J.W. (1983), *Health and Daily Living Form Manual.* Palo Alto, CA: Social Ecology Laboratory, Veterans Administration and Stanford University Medical Center.

Morris, D.B. (1986), The languages of pain. In: *Exploring the Concept of Mind*, ed. R.M. Caplan. Iowa City: University of Iowa Press, pp. 89–99.

Paris, S.G., & Lindauer, B.K. (1982), The development of cognitive skills during childhood. In: *Handbook of Developmental Psychology*, ed. B.B. Wolman. Englewood Cliffs, NJ: Prentice-Hall, pp. 333–349.

Parkes, K.R. (1984), Locus of control, cognitive appraisal, and coping in stressful episodes. *J. Pers. & Soc. Psychol.*, 46/3:655–668.

Patrick, C.J., Craig, K.D., & Prkachin, K.M. (1986), Observer judgments of acute pain: Facial action determinants. *J. Pers. Soc. Psychol.*, 50/6:1291–1298.

Payne, B., & Norfleet, M.A. (1986), Chronic pain and the family: A review. *Pain*, 26:1–22.

Pearlin, L.I., & Schooler, C. (1978), The structure of coping. *J. Health & Soc. Behav.*, 19:2–21.

———Leiberman, M.A., Menaghan, E.G., & Mullan, J.T. (1981), The stress process. *J. Health & Soc. Behav.*, 2:337–356.

Rahe, R.H. (1974), The pathway between subjects' recent life changes and their near-future illness reports. In: *Stressful Life Events: Their Nature and Effects*, eds. B. Dohrenwend & B. Dohrenwend. New York: John Wiley.

Reading, A.E. (1982), A comparison of the McGill Pain Questionnaire in chronic and acute pain. *Pain*, 13:185–192.

Rosenstiel, A.K., & Keefe, F.J. (1983), The use of coping strategies in chronic low back pain patients: Relationship to patient characteristics and current adjustment. *Pain*, 17:33–44.

Rybstein-Blinchik, E. (1979), Effects of different cognitive strategies on the chronic pain experience. *J. Behav. Med.*, 2:93–102.

Scarry, E. (1985). *The Body in Pain.* New York: Oxford University Press.

Scheir, M.F., Weintraub, J.K., & Carver, C.S. (1986), Coping with stress: Divergent strategies of optimists and pessimists. *J. Pers. & Soc. Psychol.*, 51/6:1257–1264.

Schweiger, A., & Parducci, A. (1981), Nocebo: The psychologic induction of pain. *Pav. J. Biolog. Sci.*, 16/3:140–143.

Spanos, N.P., Horton C., & Chaves, J.F. (1975), The effects of two cognitive strategies on pain thresholds. *J. Abnorm. Psychol.*, 84:677–681.

Stone, A.A., & Neale, J.M. (1984), New measure of daily coping: Development and preliminary results. *J. Pers. & Soc. Psychol.*, 46/4:892–906.

Swanson, D.W., Maruta, T., & Wolff, V.A. (1986), Ancient pain, *Pain*, 25:383–387.

Tamsen, A., Sakurada, T., Wahlstrom, A., Terenius, L., & Hartvig, P. (1982), Postoperative demand for analgesics in relation to individual levels of endorphins and substance P in cerebrospinal fluid. *Pain*, 13:171–183.

Taylor, S.E. (1983), Adjustment to threatening events: A theory of cognitive adaptation, *Amer. Psycholog.*, November:1161–1172.

Turk, D.C., & Rudy, T.E. (1986), Assessment of cognitive factors in chronic pain: A worthwhile enterprise? *J. Consult. & Clin. Psychol.*, 54:760–768.

Turner, J.A., & Clancy, S. (1986), Strategies for coping with chronic low back pain: Relationship to pain and disability. *Pain*, 24:355–364.

Vaillant, G.E. (1977). *Adaptation to Life*. Boston: Little, Brown.

Vitaliano, P.P., Maiuro, R.D., Russo, J., & Becker, J. (1987), Raw versus relative scores in the assessment of coping strategies. *J. Behav. Med.*, 10/1:1–17.

———Russo, J., Carr, J., Maiuro, R., & Becker, J. (1985), The ways of coping checklist: Revision and psychometric properties. *Multivar. Behav. Res.*, 20:3–26.

Wilson, J.F. (1981), Behavioral preparation for surgery: Benefit or harm? *J. Behav. Med.*, 4/1:79–102.

———(1982), Recovery from surgery and scores on the defense mechanisms inventory. *J. Pers. Assess.*, 46/3:312–319.

———Bennet, R. (1984), Coping styles, medication use, and pain scores in patients using patient–controlled analgesia for postoperative pain. *Anesthesiol.*, 61/3A:A193.

Winer, B.J. (1971). *Statistical Principles of Experimental Design*, 2nd ed. New York: McGraw-Hill.

Woodforde, J.M., & Merskey, H. (1972), Personality traits of patients with chronic pain. *J. Psychosom. Res.*, 16:167–172.

Zelinski, E.M., Gilewski, M.J., & Thompson, L.W. (1980), Do laboratory tests relate to self-assessment of memory ability in the young and old? In: *New Directions in Memory and Aging*, eds. L.W. Poon, J.L. Fozard, L.S. Cermak, D. Arenberg, & L.W. Thompson. Hillsdale, NJ: Lawrence Erlbaum, pp. 519–540.

20

The Multidisciplinary Chronic Pain Treatment Team

NANCI I. MOORE, PH.D.

INTRODUCTION

While numerous articles have been written about the effectiveness of the multidisciplinary team in the treatment of chronic pain (Greenhoot and Sternbach, 1977; Newman, Seres, Yospe, and Garlington, 1978; Dolce, Crocker, and Doleys, 1986), there is considerable difference in the ways in which the teams are constituted and little description of the functioning of the team itself. Almost all such teams include a physician and psychologist, yet, in spite of considerable writing about the role of the family in the dynamics of chronic pain problems (Fordyce, 1976; Waring, 1982; Turk, Meichenbaum, and Genest, 1983), not all teams include a social worker or other specified family therapist. While inpatient treatment is frequently recommended (Fordyce, 1976) and the role of physical therapists is occasionally described (Newman et al., 1978; Turk et al., 1983), the role of the nursing staff is often not mentioned and/or there is no designated nursing member of the team.

Perhaps even more importantly, the dynamics of the interactions of the pain team members are rarely mentioned, and there is only scant information concerning the relationship of the team to ward staff or staff of other hospital programs.

The purpose of this chapter is to describe the disciplines to be considered in constituting a multidisciplinary pain treatment team when a component of the treatment program consists of an inpatient stay. The problems encountered in interdisciplinary communications and potential conflicts among the disciplines represented will also be explored briefly.

In the following descriptions of disciplines, it should be noted that there is considerable overlap in functions. For example, individual, family, or group therapy may be done by a psychiatrist, a psychologist, a social worker, or occasionally a nurse; transcutaneous electrical nerve stimulation (TENS) units may be employed by a neurosurgeon, a physiatrist, a physical therapist, or an occupational therapist; nutritional assessments may be done by a physician or a dietitian; relaxation therapy (whether biofeedback-assisted, or not) may be done by a psychologist (or psychology technician), social worker, physical therapist, or nurse. These areas of overlap are frequently precisely those areas where conflict may occur, and the training and qualifications of the individual team members privileged to perform these procedures must be thoroughly explained to the members of the team.

Psychologist

While much has been written about the role of the psychologist in the evaluation and treatment (or management) of chronic pain (Turk et al., 1983), little has been said about the role of the psychologist within the team itself. Because of the usual training in both individual and group dynamics, the psychologist may well be the team member best suited to assist the team with team building, communication skills, facilitation in uncovering team conflicts, and conflict resolution. The psychologist need not be the team leader to fulfill this function and, in fact, might not be in an optimal position to perform this function if he or she is the team leader. It is important, though, that someone on the team, be it psychologist, psychiatrist, or social worker, be selected and recognized by the team for their expertise in the areas of team building and conflict resolution.

Such an individual is also most valuable in working with the ward staff to develop a consistent treatment plan (e.g., ignoring pain behaviors, giving attention to health behaviors) to be implemented by the ward staff. No inpatient pain team program can expect to be successful without the cooperation of the ward staff, and such cooperation is rarely gained by simply expecting them to follow orders.

Specific training in behavioral and cognitive behavioral approaches to chronic pain management is, of course, also essential for the psychologist not only to employ directly with the patients, but to demonstrate to each professional who is also working with the patient. Additional skills, such as individual therapy, group therapy, biofeedback, hypnotherapy, and family therapy are valuable tools for the pain team psychologist to have but are actually secondary to team-building skills and specific behavioral and cognitive behavioral skills applicable to the chronic pain patient.

In a recent study (1985), Hickling, Sison, and Holtz surveyed a number of multidisciplinary pain clinics. They described the psychologist's role as consisting of psychotherapy, evaluation, administration, supervision, research, teaching, consultation, and public relations. Primary interventions employed by these psychologists included relaxation therapy, behavioral programming, operant conditioning, individual psychotherapy, electromyography (EMG) biofeedback, group therapy, temperature biofeedback, autogenic therapy, couples therapy, family therapy, and hypnotherapy (listed in descending order of frequency of reported use). Keefe and Bradley (1984) list operant conditioning, self-management techniques (e.g., biofeedback and relaxation therapy, cognitive behavioral interventions), and multimodal approaches. Finally, Moore and Chaney (1985) describe individuals and couples groups in which the group participants are taught Melzack's (1973) gate-control concepts of pain, problem solving, relaxation, controlled breathing and guided imagery, operant components of chronic pain, attention distraction techniques, pain-reinterpretations strategies, assertiveness training, and active listening.

Fey and Fordyce (1983) describe a multidisciplinary pain

treatment program that includes vocational assessment and simulated work stations, as well as the more usual relaxation therapy, biofeedback, hypnosis, and cognitive behavioral strategies.

While the above articles are not intended to exhaust the literature on psychologists' roles and functions in the multidisciplinary treatment of chronic pain, they are intended as illustrations of the kinds of things psychologists do in such settings.

The Physician

The specific specialty of the physician member(s) of the team is not nearly as important as the individual physician's interest and knowledge of both the physiology and psychology of pain. Interns, and even residents, often seem to believe that pain is a "sensation"; that there is some point-by-point correlation between physical damage and the intensity of pain. They frequently need to be taught that pain is a perception mediated by higher cortical processes and with multiple intervening variables. When physicians in training are assigned to, or volunteer for, the pain team they must be supervised by a more permanent pain team member, preferably a physician. In other words, it is crucial that the physician members of the pain team not include only interns and residents, but experienced practitioners too.

Physicians in many specialties are well trained in the evaluation and treatment of chronic pain, in particular, neurologists, neurosurgeons, anesthesiologists, psychiatrists, and physiatrists. Each tends, naturally, to approach the problem from the viewpoint of his or her own specialty. This may take place to such a degree that it is frequently helpful to have more than one physician team member. Anesthesiologists are quite a valuable asset to the multidisciplinary pain team. They are frequently the team member with the most specific training in the medical management of chronic pain (Bach, Carl, Ravlo, Crawford, and Werner, 1986; Carl, Crawford, Ravlo, and Bach, 1986; Srikantha, Choi, and Wu, 1986). Specific modalities employed include diagnostic and therapeutic "nerve blocks," electrical stimulation and, occasionally, acupuncture.

However, for general medical management of the inpatient, combined with specific training in neurophysiology and pharmacology, a neurologist, neurosurgeon, or psychiatrist is generally needed. In recent years, neurosurgeons have written a good deal about the treatment and management of chronic pain. Gildenberg (1984) has outlined an approach to be employed by any primary physician which includes such things as working with the spouse or caretaker, withdrawal from pain medications, management of depression, physical exercise, relaxation training, TENS, possible ablation procedures, and trigger point blocks. Several neurosurgeons (Long, 1983; Epstein, 1985) stress the importance of psychosocial assessment, behavior modification, and stress management. They then continue to discuss the use of TENS, intracranial stimulation, opiate infusion, dorsal column stimulation (Yingling and Hosobuchi, 1986), cordotomy and rhizotomy (Mullan, 1983; Saris, Silver, Vieira, and Nashold, 1986), and preoperative withdrawal from pain medications. Richardson (1983), in particular, stresses the importance of extensive evaluation and rehabilitation in a multidisciplinary pain unit prior to any consideration of operative interventions for pain.

Flexner (1985) also states that pain management should be accomplished in a multidisciplinary setting. In his case he recommends a team comprised of internists, surgeons, orthopedists, anesthesiologists, psychologists, psychiatrists, social workers, nurses, and physical therapists. He describes the role of the pain team physician as a thorough evaluation of the causes of the pain (skeletal, nervous system, viscera, tissue; necrosis, infection, ischemia; tension, anxiety, apprehension, depression), gathering information regarding the history and pattern of the pain, a physical examination (including neurological examination, thorough laboratory and radiologic studies, routine chemistry, EMG, and cystometry), administration of pain questionnaires (including the effect of the pain on activities of daily living [ADLS]), and differential nerve blocks. Only then is the physician in a position to make decisions regarding the use of analgesics (including route of administration as well as dosage), use of TENS, neurolytic blocks, epidural catheters, or neurosurgical procedures (e.g., cordotomies, rhizotomies, myelotomies, cranial nerve sections).

Obviously, the role of the physician team members will depend to some degree on where the patient is housed. For example, if the pain team beds are on neurology, the neurologist on the pain team may be the patient's primary care physician (or be supervising the patient's primary physician) while the other team physicians are acting in a consultant capacity. Conversely, if the beds are on medicine, the internist would be consultant. While it is this writer's belief that chronic pain patients, particularly when lacking any psychiatric diagnosis (other than, perhaps, chronic pain syndrome), should not be housed on psychiatric units, a number of pain programs are housed on the psychiatry service. Duke Medical Center (Houpt, Keefe, and Snipes, 1984) has a fifteen-bed inpatient pain program housed on the psychiatry service. The team consists of a psychiatrist, who is the medical director; a psychologist who coordinates the pain management program; a staff psychiatrist, who is the patient's primary physician and consults with anesthesiology, neurosurgery, and internal medicine; and psychiatric nurses. During the assessment phase, the psychiatrist is responsible for directly assessing the patient's intrapsychic and interpersonal dynamics, need for psychotropic medications, and possibility of addiction. He or she is also responsible for consulting with other specialties (anesthesiology, neurosurgery, orthopedics) regarding such modalities as nerve blocks, transcutaneous or implanted neurostimulators, or surgical procedures. During the treatment phase, the psychiatrist coordinates the overall care of the patient, prescribes psychotropic medications if indicated, performs individual and/or family therapy, and detoxifies the patient (if needed) employing a pain cocktail. Reich, Steward, Tupin, and Rosenblatt (1985) report on the activities of their multidisciplinary pain clinic with a slightly different team composition (medicine, anesthesiology, neurosurgery, neurology, psychiatry, psychology, clinical pharmacology, and medical social work).

When the pain team is not located on a psychiatric unit, the role of the psychiatrist on the pain team (where this individual is not the designated team builder or family therapist) is more like that of the consultation liaison psychiatrist. Depression, anger, and hostility are frequent accompaniments or consequences of chronic pain and may be treated effectively with psychotropic medications and/or psychotherapy. Psychiatrists, too, may be more familiar with designing detoxification schedules and suggesting alternate medications to deal with the symptoms of medication and/or alcohol withdrawal. They may also be more prepared to recognize when pain is an expression of underlying psychopathology (similar to what is occasionally found in sexual dysfunction in severe depressives, schizophrenics, or phobics).

Any physician, regardless of discipline, with specialized training in the evaluation and treatment of chronic pain is of greater value to the pain team than the most skillful neurosurgeon or talented neurologist who has not received such training. Barring the availability of such a physician, the next best individual is a physician who is willing to *learn* about chronic pain, perhaps even from a nonphysician.

The Social Worker

Although there are many well-known psychologists and psychiatrists who are family therapists and systems theorists (Minuchin and Barcai, 1972; Ackerman, 1972; Framo, 1972; Sager and Kaplan, 1972), the team member most likely to have had specific training and experience in family therapy is the social worker. The role of family dynamics in the maintenance of chronic pain problems is also well known (Waring, 1982; Roy, 1984). Yet, it is surprising how many pain teams do not have family assessment, let alone family therapy, as a routine part of their treatment program. Even more difficult to find is a pain team with a social worker specifically trained in analyzing the family dynamics which reinforce the chronic pain behaviors and undermine health behaviors. (Hickling et al.'s [1985] survey, mentioned earlier, found that almost 44 percent of the teams surveyed did not have a social worker as part of their team.) The case examples which could be given are too numerous and varied to even begin to cover here, however, see chapter 22. Relapse prevention is nearly impossible without working with the significant others of the identified pain patient. This is particularly true when the pain problem has persisted for a number of years or is embedded in a context of substance abuse, child abuse, spouse abuse, or psychopathology.

Roy (1981) describes the role of the social worker in the assessment and treatment of chronic pain problems. He stresses the importance of a thorough psychosocial assessment including specific exploration of the role that pain has played in the patient's life. In addition to the individual's psychological reaction to chronic pain (e.g., depression, anxiety), Dr. Roy suggests exploring the effect of the patient's pain problem on the performance of social roles (e.g., spouse, parent, worker) and an exploration of current family dynamics (e.g., the family's attitudes toward, and reaction to, the patient's pain behavior). The exploration of the patient's developmental history should include the patient's past experiences with pain, pain problems in other members of the patient's family of origin, and any history of physical or emotional abuse. Following this assessment, the social worker attempts to address the pain problem in psychosocial terms; for example, is the problem related to a life change, family problems, or is this a pain prone individual? The social worker's treatment options include individual psychotherapy or casework of a "client-centered, short-term, education, and problem-solving" nature (Roy, 1981, p. 60), conjoint marital therapy, or family therapy.

In addition to the crucial role of the social worker in family assessment and therapy, this individual might also be the best-trained team member in team building or conflict resolution. Finally, there is the traditional, valuable knowledge of social workers with regard to occupational and financial status, and community resources. Frequently, chronic pain problems have resulted in loss of employment and financial stresses which, in turn, exacerbate the chronic pain problem, and the social worker is generally the team member best equipped to address these issues. Community service specialists who assist the patient in dealing with a variety of community resources, including Social Security, Workman's Compensation, State Vocational Rehabilitation, and courts and lawyers, are frequently social workers by training.

The Nurse

As mentioned earlier, an inpatient pain team program can rarely if ever be successful without the cooperation of the ward staff. While the pain team's designated team builder may be helpful in gaining this cooperation in individual cases, the nurse pain team member (ideally, the head nurse of the ward that houses the pain team patients) is the most logical person for bridging the gap between the pain team and the ward staff. In particular, this person must be successful in counteracting the tendency to see these often difficult, frustrating, and/or manipulative patients as malingerers whose pain behaviors are all put on or entirely attention-seeking behavior. Pain patients are frequently demanding and irritating. In addition, it goes against almost all medical training to ignore pain behaviors and spend time with patients who are not in any distress, particularly, on a busy medical ward.

Often, too, when nursing notes are relegated to the back of the chart where, nurses suspect, they are never read, nurses feel devalued and taken for granted. They perceive requests to treat particular patients differently, perhaps rightfully, as unwelcome intrusions and extra burdens. Thus, the importance of the role of the head nurse (who, one hopes, is specially trained in the treatment of chronic pain) cannot be underestimated in helping the ward staff to understand the dynamics and treatment of chronic pain.

Finally, there is no better way to observe baseline behaviors and progress than by reading the nursing notes (which should be part of integrated progress notes on any ward that has a multidisciplinary team). If a patient says he is not sleeping, the nursing staff can chart whether this is an accurate self-perception. Is the patient being active, staying out of bed, socializing in a relaxed fashion with other patients, or sitting tensely in isolation? All of this information can be communicated by the ward staff if they are convinced that their input is valued and important to the treatment plan. Without such a sense of being valued, nursing notes may well, indeed, be "chatter charting" as some other professionals contend.

Houpt et al., (1984) describe the nurse's role in the assessment of the pain patient in terms of making direct behavioral observations of the patient's pain behaviors, drug usage, and interpersonal interactions, and then comparing these observations to the patient's own activity diary. In treatment, ward nursing staff actively encourage the patient in problem solving, improving communication skills, and understanding the relationship between stress and pain. They actively reward desired behaviors and discourage undesired ones. Fey and Fordyce (1983) also stress the important role that the nursing staff play in an inpatient pain team setting in reducing the social attention and reinforcement contingent upon pain behavior.

The recent National Institutes of Health Consensus Development conference on multidisciplinary management of pain (1987) specifically addressed the role of the nurse in such teams. They highlighted the role of the generally trained nurse in facilitating communication between the patient and family and other members of the team, and in encouraging the patient to participate in the decision-making process. They also suggest that the nurse is in an optimal position for linking up the patient with community health, public health, or home health care resources post discharge. In addition to preop patient education, the nurse may plan individual medication schedules based on individual preferences and activity schedules and implement nonpharmacological treatment methods during acutely painful events. The nurse with specialized training may also be responsible for the titration of analgesics, assessment and participation in the use of both pharmacological and nonpharmacological modalities, and education of, and consultation with, the other members of the nursing staff.

PHARMACY

Patients with chronic medical problems, including chronic pain, often come to the pain team on a bewildering array of medications: anti-inflammatory agents, narcotics or narcotic-like medications, antidepressants, antihypertensives, "seizure" medications, antianginals, antianxiety agents, laxatives, and antacids, to name but a few. The busy physician can rarely keep up with the vast array of pharmaceuticals while still treating patients and keeping abreast of new developments in his or her specialty. But, the pharmacist's full-time job is to be knowledgeable about pharmaceuticals. Often, it is the pharmacist member of the pain team who can suggest a new medication, dosage schedule, or route of administration to be attempted by the team or point out how one medication the patient is taking may be counteracting or adversely affecting the action of another (Swerdlow, 1984; Montastruc, Tran, Blanc, Charlet, David, Mansat, Cotonat, Patacq-Sapijanskas, Guiraud-Chaumeil, Rascol, and Montastruc, 1985).

Unfortunately, the staff of an active inpatient pharmacy may often not have the time or resources to develop individually tailored pain cocktails. But, where this is possible, it is a powerful mode of treatment involving detoxification and/or adjustment of relative dosages. The use of such a cocktail has been described elsewhere (Fordyce, 1976) and will not be discussed here except to mention that pain relief is often associated with the patient's perception of the size or strength of the medication. This association is best dealt with via the pain cocktail.

The pharmacist on the Ohio State University Hospital's pain management service (Kientz, Fitzsimmons, and Schneider, 1983) meets with the patient to negotiate a contract for stepwise decreases in analgesic and sedative drugs. The pharmacist also holds classes on more effective use of nonprescription drugs, and encourages family education and involvement.

REHABILITATION MEDICINE

Few descriptions of multidisciplinary pain teams omit the role of the physiatrist or the physical therapist (Doleys, Dolce,

Doleys, Crocker, and Wolfe, 1986; Guck, Meilman, Skultety, and Dowd, 1986). In addition to evaluation of strength, flexibility, and range of motion, the physical therapist possesses an impressive arsenal of effective pain treatment modalities, not the least of which are strengthening and flexion exercises, ultrasound, dry and moist heat, whirlpool, and TENS. Gait-training and conditioning exercises can increase independence and, frequently, directly decrease pain caused by improper adaptation to an injury. Often, too, it is the physiatrist or physical therapist who detects problems with wheelchairs, wheelchair seat cushions, braces, or other assistive devices that, in fact, either account for or exacerbate the chronic pain problem.

At a minimum, descriptions of pain team functioning generally mention establishing baseline physical activity levels and attempting to increase these levels (Fey and Fordyce, 1983). Increase in physical activity may be accomplished through walking, bicycling, calisthenics and mat exercises, and other general physical conditioning activities (Beckman and Axtell, 1985). However, in addition to such general physical activities, many programs (Houpt et al., 1984) evaluate posture, mobility, and muscle strength, and design individualized programs for patients including aerobic exercises, exercises to reverse the effects of pain-avoidance posturing, flexion and/or extension exercises, heat, ultrasound, TENS, and patient education.

In a 1984 survey of 263 multidisciplinary pain treatment centers, Doliber found that the most common treatments employed by physical therapists were individualized exercise programs, relaxation training, TENS, instruction in body mechanics, and biofeedback. Other treatments by physical therapists included group exercise, mobilization, hot packs, cold packs, deep muscle massage, ice massage, whirlpool, manipulation, therapeutic pool, and paraffin treatments. Least frequently used modalities were acutherapy, electrical nerve stimulation, gait training, traction, ultrasound, education in kinesiology, aerobic conditioning, leisure counseling, or electrical muscle stimulation. Most physical therapists responding reported meeting with family members of patients and conducting family education as well as teaching classes for patients on physical therapy. Other descriptions of physical therapy and pain control can be found in Graziano (1985) and Sikorski (1985).

Few descriptions of pain teams include the role of the occupational therapist. Yet, in addition to designing diversional activities (i.e., activities to "divert" the patient's attention from the pain), the occupational therapist assesses the patient's ability to independently perform ADLS and can suggest assistive devices to increase the patient's independence. Such increased independence (although occasionally resisted by the caregiver) frequently elevates mood and/or directly reduces pain perception.

A brief description of the role of occupational therapy (OT) in chronic pain management appeared in *Hospital Practice* (Borrelli and Warfield, 1986). In addition to assessing ADLS, the occupational therapist educates patients in modification of movement patterns and in the selection and use of a wide range of assistive devices (e.g., dressing sticks and stocking aids, built-up handles on utensils, raised toilet seats, reachers, back supports, tub chairs, and grab bars). They may administer retrograde massage and passive and active range-of-motion exercises. They may make recommendations for static or dynamic splints, contour pillows, or neck collars. They frequently teach joint protection (e.g., for arthritics).

Flower, Naxon, Jones, and Mooney (1981) describe a very thorough occupational therapy (OT) program for the management of chronic pain on the Orthopedic Spine Unit at VA Medical Center, Dallas. The initial OT evaluation consists of an assessment of daily vocational and home activities that may contribute to the patient's pain. Physically stressful activities are then reproduced, and physical responses, body mechanics, activity tolerance, pain reporting, and emotional responses are observed. During this phase education of the patient is begun in anatomy of the spine, techniques of relaxation, good body mechanics, and posture. The initial phase of OT treatment includes group OT (primarily education and demonstration of body mechanics and progressive muscle relaxation) and two hours of individual OT daily. During these latter sessions, patients engage in leatherworking or small woodworking projects with the goals of increasing tolerance to work-related activities, reducing tension, and monitoring body mechanics.

Phase II of the program is conducted in a day treatment center setting. Occupational therapy evaluation focuses on frustration tolerance, organizational ability, levels of depression, anxiety, hostility, and dependency, and body image. In daily OT sessions goals are to improve the patient's ability to responsibly interact with others, to positively reinforce new, healthy behaviors (including assertiveness), to increase work tolerance; planning for home and community activities; and to reduce pain behaviors through nonreinforcement. Walking exercises, relaxation training, and body mechanics class are continued from Phase I.

Recreation Therapy

Few articles mention the role of leisure time activities in the maintenance or the reduction of chronic pain. Yet, many patients give up leisure time activities (except watching TV) altogether or, conversely, persist in attempting leisure time activities which aggravate their pain problems (e.g., bowling, basketball, canoeing, bicycling). They do so because they are unaware of how to develop alternative satisfying activities, are unwilling to learn new activities, or refuse to accept their physical limitations. It is in this area that a skilled recreational therapist, knowledgeable in the area of sports physiology and disability, can make a significant contribution to the quality of life of the chronic pain patient.

Houpt et al.'s (1984) description of their multidisciplinary pain program illustrates the role that a recreation therapist can play in such a program. The recreational therapist assesses the patient's use of leisure time outside of the hospital and observes the patient's pursuit of recreational activities within the hospital. The recreational therapist then attempts to increase the patient's involvement in pleasant activities and to assist the patient in developing physical activities to aid in tension release, weight control, or general fitness.

DIETETICS

Low back pain patients, in particular, are frequently found to be obese. Headache and neck pain patients frequently consume excess caffeine. Many self-medicating patients are unaware of toxic levels of vitamin supplements and most patients are unaware of drug/food interactions. Yet, it is rare to find a dietitian member of a pain team. A thorough nutritional assessment by a qualified dietitian should be a standard part of every chronic pain assessment with particular attention to ideal body weight and its relationship to the chronic pain problem, eating patterns and food preferences, and adequacy of diet. Often, along with exercise, weight loss may be the most important aspect of pain control for the majority of low back pain sufferers.

Warfield and Stein (1983), in their column "The Pain Clinic" in *Hospital Practice*, point out that obesity is a frequent complication of chronic pain treatment and, for this reason if no other, "nutritional instruction often must be part of the treatment plan for the chronic pain patient" (p. 100). They also point out that a number of painful syndromes can be influenced by dietary changes. For example, migraine sufferers are usually instructed to avoid caffeine (coffee, tea, chocolate) and alcohol. A possible link has been established between dysmenorrhea and increased salt intake. Further, research (Seltzer, 1985; Millinger, 1986) has demonstrated that some maxillofacial pain sufferers may benefit from daily tryptophan supplements and a diet consisting of 80 percent carbohydrates, 10 percent protein, and 10 percent fat content.

INTERDISCIPLINARY COMMUNICATION

Given the multiplicity of the disciplines represented on the chronic pain treatment team, it is readily understandable that some common core of beliefs, values, and knowledge must be established. Ideally, all team members will regard the perception of pain by its sufferer as a complex phenomenon affected by social status, ethnicity, family dynamics, occupational status, and individual dynamics (to name but a few factors). The belief in a direct correlation between degree of anatomical "damage" and intensity of perceived pain should be strongly discouraged. Whenever possible, the team should have shared training by "outside experts" in the treatment of chronic pain (in medical settings, the biblical observation that a prophet is without honor in his own land was never truer). Where this is not possible, the team members, individually trained in their own specialty's approach to the treatment of chronic pain, are well advised to set up a number of meetings for the purpose of sharing their expertise with each other prior to sharing it with patients. It is to be hoped that, at this point, team members will begin to develop a mutual respect for each other's areas of expertise. Such respect will greatly reduce the occurrence of many communication difficulties and potential conflicts.

However, such difficulties and conflicts are bound to occur and are best regarded as a normal stage of team development. They will not be prevented by the team leader declaring that team meetings are to be "professional," to focus on the needs of the patient, and are not to involve personal interactions. It does not seem to be possible for persons (no matter what their professional identification) to continually interact with each other without such interactions being personal. Most professionals, having spent long years in training, are closely identified (and ego-involved) with their disciplines, and a perceived slight to their field of expertise can rarely be dismissed by advising the team member not to take it personally. Such instructions only serve to force the conflicts underground where they are considerably more difficult to resolve. Unresolved conflicts have a way of forming the basis of additional, more difficult conflicts. Thus, team members need to be encouraged to clarify communications, to ask questions, and to voice their feelings. The identified team builder is thereby enabled to function.

However, many communication problems are inevitable in a multidisciplinary team. The team members have spent many years learning the specialized terms and jargon of their field. Once it is agreed that no member's specialized jargon is superior to any of the others, team members can feel free to ask for definitions of terms and to begin to establish a shared language. Here, too, the nurse team member may be of valuable assistance since she may have many years experience in interpreting the jargon of a number of medical and health-related specialists to patients. A communications skills training exercise called nondefensive listening can be employed with considerable benefit in the early stages of team building. Learning that differing opinions do not necessarily mean that the team member's input is not valuable is frequently difficult in multidisciplinary team functioning. When the team leader is also the physician responsible for writing orders during the patient's hospital stay, this may present considerable difficulty. For example, if the anesthesiology member of the team feels a trial of diagnostic blocks is indicated and the neurosurgeon team member disagrees and refuses to write an order, this conflict can only be dealt with by a discussion of both physicians' opinions in a team meeting. If the neurosurgeon simply omits the referral, all team members may be affected, assuming that the inpatient physician has veto power over team decisions. This may well be true even if the two physicians satisfactorily clarify their difference of opinion outside the team meeting since the rest of the team is kept in the dark. It is most important that all team members are knowledgeable about what is being done with the patient and why. With such knowledge, even when they may not be in total agreement, team members can act professionally and carry out a unified treatment plan. Without such knowledge, personal conflicts or even covert sabotage of the treatment plan, may well occur.

Conflict Resolution

All conflicts among team members, either personal or professional, are best dealt with within a team meeting. If not in a regularly scheduled administrative meeting or a more frequently held treatment planning meeting, then at a specially convened meeting of all available team members (including, of course, *both* parties to the conflict). However, this is not intended to condone crisis management. Whenever a team has frequent crises requiring special team meetings, a careful analysis needs to be done of team composition, team functioning and process, and (in particular) formal (and informal) team leadership. (The designated team leader is often not the person the team looks to for leadership.) The designated expert in team building is generally the team member who can perform this function. In particular, the team builder needs to be alert for the possibility that the formal, or informal, team leader is a crisis manager, one who manages by creating crises (or "allowing" crises to occur) which he or she is able to resolve, thereby demonstrating leadership. Many people in the helping professions feel bored, restless, or dysfunctional unless they are dealing with crises, but equally many burn out in such a system. Therefore, it is important to distinguish which team conflicts require special meetings from those which can be dealt with in a regular team meeting. All team meetings need to be long enough to allow for conflict resolution. If, in spite of the efforts of the team builder, frequent conflicts continue, it may be necessary to contact an outside expert. Such experts may often be located through an affiliated university with a training program in conflict resolution. Another option might be through borrowing the team builder from another medical facility's pain team or other multidisciplinary treatment team (e.g., geriatrics evaluation unit team).

Of course, there are times when a team member may decide that she or he does not agree with the overall team philosophy and may decide to leave the team rather than find herself or himself in constant conflict with the rest of the team. In the writer's opinion, there are few people who are not "team players" (i.e., who are unable to work cooperatively with other members of a team) but there are people who are quite talented and possess considerable expertise in pain treatment who present themselves in an authoritarian manner and frequently offend other team members. Conversely, there are equally skilled individuals who feel insecure in their own abilities or defensive about their discipline's status relative to other disciplines on the team and may feel offended quite easily. While in a private facility in a large metropolitan area rich in professional resources, it might be possible to simply discharge such individuals from the pain team, for most facilities this is not possible without destroying the team.

Summary

While most chronic pain treatment teams consist of a core of physicians, psychologists, and physical therapists, numerous other professionals can make valuable contributions to the treatment of the chronic pain patient. Particularly important are the team's designated team builder and family therapist. In addition, inpatient teams are well advised to include nursing representation on the team. The ideal team would consist of two or more physician members (neurology, neurosurgery, psychiatry, etc.) of which one, if possible, should be an anesthesiologist; psychologist, social worker, nurse, physical therapist, occupational therapist, recreational therapist, pharmacist, and dietitian.

With such a variety of disciplines involved, communication problems and conflicts are bound to occur and should be perceived as a normal stage in team development. Such conflicts need to be dealt with openly in regularly scheduled team meetings. The team's designated team builder plays a crucial role in conflict resolution, thereby allowing the team to function smoothly and provide comprehensive and consistent patient care to sufferers of chronic pain.

Case Illustration

The case of Mr. H is a fictionalized case study derived from a number of cases seen by this pain team over the past six years. Mr. H was a forty-seven-year-old white male who had suffered from low back pain for over twenty years. During this period he had been treated intermittently with analgesics, minor tranquillizers, and physical therapy, but with only temporary relief. However, he was able to maintain gainful employment. Within the year preceding his referral he was diagnosed as having cancer of the thyroid which was successfully treated. Following his surgery, pain complaints increased and extended to hip and shoulder pain. Medications included thyroxine, a moderate dosage of a tricyclic antidepressant taken four times daily, and ranitidine. Mr. H was almost totally immobilized by his pain complaints, doing little other than watching TV and smoking cigarettes.

Mr. H was first screened by the psychologist. Since he had mostly been seen by private physicians and in several different private and university hospitals, he was asked to bring a copy of his medical records to the screening. Results of psychological evaluation revealed that he was well motivated and open to learning nonchemical, nonsurgical means of dealing with his pain problem. He was of average, or higher, intelligence. Personality testing indicated that he was a tense, rigid person who tended to respond to stress with a heightened and prolonged physical response which might lead to the development of physical problems (i.e., a psychophysiological stress responder). He tended to minimize or deny emotional problems. Pain complaints showed no particular pattern except that pain was relieved by rest or inactivity and exacerbated by any type of physical activity. His wife was presented as "a wonderful woman" who did anything she could to relieve his pain and suffering.

The results of the initial screening, together with available medical records, were presented at the next regularly scheduled meeting of the pain team. The internist's review of the medical records was significant for a vagotomy due to peptic ulcer disease about seven years in the past, neurological findings consistent with a possible herniated disc, and unsuccessful treatment with biofeedback-assisted relaxation therapy, in addition to the previously reported surgery for thyroid cancer. There had been no consistent follow-up of his thyroxine replacement therapy with the patient seemingly adjusting his own dosage of medication depending on his self-perceived symptoms. It was noted that the patient had refused recommended nerve blocks. The team decided to admit Mr. H for further evaluation and treatment. The internist wrote the order to admit Mr. H to an acute medicine bed for the evaluation phase (7–10 days) of a planned four-week stay.

Mr. H presented for admission accompanied by his wife, as requested. Once his admission was processed, they were met on the ward by the team's administrative coordinator. Almost from his first hour on the ward he began to complain of pain and a variety of conditions and procedures which he found annoying. He and his wife were met by the social worker and a psychosocial assessment of the couple was completed. It was noted that he largely answered the questions while his wife sat quietly out of his sight and either nodded concurrence or, occasionally, caught the social worker's eye to nonverbally indicate that she did not agree. The couple were financially secure. This was the second marriage for each and they had been married for ten years. Her fourteen-year-old son lived with them while his four children lived with his first wife and stayed with them on alternate weekends. The couple agreed that since his forced medical retirement following his diagnosis of cancer he had become increasingly disabled by his pain, to the point that he rarely left the house and was almost totally inactive. Considerably more history was revealed when the social worker met alone with the wife on a subsequent visit. The wife had been given a spouse's pain questionnaire to fill in and return. Her answers showed her to be quite responsive to her husband's pain complaints and resentful of her caretaking activities. She reported that Mr. H had a history of alcoholism and had physically abused her in the past. Added to this was a history of abuse of pain medications and tranquillizers by the patient. All of this had stopped only with his diagnosis of cancer. She believed that he was terminally ill. Her mother had died of cancer after a long debilitating illness during which Mrs. H was her primary caregiver.

During the evaluation phase, neurosurgery was consulted. Although they did not feel surgical interventions were indicated, they suggested a number of radiologic procedures to rule out bone metastases. Findings were largely normal except for some evidence of degenerative joint disease of the spine, shoulders, and hips, as well as the previously mentioned bulging disc. Laboratory results were also normal with the exception of a low thyroxine level. In addition to numerous complaints and righteous indignation by the patient about the hospital food, the dietitian's assessment revealed that Mr. H was about fifteen pounds over his ideal body weight. He refused a weight-loss diet but agreed to a diet with no added concentrated sweets and no added salt. His diet at home was deemed to be nutritionally adequate without excessive caffeine or sugar. Mr. H stated he would lose the excess poundage simply by cutting back his food portions. Neurological evaluation revealed some peripheral neuropathy bilaterally of the hands and feet. Occupational therapy assessment found him to be largely independent in performance of ADLS but in need of assistive devices such as eating utensils with enlarged, weighted handles. Diversional activities could be performed for about twenty minutes before Mr. H became restless and complained of pain. Physical therapy evaluation revealed restricted range of motion in the shoulders but good strength in the upper extremities. Some weakness of the lower extremities was also noted. A trial of EMG biofeedback showed that Mr. H was quite good at using this modality and found it helpful in reducing his pain. His previous unsuccessful trial had not included guided imagery. Recreational therapy determined that Mr. H's primary leisure time activities had included hunting, fishing, and boating. These were often with his "drinking buddies" and often included camping out. Sleeping on the ground, understandably, increased his pain complaints. Nursing staff reported that Mr. H walked rigidly and slowly but was quite active on the ward, generally being out of his room, working on small projects provided by occupational therapy, or practicing his relaxation exercises with a tape recorder provided. Although he complained that the noise and activity in his four-person room interfered with his concentration and with his sleep, he was quite friendly with the other patients in his room. Mild sleep disturbance was documented. Most significant were ward observations of his quick temper, low frustration tolerance, and his many demands for attention or special favors. Staff also noted his tendency to become righteously indignant on behalf of other patients. They were quite relieved when he was transferred to a rehabilitation bed for the remainder of his stay.

At the end of the evaluation phase, the team again met to discuss the findings and to make recommendations for treatment. It was noted that chloral hydrate had been started and cimetidine substituted for ranitidine, without consulting the team. The pharmacist pointed out the possible interactive effects of cimetidine and antidepressant medications and suggested altering the dosage schedule of the antidepressant from QID to most of the dose HS and the remainder AM. The internist concurred and discontinued chloral hydrate. Thyroxine was also increased. Mr. H had also begun to complain of epigastric distress and an EKG and upper GI series was ordered. However, cimetide was also withdrawn and ranitidine restarted.

Physical therapy recommended a trial of TENS, flexion exercises, and moist heat. Occupational therapy recommended an increase in diversional activities. Social work recommended that the internist meet with the patient and wife together to explain that Mr. H was not terminally ill. Marital therapy was also recommended. Psychology recommended a continuation of biofeedback-assisted relaxation therapy and the addition of cognitive restructuring strategies. Anesthesiology recommended a trial of nerve blocks. Nursing recommended confrontation of the patient's quick anger and low frustration tolerance and encouragement of self-reliance in place of demands for others to perform tasks he was well able to do himself.

The most effective modalities for Mr. H proved to be moist heat (which he learned to apply himself once he was provided with a moist heating pad), TENS (which he learned to apply himself, although initially trying to insist the ward staff do so), and biofeedback-assisted relaxation therapy (particularly after he was able to suggest guided imagery which he thought he would find most helpful). He was rather resistant to marital therapy, but his wife found it quite helpful and was able to relieve some of her resentment and gradually give up her caretaker role. The alteration in antidepressant dosing schedule resulted in improved sleep without undue daytime nervousness. He continued to refuse nerve blocks, having found these other modalities helpful. He became quite involved in diversional activities and was able to concentrate on these for more than an hour at a time without motor restlessness or pain complaints. Overall he reported greater than a 50 percent decrease in pain levels and demonstrated a considerable increase in activity level.

The team met again during the last week of Mr. H's stay to devise an outpatient treatment plan. Weekly visits were recommended for marital therapy with the social worker and individual psychotherapy with the psychologist (focusing on increasing frustration tolerance, decreasing anger, and improving relaxation responses). Monthly visits were recommended to the Endocrine clinic (for regular monitoring of thyroxine levels), the Medicine clinic (for monitoring of other medications), Physical Therapy (with decreasing frequency to monitor performance of exercises), Occupational Therapy (for monitoring home activities program), Recreational Therapy (for refinement and reinforcement of alternative leisure time activities), Dietetics (Mr. H had gained five pounds during his inpatient stay), and the Psychology Service (for overall coordination and monitoring of the treatment plan). Six months following discharge all gains had been stabilized and Mr. H concurred with discontinuing regularly scheduled appointments to all but Endocrine Clinic. Since pain patients often relapse after discharge from a formal pain team program a follow-up appointment was scheduled with the administrative coordinator for three months after discontinuing of regularly scheduled appointments. Mr. H agreed not to take any pain medications or undergo surgeries or other modalities for the relief of pain without first consulting with the pain team.

The particular pain team's philosophy regarding the nature and treatment of chronic pain will largely determine its composition and functioning. Therefore, the above example is intended to illustrate only one approach to evaluation and treatment. The philosophy of the team described is that different modalities may work better for one patient than another; however, emphasis is placed on teaching the patient things he or she can do to reduce pain levels rather than on things perceived by the patient as being done to him or her. A good deal of motivation, ability to learn new behaviors, willingness to make life-style changes, and freedom from such complications as active abuse of nonprescribed chemicals (such as alcohol) or psychosis is required. This team was under the administrative direction of the psychology service and was composed of a psychologist, social worker, internist, physical therapist, occupational therapist, nurse, dietitian, anesthesiologist, pharmacist, and recreational therapist.

References

Ackerman, N. W. (1972), The growing edge of family therapy. In: *Progress in Group and Family Therapy*, eds. C. Sager & H. Kaplan. New York: Brunner/Mazel.

Bach, V., Carl, P., Ravlo, O., Crawford, M. E., & Werner, M. (1986), Potentiation of epidural opiods with epidural droperidol. *Anaesthes.*, 41:1116–1119.

Beckman, C., & Axtell, L. (1985), Ambulation, activity level, and pain. *Phys. Ther.*, 65/1:1649–1657.

Borrelli, E., & Warfield, C. (1986), Occupational therapy for chronic pain. *Hosp. Pract.*, 21/8:36–37.

Carl, P., Crawford, M. E., Ravlo, O., & Bach, V. (1986), Long-term treatment with epidural opiods. *Anaesthes.*, 41:32–38.

Dolce, J., Crocker, M., & Doleys, D., (1986), Prediction of outcome among chronic pain patients. *Behav. Res. Ther.*, 24/3:313–319.

Doleys, D., Dolce, J., Doleys, A., Crocker, M. & Wolfe, S. (1986), Evaluation, narcotics, and behavioral treatment influences on pain ratings in chronic pain patients. *Arch Phys. Med. Rehabil.*, 67:456–458.

Doliber, C. (1984), Role of the physical therapist at pain treatment centers: A survey. *Phys. Ther.*, 64/6:905–909.

Epstein, J. A. (1985), Changing trends in the neurosurgical management of chronic pain. *Spine*, 10/1:100–101.

Fey, S. G., & Fordyce, W. E. (1983), Behavioral rehabilitation of the chronic pain patient. *Ann. Rev. Rehabil.*, 3:32–63.

Flexner, J. M. (1985), Management of chronic pain. *Compr. Ther.*, 11/4:6–9.

Flower, A., Naxon, E., Jones, R., & Mooney, V. (1981), An occupational therapy program for chronic back pain. *Amer. J. Occup. Ther.*, 35/4:243–248.

Fordyce, W. (1976), *Behavioral Methods for Chronic Pain and Illness*. St. Louis: C. V. Mosby.

Framo, J. L. (1972), Symptoms from a family transactional viewpoint. In: *Progress in Group and Family Therapy*, eds. C. Sager, & H. Kaplan. New York: Brunner/Mazel.

Gildenberg, P. L. (1984), Management of chronic pain. *Appl. Neurophysiol.*, 47/4–6:157–170.

Graziano, J. (1985), Retrospective analysis of acute and chronic pain control in physical therapy and rehabilitation with T.E.N.S. *Basal Facts*, 7/1:75–80.

Greenhoot, J. H., & Sternbach, R. A. (1977), Conjoint treatment of chronic pain. In: *Pain: A Source Book for Nurses and Other Health Professionals*, ed. A. Jacox. Boston: Little, Brown, pp. 295–302.

Guck, T., Meilman, P., Skultety, F. M., & Dowd, E. T. (1986), Prediction of long-term outcome of multidisciplinary pain treatment. *Arch. Phys. Med. Rehabil.*, 67:293–296.

Hickling, E. J., Sison, G. F. P., & Holtz, J. L. (1985), Role of psychologists in multidisciplinary pain clinics: A national survey. *Prof. Psychol.: Res. & Prac.*, 16:868–880.

Houpt, J., Keefe, F., & Snipes, M. (1984), The clinical specialty unit: The use of the psychiatry inpatient unit to treat chronic pain syndrome. *Gen. Hosp. Psychiat.*, 6:65–70.

Keefe, F. J., & Bradley, L. A. (1984), Behavioral and psychological approaches to the assessment and treatment of chronic pain. *Gen. Hosp. Psychiat.*, 6:49–54.

Kientz, J. E., Fitzsimmons, D. S., & Schneider, P. J. (1983), Reducing medication use in a chronic pain management program. *Amer. J. Hosp. Pharm.*, 40:2156–2158.

Long, D. M. (1983), Stimulation of the peripheral nervous system for pain control. *Clin. Neurosurg.*, 31:323–343.

Melzack, R. (1973), *The Puzzle of Pain*. New York: Basic Books.

Millinger, G. (1986), Neutral amino acid therapy for the management of chronic pain. *J. Craniomand. Prac.*, 4:157–162.

Minuchin, S., & Barcai, A. (1972), Therapeutically induced family crisis. In: *Progress in Group and Family Therapy*, eds. C. Sager & H. Kaplan. New York: Brunner/Mazel.

Montastruc, J., Tran, M., Blanc, M., Charlet, J., David, J., Mansat, M., Cotonat, J., Patacq-Sapijankas, M., Guiraud-Chaumeil, B., Rascol, A., & Monstastruc, P. (1985), Measurement of plasma levels of clomipramine in the treatment of chronic pain. *Clin. Neuropharm.*, 8/1:78–82.

Moore, J. E., & Chaney, E. F. (1985), Outpatient group treatment of chronic pain: Effects of spouse involvement. *J. Consult. Clin. Psychol.*, 53:326–334.

Mullan, S. F. (1983), Cordotomy and rhizotomy for pain. *Clin. Neurosurg.*, 31:344–350.

National Institute of Health Consensus Development Conference (1987), The integrated approach to the management of pain. *J. Pain & Symp. Mgmt.*, 2/1:35–44.

Newman, R. I., Seres, J. L., Yospe, L. P., & Garlington, B. (1978), Multidisciplinary treatment of chronic pain: Long-term follow-up of low-back pain patients. *Pain*, 4:283–292.

Reich, J., Steward, M., Tupin, J., & Rosenblatt, R. (1985), Prediction of response to treatment in chronic pain patients. *J. Clin. Psychiat.*, 46:425–427.

Richardson, D. E. (1983), Intracranial stimulation for the control of chronic pain. *Clin. Neurosurg.*, 31:317–318.

Roy, R. (1981), Social work and chronic pain. *Health & Soc. Work*, 6:54–62.

——— (1984), "I have a headache tonight": Function of pain in marriage. *Internat. J. Fam. Ther.*, 6/3:165–175.

Sager, C., & Kaplan, H., eds. (1972), *Progress in Group and Family Therapy*. New York: Brunner/Mazel.

Saris, S. C., Silver, J. M., Vieira, J. F., & Nashold, B. S. (1986), Sacrococcygeal rhizotomy for perineal pain. *Neurosurg.*, 19/5:789–793.

Seltzer, S. (1985), Pain relief by dietary manipulation and tryptophan supplements. *J. Endodon.*, 11/10:449–453.

Sikorski, J. (1985), A rationalized approach to physiotherapy for low-back pain. *Spine*, 10/6:571–579.

Srikantha, K., Choi, J., & Wu, W. (1986), Electrical stimulation of the celiac plexus for pain relief in chronic pancreatitis. *Internat. J. Acupunc. Electro-Ther. Res.*, 11:111–117.

Swerdlow, M. (1984), Anticonvulsant drugs and chronic pain. *Clin. Neuropharm.*, 7/1:51–82.

Turk, D. C., Meichenbaum, D., & Genest, M. (1983), *Pain and Behavioral Medicine*. New York: Guilford Press.

Warfield, C., & Stein, J. (1983), The nutritional treatment of pain. *Hosp. Pract.*, 18/7:100N–100P.

Waring, E. M. (1982), Conjoint marital and family therapy. In: *Chronic Pain: Psychosocial Factors in Rehabilitation*, eds. R. Roy & E. Tunks. Baltimore: Williams & Wilkins, pp. 151–165.

Yingling, C. S., & Hosobuchi, Y. (1986), Use of antidromic evoked potentials in placement of dorsal cord disc electrodes. *Appl. Neurophysiol.*, 49:36–41.

21

Using Drugs for Cancer Pain

MARGARET A. RANKIN, R.N., B.S.N., M.A.

To the general public, a diagnosis of cancer is often perceived as being synonymous with pain; one of their greatest immediate concerns is fear of unrelieved pain (Oster, Vizel, and Turgeon, 1978; Cleeland, 1984b; Cohen, Ferrer-Brechner, Pavlov, and Reading, 1985). Health professionals recognize that not all cancer patients suffer from pain, but for some it can be a serious complication. It occurs most commonly in the later stages of the disease with recurrence of the tumor or metastasis. Bonica (1978) states that by the time patients are hospitalized for cancer, approximately 60 to 80 percent suffer from severe pain.

Stjernsward, Cancer Chief of the World Health Organization (WHO), conservatively estimates that at least 3.5 million people worldwide are suffering from cancer pain daily (World Health Organization, 1985; Roller, 1986). Surveys of patients with cancer indicate that (1) 38 percent of patients in all stages of cancer experience pain (Foley, 1981); (2) 40 percent of patients in intermediate stages and 55 to 85 percent of patients in advanced or terminal stages experience moderate to severe

Acknowledgment. The two studies cited within this chapter were substudies of Federal Grant NU00467–3, Pain Alleviation Through Nursing Intervention, directed by Ada K. Jacox, Ph.D., and also funded by a 1980 Summer Research Fellowship from the University of Iowa College of Nursing.

pain (Bonica, 1982); (3) 80 percent experience more than one anatomically distinct pain (Twycross and Fairfield, 1982); (4) 73 percent of terminal patients experience sleep disruption because of pain. (Daut and Cleeland, 1982).

A questionnaire sponsored by the WHO and administered to 1000 cancer patients with pain in Israel, Japan, Brazil, India, and Sri Lanka indicated that less than 10 percent of those suffering from severe pain obtained complete relief from current treatment. In addition, 29 percent with moderate pain reported little or no relief. In a study by Cleeland (1984a), 47 percent of the patients rated their pain relief from treatment or medication on a 0 to 100 percent scale as greater than 70 percent while 13 percent reported less than 30 percent relief. This data certainly indicates that cancer pain is a major problem throughout the world.

Pain has been defined by the International Association for the Study of Pain (IASP) (1979) as "an unpleasant sensory and emotional experience associated with actual or potential tissue damage" (p. 250). It is therefore a dual phenomenon consisting of perception of the sensation followed by the patient's emotional reaction to it (Twycross, 1982). However, Sternbach (1968) emphasized that pain is an abstract concept referring to: "(1) a personal, private sensation of hurt; (2) a harmful stimulus which signals current or impending tissue damage; and (3) a pattern of responses which operate to protect the organism from harm" (p. 12). Therefore, pain serves as a feeling, stimulus, or response, which Melzack (1975) refers to respectively as the affective, sensory, and evaluative aspects of the pain experience. Pain, then, as a subjective experience can only be described by the person to whom it occurs, and others can only observe behaviors associated with that person's response to it.

Jacox and Stewart (1973) described the pain of patients with cancer as "progressive pain." This pain seems to become more extensive and intense with the physiological progression of the disease through its various stages. Also, the pain seems to be intensified psychologically because patients know that the disease causing the pain will ultimately cause their death.

Therefore, both physiological and psychological mechanisms influence the character of the pain as the disease progresses.

The pain of cancer patients has been portrayed by those who work with them in various ways. Bonica (1953) noted that the pain "becomes progressively more severe and finally develops into violent, boring, relentless, intolerable agonizing suffering, which soon demoralizes the victim and prevents him from eating, resting, or sleeping" (p. 1422). Twycross and Lack (1983) stated that the "pain is continuous and tends to get worse. This produces mental and physical exhaustion. The patient becomes demoralized, depressed, and increasingly fearful as yet another day of unrelieved suffering is anticipated. In addition, frequently the patient is incapacitated by pain, and becomes housebound or bedfast" (p. 9). Saunders (1981) indicated that for these patients: "Pain can blot out the world, cut off all true communication and perpetually renew a vicious circle of pain, fear, tension and further pain. . . . Terminal pain . . . traps the patient in a situation for which there is no reassuring explanation and to which there is no foreseeable end" (p. 219).

Hospitalized cancer patients themselves have commented about their pain to illustrate their agony and suffering:

> 1. Cancer pain is nasty pain, deep pain, like a toothache gets in there and aches and you go crazy with it. I just wish I could be free of it. It won't give up. It gets so you can't even think . . . can't concentrate, don't want anyone around, and then when alone, I didn't know what to do!
>
> 2. The mental anguish is almost unbearable!
>
> 3. It just "picks" at you constantly.
>
> 4. Sometimes I just feel like tearing things apart because I hurt so bad.
>
> 5. At its worst, it's excruciating and then you want to cry and throw things. I hate the world and everything in general!
>
> 6. The pain is so bad at night I just hate to see it coming. I don't know how I can face it. I don't know how I can stand it day after day.
>
> 7. If I have to wait too long for my pain pill, it takes longer to take effect [Rankin, 1980, p. 57].

These comments certainly confirm the previously described observations of cancer care experts.

Stages of Cancer Pain

Three stages of cancer pain have been described by Mathews, Zarro, and Osterholm (1973) to outline how the character of pain changes as the disease progresses. These are the early, intermediate, and late stages.

Early stage pain usually occurs during the diagnostic phase of the illness. It most often occurs following surgery for diagnosis or treatment of the primary lesion. As with all incisional pain, the intensity decreases markedly after the third day and eventually subsides. However, the mental stress and tension of awaiting the results of the diagnostic tests and pathology reports may add to this discomfort. This pain closely resembles acute pain since it is short term and temporary.

Intermediate stage pain usually results from cancer recurrence or metastasis. However, postoperative contractions of scars, nerve entrapment, or neuroma formation may also cause pain during this stage. Further diagnostic procedures and surgery again produce discomfort. Anxiety about the outcome may be even higher than during the early stage. Treatment varies according to the precipitating pathology and stage of the disease. The pain for some may again subside, but for others it may require palliative treatment with radiation, chemotherapy, neurosurgery, or analgesics.

These palliative methods may even add to the patient's discomfort. For instance, patients receiving radiation to the pelvis may develop the burning discomfort of cystitis secondary to radiation. For severely emaciated patients, simply lying on the hard table to receive the radiation treatments may cause extreme discomfort. Patients receiving intravenous chemotherapy often dread the discomfort precipitated by repeated venous punctures, side effects of the drugs, or the drug itself. For example, patients receiving Vinblastine sometimes report pain in the original tumor site while receiving that chemotherapeutic agent (Lucas and Huang, 1977). Neurosurgical prodecures sometimes produce deafferentation type pain which seems to be extremely difficult to control (Foley, 1985). Thus, the characteristics of intermediate stage pain may resemble temporary acute pain, the long-enduring qualities of chronic pain, or a mixture of the two.

Late stage pain coincides with the terminal stage of the illness when treatment methods no longer affect the progress of the disease. During this stage, patients often experience both anxiety and depression as they become more debilitated and realize that death is imminent. Continuous pain overwhelms them and seems to rule their lives. It interferes with all their normal activities and prevents them from enjoying living. Thus, this stage of pain is consistent with chronic, intractable pain because it persists and remains refractory to treatment. Symptomatic methods to relieve the distress and narcotic analgesics to control the pain are the only treatment approaches remaining.

Pain Syndromes

While collecting data from cancer patients at Memorial Sloan-Kettering Cancer Center, Foley (1979) distinguished three major pain syndromes according to etiology. Patients may have pain (1) associated with the malignant tumor; (2) associated with cancer therapy; or (3) be unrelated to either the tumor or its therapy. The number of patients affected by each syndrome varies with the setting. For example, approximately 78 percent of hospitalized patients and 62 percent of patients in the outpatient clinic suffered pain associated with direct tumor growth. Only 19 percent of hospitalized patients and 28 percent of clinic patients were afflicted with pain from cancer therapy. Fewer patients complained of pain unrelated to either cancer or cancer therapy since only 3 percent of hospitalized and 10 percent of clinic patients fell into this category (Foley, 1982).

Pain Associated with Tumor

Pain associated with the tumor can result from both physiological and psychological factors. Five physiological mechanisms produce pain: (1) bone invasion and destruction; (2) nerve infiltration or compression; (3) obstruction of a viscus or vessel; (4) infiltration or distention of integument or tissue; (5) inflammation, infection, and necrosis of tissue (Bonica, 1953, 1982; Derrick, 1972; Murphy, 1973; Parker, 1974). The psychological component of cancer pain depends upon the perception of threat or stress and the individual's subsequent reaction to it (Lazarus, 1966). Both physiological mechanisms and psychological factors will be discussed further in the following paragraphs.

Physiological Mechanisms. Bone destruction by tumor infiltration is the most common physiological cause of pain in patients with cancer, and may occur from either direct primary invasion or metastasis (Foley, 1979, 1981). Metastatic bone lesions are often secondary to primary carcinomas of the breast, lung, prostate, kidney, bowel, and lymphoid tissue (Parker, 1974; Twycross, 1978). The usual bones involved are the spine, pelvis, and long bones (Foley, 1981). According to Twycross (1978), bone metastases produce a prostaglandin which causes bone resorption and lowers the pain threshold by sensitizing free nerve endings. Bone destruction may lead to pathological fractures without displacement which then cause increased sensitiveness over the area or produce sharp, continuous, lancinating pain (Bonica, 1953; Charkes, Durant, and Barry, 1972). The pain often becomes more evident upon movement and ambulation. When radiation is used to treat it, the pain intensity usually decreases by the fourth day of treatment. Because dramatic resolution of the pain often occurs with appropriate treatment, this pain is similar to acute pain (Foley, 1982).

Infiltration or compression of nerve tissue by tumor may occur at any level of the nervous system; that is, peripheral nerves, plexus, spinal cord, or meninges. Thus, the sacral plexus may become involved from metastatic spread from the cervix or the brachial plexus secondary to carcinoma of the breast. Pain sensations vary considerably with location of the tumor (Foley, 1981). For instance, meningeal infiltration causes headache (Foley, 1981), while infiltration or compression of peripheral nerves or nerve plexus produces continuous, sharp, stabbing pain (Bonica, 1953) or a constant, burning sensation (Foley, 1979). Hyperesthesia, paresthesia, and dysesthesia may result (Bonica, 1953; Foley, 1979). If early treatment is not instituted, irreversible nerve damage may occur, pain may persist in spite of eradication of the primary tumor, and management of this chronic pain may be difficult (Foley, 1982).

Obstruction of a viscus, or hollow organ, may occur when an organ lumen becomes obstructed by tumor growth (Bonica, 1982). Thus, if the gastrointestinal or genitourinary tract becomes obstructed, severe, colicky, crampy abdominal pain is produced which may radiate to the shoulder or groin (Parker, 1974; Foley, 1981). The pain is often accompanied by significant dysfunctional symptoms in the affected system (Foley, 1981).

Obstruction of a vessel, like a vein, artery, or lymphatic channel, may result in venous engorgement, arterial ischemia, or edema. For instance, arm edema may occur secondary to axillary metastasis from breast cancer, or leg edema may be secondary to intrapelvic tumors. The subsequent pain is characterized by a dull, diffuse, burning, and aching sensation (Bonica, 1953, 1982).

Infiltration or distention of integument, fascia, or tissue occurs when skin or tissue is tightly stretched from underlying tumor growth, as from a carcinoma of the neck, or when ascites and tumor distend the abdomen. It produces localized, dull, aching pain which becomes more severe as the tumor increases in size (Bonica, 1953, 1982).

Inflammation, which initiates redness, edema, pain, heat, and loss of function, may progress to necrosis and sloughing of tissue. The pain of inflammation begins as very sensitive, tenderness to touch, but it may become excruciating with actual necrosis and sloughing of tissue (Bonica, 1953, 1982). Therefore, pain during dressing changes may be especially severe.

Psychological Factors. As stated previously, the psychological component of cancer pain is associated with individuals' perceptions of threat or stress and their reactions to it (Lazarus, 1966). Thus how people react, or cope, with their pain depends upon their perception of (1) how threatening it is to their lives and (2) their resources and capabilities to successfully meet the demands of the situation (Lazarus and Folkman, 1984). Both personality characteristics and past experience influence the interpretation of threat and appraisal of coping resources. Because the threat configuration varies with the stage of the illness, patients coping responses likewise vary. Thus, it is their interpretation of pain as a stressor which produces the reactive or affective component of pain. Patients may refer to this aspect as distress, suffering, or "mental anguish." According to Lamerton (1973), "These mental pains may be at least as bad as the physical ones" (p. 57). However, any physical distress only serves to enhance the mental suffering (Saunders, 1981).

Cassell (1983) defines this suffering component as severe distress associated with events which (1) threaten the intactness or wholeness of people, and (2) continue until the threat is gone or the integrity of the person is otherwise restored. He states:

> Patients may tolerate severe pain without considering themselves to be suffering, if they know the source of the pain, that it can be controlled, and that it will come to an end. However, even apparently minor pain or other symptoms may cause suffering if they are believed to have a dire cause (e.g., a malignant neoplasm), if they are viewed as never-ending, or if patients consider the symptom (and themselves) to be beyond help, or if their condition is considered hopeless [p. 522].

Continuous pain from cancer which interferes with peoples' life-styles could definitely threaten their sense of wholeness to provoke the suffering that Cassell describes.

Volicer and Bohannon (1975) designed a study asking 261 medical and surgical patients to rank order forty-nine events perceived as stressful in the hospital setting. The events were ranked from least to most stressful so that items creating the most stress had the highest number values. Results indicated the following: "Not getting relief from pain medications" was ranked fortieth; "Not getting pain medications when you need it" was forty-second; "Knowing you have a serious illness" was forty-sixth, and "Thinking you might have cancer" was forty-eighth. This implies that cancer patients with inadequately relieved pain perceive their situation as highly stressful and probably suffer severe distress.

Engel (1962) lists three categories of psychological stressors: (1) injury or threatened injury; (2 loss or threatened loss; and (3) frustration of drives. A patient with cancer accompanied by pain may experience any or all of these stressors (Shawver, 1977).

With injury or threatened injury, it is the ambiguity associated with the new diagnosis of cancer, the diagnostic tests, and treatment modalities which patients perceive as threatening. Fear and anxiety are aroused about effects the disease may have on their life-style or relationship with others. When treatment begins, body image may be threatened by radical surgery or side effects from radiation or chemotherapy. Patients often fear personal disfigurement, progressive deterioration, a painful death, or abandonment by family and friends. They are especially concerned about their ability to cope with the whole situation. The resulting fear and anxiety only seem to potentiate already-perceived pain (Rankin, 1980). According to Saunders (1981), "Any illness causes anxiety and one that becomes more serious in spite of a variety of treatments until it is patently life-threatening will engender many fears" (p. 233).

Loss or threatened loss in those with cancer produces a reactive depression with feelings of despair, helplessness, and hopelessness. The loss may be of a body part as with a leg amputation, radical mastectomy, or colostomy. Loss of the wage-earner role or loss of a job may disrupt patients' lives and lead to decreased self-esteem. The subsequent loss of income when medical bills are increasing produces additional stress. Loss of energy due to the progressing disease leads to fatigue and decreased strength to cope with persistent, physical pain (Shawver, 1977). However, the ultimate loss threatening patients is loss of life from this progressive disease causing their pain.

Frustration of drives may add to the depression and thus

increase physical pain. Personal satisfaction of needs may be impossible because of patients' deteriorated physical condition or environmental restrictions. Thus, sexual needs may remain unmet because of isolation from spouse or lack of privacy in the hospital. Also contact with immediate family members may be hindered because of hospital rules which prohibit visits from small children. Other unsatisfied needs may include: getting uninterrupted sleep at night; eating because of nausea induced from radiation or chemotherapy; engaging in gratifying or pleasurable activities like hobbies or sports; socializing with friends; participating in family activities and decisions; and maintaining personal grooming standards. Frustration of these needs contribute to decreased self-esteem and added distress because personal sources of pleasure are being neglected (Senescu, 1963).

Pain Associated with Therapy

Pain associated with therapy is the second major cancer-pain syndrome which Foley described. Pain may occur during, or as a result of surgery, radiation, or chemotherapy. Each of these therapeutic modalities is associated with characteristic pain patterns and clinical presentations (Foley, 1982).

Postsurgical pain syndromes result from interruption of sensory nerves during such surgical procedures as mastectomies, thoracotomies, radical neck dissections, and limb amputations. Pain begins approximately four to six weeks after surgery when incisional discomfort is no longer a factor. Typically, it begins as acute, lancinating pain which then dissolves into burning dysesthetic or hyperesthetic pain in the area of sensory loss. It is believed to be caused by the development of a traumatic neuroma (Foley, 1981).

Pain following radiation may result from (1) fibrosis of surrounding connective tissue which causes secondary injury to nerves like the brachial and lumbar plexus; (2) damage to the spinal cord: or (3) radiation-induced peripheral nerve tumors. Pain develops after sensory and motor changes occur, and paresthesias and dysesthesias are common (Foley, 1979, 1981).

Pain following chemotherapy may occur for several reasons. (1) Peripheral neuropathy, precipitated by Vincristine or Vinblastine administration, can produce dysesthesias, usually localized to the hands and feet. The burning pain is often exacerbated by superficial stimuli. (2) Pseudorheumatism, resulting from steroid withdrawal, causes diffuse myalgias and arthralgias. (3) Aseptic necrosis of bones, like the head of the humerus or femur, may occur secondary to chronic steroid therapy and causes limited joint movement because of pain. (4) Postherpetic neuralgia probably occurs secondary to the depressed immune system caused by chemotherapeutic agents. Three types of pain sensations are typical: continuous burning pain in the area of sensory loss, painful dysesthesias, and intermittent shocklike pain (Foley, 1981).

Pain Unrelated to Tumor or Therapy

The third major pain syndrome observed in cancer patients is unrelated to either the cancer or its therapy. Patients often suffer pain from other chronic conditions, such as diabetic neuropathy, rheumatoid arthritis, degenerative disc disease, and aortic aneurysms (Foley, 1981, 1982). Correct identification of nonmalignant sources of pain may considerably reduce threat and stress for patients as well as assure more appropriate treatment of the pain.

Medical Approaches to Cancer Pain

Primary, palliative, and symptomatic medical approaches are used for treating pain from cancer (Bolund, 1982; Murphy, 1973; Sanford and Patrick, 1977). While the purpose of both primary and palliative methods is to treat the cause of the pain, the purpose of symptomatic methods is to merely control the pain. Because primary treatment is aimed at removing the tumor to promote a cure, it is indicated in early stage pain. Palliative procedures are used when removal or destruction of the tumor is not feasible because of the extensiveness of the neoplasm or its location. Thus procedures like radiation, chemotherapy, hormonal therapy, and ablation of endocrine glands increase comfort by decreasing tumor size or controlling cell replication. They are indicated during intermediate stage pain. Symptomatic methods are instituted when all treatment methods for controlling tumor growth have been exhausted. They are implemented during late stage pain to simply relieve the pain. Consequently, analgesics provide the main treatment although neurosurgery and nerve blocks may sometimes be helpful. The goal of symptomatic treatment for these terminally ill patients is quality of life by maintaining function as long as possible and keeping them comfortable until they die (Inturrisi, 1984).

Prescription and Administration of Analgesics

Analgesics, used symptomatically, act either to reduce the painful stimulus or to reduce the perception of the painful stimulus. Their action, which varies with the drug, occurs either peripherally at the receptor site or centrally in the brain (American College of Physicians, 1983). Rogers (1977) stated: "In patients with pain due to cancer, when all modalities used in an attempt to control disease and pain have failed, drugs may be the one method left to alleviate pain and suffering" (p. 39). Both Twycross (1975, 1984) and Saunders (1976, 1981) have strongly advocated preventing pain by administering narcotics at regularly scheduled intervals to maintain constant analgesic blood levels. Saunders (1976) explained that if patients receive prompt relief of pain from the beginning and know that they can rely on their next dose arriving on time, they do not increase their own pain by fear and tension.

However, health professionals have often been reluctant to prescribe and administer medications, especially narcotics, at regular intervals because of concern about the development of dependence and tolerance. Hackett (1971) listed several prejudices physicians exhibit toward prescribing narcotics for patients with pain. First, narcotic doses are seldom individualized, with consideration given to body weight and acquired drug tolerances. Second, doses are frequently inadequate for controlling or relieving pain because of concern about addiction.

Therefore, patients are often undermedicated and suffer needlessly.

Most physicians continue to write orders for analgesics to be given on a PRN basis, or as necessary for patients' pain. Nurses are then expected to use their judgment about actually administering the medication. Subsequently, most nurses administer them cautiously because they have been educated to use narcotic analgesics judiciously to prevent addiction. The fact that physicians conservatively order narcotics because of their own concern for addiction seems to reinforce the nurses' conservative administration policy. Consequently, nurses have sometimes appeared reluctant to administer analgesics, both narcotic and nonnarcotic, to advanced and terminal cancer patients suffering severe pain. Shawver (1977) states that nurses may withhold medications for thirty to forty-five minutes until a prescribed four-hour interval expires because they are overly concerned about addicting these patients. Because nurses fail to evaluate the effectiveness of analgesic doses and administration intervals, patients become more irritable and anxious as their pain increases.

McCaffery (1979) observed that three factors contribute to nurses' undertreatment of patients' pain: (1) fear of causing respiratory depression; (2) fear of causing addiction; and (3) failure to use (or lack of) basic pharmacologic knowledge. Nurses are especially frightened when giving increasingly larger doses of narcotics to cancer patients. They fear that the dose they administer may "kill" the patient because of respiratory depression and thus be the "last dose" the patient receives.

Degner, Fujii, and Levitt (1982) cited several factors which concerned nurses participating in a planned program to change narcotic administration to cancer patients suffering pain. Nurses were concerned about (1) giving narcotics on a regular basis to patients who did not ask for them; (2) increasing the narcotic dosage when the patients did not have clinical evidence of disease progression; (3) producing respiratory depression; and (4) making the patient too sleepy.

Fox (1982) surveyed seventy-two nurses about their knowledge, attitudes, and management of cancer pain during terminal illness. Results indicated that nurses understood malignant pain but lacked knowledge of therapeutic principles and strategies of intervening appropriately.

Other factors which have been noted to influence nurses' perceptions of patients' pain and their subsequent decisions to administer PRN analgesics include: (1) difficulty in assessing pain and (2) their own beliefs about suffering. Jacox (1979) suggested that nurses and health professionals "gradually become less sensitive to patients' complaints of pain, particularly if they are in a situation where pain is difficult to alleviate" (p. 900). Certainly the pain associated with cancer is often difficult to alleviate, and nurses may therefore, undermedicate these patients. Davitz and Davitz (1980), from numerous studies, found that cultural factors like social class, religion, and ethnic background play a role in nurses' inferences of patients' pain. Although their study was limited to nurses, one wonders if these same cultural factors may affect physicians' perceptions of pain and their subsequent policies for prescribing analgesics.

Studies of Analgesic Treatment of Cancer Pain

Various aspects of analgesic treatment of cancer pain have been studied. Marks and Sachar (1973) investigated the use of the narcotic Demerol (meperidine) in treating hospitalized medical patients and found that physicians seldom prescribe it at the recommended therapeutic level of 100 mg every three hours. Furthermore, the nursing staff actually administered less medication than was prescribed PRN for the patients. Interviews with the affected patients revealed that 73 percent remained in moderate to severe pain as a result of less than optimal doses of medication. Questionnaires to house staff physicians revealed that for patients with pain from terminal metastatic cancer, physicians (1) undermedicated patients in pain because they lacked knowledge about narcotics and feared producing addiction; and (2) overestimated the addiction potential of Demerol (meperidine). The greater the physician's estimate of potential addiction, the lower were the doses of medication prescribed for these patients.

Charap (1978) surveyed the knowledge, attitude, and experience of surgical residents, neoplastic fellows, and nurses in treating pain in terminally ill patients. Results indicated that (1) approximately half of the total group believed that prescribing pain medications on a PRN basis minimized development of tolerance and inadvertent overdosing; (2) the majority of neoplastic fellows and nurses selected complete relief of pain as their intended goal, but most surgical residents preferred the option "enough pain relief so that . . . pain is noticed but is not distressing"; (3) both surgical residents and nurses believed that most patients are overmedicated rather than undermedicated. Charap concluded that the majority of the total group demonstrated limited understanding of the implications of long-term narcotic use and lacked knowledge of current pain management techniques for the terminally ill.

Grier, Howard, and Cohen (1979) analyzed nurses' choices of analgesic–medication doses for two patients described in vignettes as suffering severe pain from terminal malignancies. They found that nurses overestimated the probability of addiction with these medications when using an intuitive rather than quantitative process for decision making. When nurses used a quantitative decision-making process, they selected analgesic medication doses which were more goal-related, but their goals apparently were to minimize side effects rather than to maximize comfort.

In two vignettes which varied only for the sex of the patient, Cohen (1980) found that nurses selected less medication for female patients than male patients. When a dosage range for Demerol (meperidine) was ordered for patients diagnosed as having inoperable, terminal malignancy with bone metastasis, 64 percent of the nurses selected choices giving the same amount or less to a female patient whose severe pain was unrelieved by the dose administered four hours earlier, while 35 percent selected this choice for the corresponding male patient. Another finding was that nurses consistently selected the lowest dose of the range available even when it did not produce adequate pain relief.

The results of Pilowsky and Bond's (1969) study indicated that female cancer patients being treated with radiation were more likely to receive analgesic drugs and to receive stronger narcotic analgesics upon staff initiative than were corresponding male patients. Also, nursing staff tended not to give stronger analgesics to elderly patients with this diagnosis and were less likely to initiate analgesics to them.

When Hunt, Stollar, Littlejohns, Twycross, and Vere (1977), interviewed eight patients with pain and ten of their nurses, they found that the degree of pain relief obtained from medications by patients was overestimated by six of the nurses. Patients and nurses agreed about the amount of relief obtained in only two cases. Other survey findings indicated that nurses seldom used PRN analgesics, even though patients, most of whom had cancer, were known to have pain. They relied upon patients to complain of pain, ask for analgesics, or admit to needing them during regular drug rounds.

Jacox and Rogers (1981) emphasized that "inadequate knowledge of the pharmacology of analgesics and the misconceptions and attitudes of those health care professionals who are involved in the care of people who have pain caused by cancer," are largely responsible for the failure of analgesics to control pain (p. 394). These studies seem to indicate that both physicians and nurses have been remiss in symptomatic treatment and care of patients with cancer pain.

Two studies were undertaken to further explore the symptomatic treatment of cancer pain. The first study investigated the use of drugs for pain control. The second study assessed nurses' perceptions, practices, and concerns in managing patients' cancer pain with drugs.

Use of Drugs for Pain with Cancer Patients

Purpose

The purpose of this study was to investigate the drugs used for pain control with patients suffering from advanced and terminal cancer.* The questions addressed were: (1) Is there a

*This was a substudy of Pain Alleviation Through Nursing Intervention funded by Federal Grant NU00467-3 which was supervised by Project Director Ada Jacox and late Assistant Project Director Mary L. Stewart.

relationship between the intensity of the patient's pain and the distress caused by the pain? (2) Is there a relationship between interference with activities of living because of the pain and either pain intensity or pain distress? (3) Is either the patient's pain intensity or pain distress related to the analgesic regime? (4) Is the use of a psychotropic drug related to either the patient's pain intensity or pain distress? (5) Is the use of a bedtime sedative related to either the patient's pain intensity or pain distress (Rankin, 1982, p. 182)?

Methodology

This descriptive study was conducted at a midwestern university teaching hospital with a 1053-bed capacity to examine patients' perceptions of pain from advanced or terminal cancer and their prescribed analgesic medications.

Subjects. During a thirty-three-week period, forty patients consented to participate in this study. The sample, who met the criteria of suffering pain from advanced or terminal cancer, consisted of twenty-nine (72.5%) females and eleven (27.5) males ranging in age from twenty to seventy-five, with an average age of fifty-three. Total days of participation ranged from 2 to 14 with a mean of 5.86 days.

All patients had cancer with either diagnosed metastatic invasion into the surrounding tissue from the original site or distant tissue metastasis to lymph nodes, lung, liver, bone, brain, or kidneys. Three patients had distant metastasis to four distinct tissue sites. Others demonstrated metastasis to only bone tissue, but several bony areas were involved. Primary lesions involved thirteen different sites with ten from the breast, seven in the uterus, and six in the lung.

Instruments. Pain, as operationally defined for this study, was any discomfort described as pain by the patient in verbal statements when interviewed and indicated on pain scales and word checklists.

The interview form included seventeen structured questions asking patients to describe their pain, its onset, duration, and severity. Additional questions inquired if medication was being received for pain, how frequently it was required, and its effectiveness in relieving or reducing pain.

Pain scales were used to assess patients' pain intensity and distress. Pain intensity refers to the magnitude of the sensory component of the pain experience. Pain distress denotes the bothersome nature of the pain and thus the psychological reaction or response to the physical sensation (Johnson and Rice, 1974). For this study, pain intensity was operationally defined as the severity of the physical sensation of pain on a 0 to 100 scale with anchor words of *no pain, moderate pain,* and *unbearable pain* at the respective 0, 50, and 100-number intervals. Three pain intensity scales were included on the form for the patient to record "current" pain, "worst" pain in the past twenty four hours, and "average" or usual pain experienced. Pain distress was operationally defined as feelings resulting from, or in response to how bothersome the pain sensation was perceived to be on a 0 to 100 scale. Anchor words of *no distress, slightly distressing, moderately distressing, very distressing,* and *extremely distressing* were coordinated with respective number values of 0, 25, 50, 75, and 100. This was Stewart's (1977) adaptation of Johnson's distress scale.

Because the reliability of an instrument depends upon the consistency with which it measures over time, it is difficult to establish a reliability coefficient for a tool measuring clinical pain which may vary drastically in intensity and distress from day to day as well as within one day. Johnson (1973) was able to demonstrate, however, that individuals could separately rate the sensation and distress components of pain and that the two do not have a "one-to-one relationship."

A checklist of thirty-four pain adjectives upon which patients could indicate words that best described their pain was used as a second pain assessment tool. It was an eclectic list, but seventeen words were included from the McGill Pain Questionnaire.

The ten-item pain relief questionnaire asked patients

whether (1) pain relief from prescribed medications had been adequate; (2) pain disturbed their sleep or other activities like visiting, reading, watching TV, or physical activity; (3) pain had ever been severe enough to cause crying, irritability, anxiety, or depression.

A medication record was used to record analgesics, bedtime sedatives, and psychotropic drugs prescribed for the patients. The times that the medications were actually administered were recorded upon it daily.

Procedure. To select patients to participate in the study, kardexes on each adult nursing unit were reviewed for those with a diagnosis of cancer and analgesic medication ordered. Only patients with metastasis, as verified on their medical record, were seen and asked if they had pain associated with their illness. Those who answered affirmatively and were willing to participate were then interviewed by the investigator. After the interview, patients were asked to indicate their pain on pain scales. Thereafter daily pain scale responses were obtained by the investigator. Patients were asked to complete the checklist of pain adjectives a few days after the initial interview, and the pain relief questionnaire within one week of the interview. The medication record was updated daily. Although patients were followed daily during their entire hospitalization, only the first fourteen days were analyzed for this study since the total number of days of participation ranged from two to forty-three.

Results

Description of Pain. Pain characteristics: These patients with advanced and terminal cancer had been suffering pain for 1 to 96 months, with a mean of 12.5 and a standard deviation of 19.4 months. For half of the patients, pain had existed for 1 to 4 months (Table 21.1). Some pain was experienced daily for all forty patients. Ninety percent categorized their pain as moderate to very bad or very bad to excruciating (Table 21.2).

TABLE 21.1
DURATION OF PAIN

Months of Pain	Number	Percent
1–4	20	50.0
5–8	13	32.5
9–12	4	10.0
13 or more	3	7.5
TOTAL	40	100.0

TABLE 21.2
INITIAL ESTIMATE OF PAIN SEVERITY

Estimate of Pain Severity	N	Percent
Mild to Moderate	4	10.0
Moderate to Very Bad	23	57.5
Very Bad to Excruciating	12	30.0
Across all categories	1	2.5
TOTAL	40	100.0

Pain scales: As seen in Table 21.3, the patients' perception of their pain intensity on daily pain scales varied for current, average, and worst pain in the past twenty-four hours. Current and average pain were approximately the same (slightly below fifty or moderately intense pain) while pain at its worst was obviously above the moderate level. Distress, as perceived by the thirty-one patients completing this scale, was perceived to be moderately distressing.

Jacox (1976) analyzed separately the pain intensity and distress scores for the eight patients who died while participating in this study. During the last two weeks prior to death, their mean average pain intensity was 66.9 and mean worst pain was 81. Half of the group reported pain between 80 and 100 (very bad to excruciating) at least half of the time. None of the patients indicated pain lower than 50 (moderate pain) and six

TABLE 21.3

RANGE, MEAN, AND STANDARD DEVIATION FOR PAIN INTENSITY AND DISTRESS

Pain	Range	$\overline{X}$	S.D.
Intensity (n = 40)			
Current	5 – 86.3	42.5	20.5
Worst	27 – 100	62.9	19.5
Average	9.6 – 85.5	47.8	18.2
Distress (n = 31)	8.8 – 87.5	50.5	20.1

never scored lower than 75. For three of these patients, the mean distress level was 69. It was concluded that these dying patients "experienced great amounts of unrelieved pain."

To evaluate the first question, Pearson correlation coefficients were used to evaluate the relationship between pain intensity and the distress caused by the pain. For the thirty-one cancer patients completing pain distress scales, high correlations existed between distress and all three measures of pain intensity with p = 0.001 (Table 21.4).

TABLE 21.4

PEARSON CORRELATION BETWEEN PAIN INTENSITY AND DISTRESS (N = 31)

	Intensity					
	Current		Worst		Average	
	r	p	r	p	r	p
Distress	0.8052	0.001	0.8153	0.001	0.8222	0.001

Pain adjectives: Table 21.5 illustrates the pain adjectives chosen by patients to describe their pain. Patients might have difficulty finding the right words to describe their pain, but would recognize immediately those words that appropriately described it. Of the nine most frequently chosen words, six are also on the McGill Pain Questionnaire which uses twenty groups of words categorized as sensory, affective, evaluative, and miscellaneous. According to Melzack (1975), sensory words describe qualities of the sensation in terms of temporal, spatial, pressure, and thermal properties. *Sharp* and *sore* fit the sensory category. Affective words describe the pain experience in terms of emotional response, like tension, fear, and autonomic properties; *tiring* fits this category. Evaluative words describe the "subjective overall intensity of the pain experience" so *miserable, troublesome,* and *unbearable* are three of the five words in this category. Using Melzack's operational definitions, the words *persistent* and *strong* would probably be classified as sensory and "depressing" as affective.

TABLE 21.5

PAIN ADJECTIVES CHOSEN

Rank Order	Word	Percent Who Chose
1	Persistent	70.3
	Miserable	70.3
2	Tiring	64.9
	Depressing	64.9
	Strong	64.9
3	Troublesome	62.2
4	Sharp	59.5
	Sore	59.5
5	Unbearable	51.4

Interference with living: To analyze the second question, concerning a relationship between interference with living and either pain intensity or distress, several tests were used. Difficulty with sleeping, concentrating, physical movement, emotional reactions, and irritability because of the pain were each examined separately and also as a total interference with living classification.

Responses from twenty-five people about difficulty sleeping at night because of pain indicated that six (24%) had no difficulty, six (24%) had some difficulty, six (24%) had moderate difficulty, and seven (28%) had considerable difficulty. However, analysis of variance of these sleep difficulty groups for current, worst, and average pain intensity and pain distress indicated no significant difference at $p = 0.05$.

In terms of difficulty concentrating because of the pain, ten (40%) denied any problems, seven (28%) sometimes had trouble, and eight (32%) often had trouble. Again, analysis of variance of these differing concentration groups for current, worst, and average pain intensity and pain distress produced no differences reaching $p = 0.05$.

With physical movement, twenty-one (84%) patients had difficulty moving because of the pain while four (16%) had no difficulty. On 2-tail t-test, a significant difference existed between the two groups for only current pain intensity with $p = 0.047$. Pain was severe enough to cause crying in eighteen (82%) of the twenty-two who responded to this item. On 2-tail t-test, the two groups differed significantly ($p = 0.044$) for only the pain distress level of measurement.

Both anxiety and depression were reported as resulting from pain by some patients. Pain caused anxiety in nineteen (83%) of twenty-three patients and depression in twenty-one (88%) of twenty-four patients responding to these items. In neither case did a significant difference exist between groups in terms of pain intensity or pain distress on t-test.

Pain caused irritability in twenty (80%) of twenty-five patients, and t-test revealed a significant difference between the two groups for current, worst, and average pain intensity (Table 21.6). The difference between the two groups reached $p = 0.06$ for pain distress.

A total interference with living classification was devised based upon responses to questions about sleep, concentration, mobility, crying, anxiety, depression, and irritability. According to these criteria, the twenty-five participating patients were classified as follows: six (24%) had slight interference with living because of the pain, sixteen (64%) had moderate interference, and three (12%) had severe interference. Analysis of variance revealed no difference existed at $p = 0.05$ among the three groups in terms of the variables of pain intensity and distress. However, 76 percent of this group reported symptoms consistent with moderate to severe interference with living.

TABLE 21.6

COMPARISON OF MEAN PAIN INTENSITY AND DISTRESS SCORES FOR PATIENTS DESCRIBING IRRITABILITY USING T-TEST

	n	x̄	S.D.	T Value	D.F.	2 Tail p
Pain Intensity Current						
Irritable	20	41.641	18.824	−2.17	23	0.0041
Not Irritable	5	22.550	10.024			
Pain Intensity Worst						
Irritable	20	61.832	17.843	−2.38	23	0.026
Not Irritable	5	41.356	13.964			
Pain Intensity Average						
Irritable	20	46.704	16.588	−2.53	23	0.019
Not Irritable	5	26.796	10.768			
Distress						
Irritable	20	52.967	20.553	−1.98	23	0.060
Not Irritable	5	32.588	20.943			

Description of Drugs

Analgesics: During this thirty-three-week period while data were being collected, 151 analgesic drugs and combinations were ordered for these forty patients. During their fourteen-day observation period, only eight (5%) were ordered to be given at specific intervals rather than PRN. This meant that only six (15%) of these patients received drugs at regular intervals rather than PRN. The six most commonly ordered analgesic drugs by drug classification were: Tylenol (acetaminophen), codeine, morphine, Demerol (meperidine), Dilaudid (hydromorphone), and Darvon (propoxyphene). This group comprised 88 percent of all the drugs ordered (Table 21.7). Tylenol (acetaminophen) with either codeine or Darvon (propoxyphene) was the most frequently ordered combination (Table 21.8). Methadone, an analgesic suggested for cancer patients because of its long duration of action in oral form, was ordered only seven times.

All patients were receiving some medication to control their pain, but only twelve (30%) reported that the medication

TABLE 21.7

TOTAL DRUG ORDERS BY DRUG CLASSIFICATION

Rank	Drug	Number of Order
1	Tylenol (acetaminophen)	31
2	Codeine	30
3	Morphine	24
4	Demerol (meperidine)	22
5	Dilaudid (hydromorphone)	15
6	Darvon (propoxyphene)	11
7	Methadone	7
8	ASA	5
9	Powdered Opium	2
	Talwin (pentazocine)	2
10	Percodan (oxycodone)	1
	L-Dopa (levodopa)	1
		TOTAL 151

completely relieved their pain. The remaining twenty-eight (70%) reported that the medication reduced the severity of their pain but did not completely relieve it. According to Table 21.9, 78 percent of the patients received pain relief for less than four hours. However, as Table 21.10 illustrates, the most frequently prescribed medication administration schedule was every four hours.

When asked if they usually received their medication right away or sometimes had to wait, nine (22.5%) said no, nineteen (47.5%) said yes, and twelve (30%) said sometimes. The estimated length of the wait was between five to twenty minutes for seventeen, between twenty to forty-five minutes for seven, and one to two hours for three. However, many patients commented that the time of the wait was difficult to estimate because "10 minutes can seem like an hour when you're having pain." As Table 21.11 indicates, 40 percent of the patients would have preferred some change in their analgesic regime. Of the forty patients, thirty-eight (95%) "actively" requested pain medication when needed while only two (5%) "passively" waited for the nurse to offer or bring the medication.

TABLE 21.8

SINGLE AND COMBINATION DRUG ORDERS

Rank	Drug and Drug Combinations	Number of Orders
1	Codeine	23
	Morphine	23
2	Tylenol (acetaminophen)	21
3	Demerol (meperidine)	17
4	Dilaudid (hydromorphone)	15
5	Tylenol (acetaminophen) Combinations (with codeine 5 and Darvon (propoxyphene) 5)	10
6	Codeine Combinations (with APC 1 and Tylenol (acetaminophen) 6)	7
7	Methadone	6
	Darvon (propoxyphene) Combinations (with ASA 1 and Tylenol (acetaminophen) 5)	6
8	Darvon (propoxyphene)	5
	Demerol (meperidine) Combinations (with Vistaril (hydroxyzine) 3 and Phenergan (promethazine) 2)	5
9	ASA	4
10	Powdered Opium	2
	Talwin (pentazocine)	2
11	ASA Combination (Darvon)	1
	Methadone with Phergan (promethazine)	1
	Morphine with Vistaril (hydroxyzine)	1
	Percodan (oxcycodone)	1
	L-Dopa (levodopa)	1
		TOTAL 151

Responding to a question which asked if they perceived being given drugs for pain as harmful or that they should not take them too often, twenty-four (60%) patients replied yes and sixteen (40%) replied no. When asked if they had been reluctant to take medication even when uncomfortable or in pain, twelve (30%) responded yes and twenty-eight (70%) no. One wonders if that half of the group who perceived drugs as potentially harmful to their health might also be reluctant to take pain medication even when uncomfortable and thus suffer more pain than necessary.

TABLE 21.9

DURATION OF MEDICATIONS' ANALGESIC EFFECT

Duration of Analgesia	Number	Percent
Less than 1 hour	1	2.5
More than 1, Less than 2 hours	6	15.0
More than 2, Less than 3 hours	10	25.0
More than 3, Less than 4 hours	14	35.0
More than 4, Less than 5 hours	3	7.5
More than 5, Less than 6 hours	0	0.0
More than 6, Less than 7 hours	1	2.5
More than 7, Less than 9 hours	2	5.0
Unknown	3	7.5
TOTAL	40	100.0

TABLE 21.10

PRESCRIBED MEDICATION ADMINISTRATION SCHEDULES

Schedule		Number	Percent
4 hours or longer		84	56
q 4 h	73		
q 4–6 h	7		
q 6 h	3		
q 8 h	1		
Total	84		
range of 2.5 to 4 hours		25	17
q 3–4 h	23		
q 2.5–4.5	2		
Total	25		
3 hours or less		39	26
q 3 h	27		
q 2 h	8		
q 2–3 h	2		
q h	2		
Total	39		
Miscellaneous		3	1
	TOTAL	151	100

TABLE 21.11

PREFERENCE FOR ANALGESIC REGIME CHANGE

Preference For Change	Number	Percent
No Change	18	45.0
More Often	6	15.0
Stronger	6	15.0
Both More Often and Stronger	3	7.5
Faster Onset	1	2.5
Not Applicable	6	15.0
TOTAL	40	100.0

Analgesic regime score: To evaluate the third question, whether the patients' pain was related to the analgesic regime, an analgesic regime score was figured. To determine this:

> [A] chart of drugs grouped according to similar therapeutic effect in a hierarchy of least to most potent formed the basis of this score. Each group was numbered consecutively from 1 to 9 with 1 indicating the least potent group composed of aspirin and Tylenol. Each patient's analgesic regime score was figured accordingly: (1) If a patient's analgesic regime included drugs from several categories, the numbers of the categories were added together and divided by the number of categories to get an average category score (ACS). (2) This average category score was multiplied by the total number of doses of analgesia given per day (TD/D) to obtain the amount of drug-per-day score (D/D). ACS X TD/D = D/D. (3) Next, each patient's amount of drug-per-day scores were added together for the days he/she participated in the study, and then divided by the number of patient days (PD). The resulting quotient was the analgesic regime score (ARS). (D/D1 + D/D2 + D/D3 . . . D/DT/PD = ARS [(Rankin, 1982, pp. 186–187)].

To determine if a relationship existed between the patients' pain and the analgesic regime, Pearson correlation coefficients were figured. These were figured per patient day and per patient for the three pain intensity scores as well as the distress score. When figured per patient day, the D/D scores were used with the patient's current, worst, and average pain intensity scores and the distress score for that corresponding day. All correlations were statistically significant with p = 0.001 on a 2-tail test. When figured per patient, ARS was used with means of the patients' current, worst, and average pain intensity scores and the distress score. These correlations also reached statistical significance but at different levels (Table 21.12). These results could indicate that the patients' daily perceptions of pain intensity and distress were influenced by their analgesic regimes, or it could simply indicate that those patients with higher levels of pain and distress had higher analgesic regime scores.

TABLE 21.12

CORRELATION OF ANALGESIC REGIME SCORE (ARS) WITH PAIN INTENSITY AND DISTRESS*

ARS Per Patient Day			ARS Per Patient		
	r	p		r	p
Intensity (N = 340)			(N = 39)		
Current	0.3692	0.001		0.4134	0.009
Worst	0.4291	0.001		0.4834	0.002
Average	0.4331	0.001		0.5043	0.001
Distress (N = 233)					
	0.2469	0.001	(N = 31)	0.4196	0.019

* = 2-tail test

Psychotropic drugs: Combining analgesics with psychotropic drugs has been recommended because of the anxiety and depression which accompany pain and cancer. Of the forty patients in this study, twenty-three (58%) had psychotropic drugs ordered. Valium (diazepam) was the psychotropic drug ordered most frequently, and it was usually ordered three times a day. Librium (chlodiazepoxide), Elavil (amitriptyline), and Thorazine (chlorpromazine) were the other psychotropic drugs ordered. When these drugs were ordered PRN, they were often not given.

To analyze the fourth question; one-way analysis of variance was used to determine if a statistical difference in pain intensity or distress existed among patient groups who received psychotropic drugs, those who did not receive any doses from their PRN order, and those for whom no psychotropic drugs were ordered. Using the 0.05 probability level for analysis of the difference between groups on pain intensity, the group for whom no psychotropic drugs were ordered was found to differ from both the group who received psychotropic drugs and those who did not receive any doses. The three groups mean pain intensity scores appear in Table 21.13. The group for whom no psychotropic drugs were ordered had lower mean pain intensity scores than the other two.

Also, as seen in Table 21.13, the mean distress score was lower for the group who had no psychotropic drugs ordered than for the group who received no doses. This indicates that the group with no order and the group receiving psychotropic drugs had less distress than the group not receiving any doses from their PRN order (see Table 21.14 for ANOVA results).

TABLE 21.13

MEANS AND STANDARD DEVIATIONS OF PAIN INTENSITY AND DISTRESS IN RELATION TO PSYCHOTROPIC DRUG USE

Psychotropic Drug Use	Current (n=40)		Worst (n = 40)		Average (n = 40)		Distress (n = 31)	
	Mean	S.D.	Mean	S.D.	Mean	S.D.	Mean	S.D.
Given	47.5	25.1	70.7	22.7	51.7	23.1	46.9	26.7
Not given	48.8	27.7	65.5	26.3	55.6	25.3	53.9	27.2
Not Ordered	33.6*	26.7	55.0*	28.5	39.7*	22.5	41.6**	28.1

*Differs from both groups at 0.05 probability level
**Differs from "not given" group at 0.05 probability level

Bedtime sedatives: For the fifth question, one-way analysis of variance was also used to see if a difference in pain intensity or distress existed among patient groups given bedtime sedatives, those not given PRN bedtime sedatives, and those for whom no

TABLE 21.14

ANOVA SUMMARY TABLE FOR PSYCHOTROPIC DRUG USE BY PAIN INTENSITY AND DISTRESS

Source of Variation	D.F.	S.S.	M.S.	F Ratio	p
		Current (n = 40)			
Between Groups	2	17 629.8125	8814.9063	12.512	0.0001
Within Groups	337	237 423.0	704.5193		
Total	339	255 052.8125			
		Worst (n = 40)			
Between Groups	2	15 557.0	7779.5000	10.792	0.0001
Within Groups	337	242 894.0	720.7537		
Total	339	258 451.0			
		Average (n = 40)			
Between Groups	2	16 659.9375	8329.9688	15.444	0.0001
Within Groups	337	181 771.7500	539.3818		
Total	339	198 431.6875			
		Distress (n = 31)			
Between Groups	2	5 300.4375	2650.2188	3.470	0.032
Within Groups	230	175 647.9375	763.6865		
Total	232	180 948.3750			

bedtime sedatives were ordered. When the pain intensity difference between groups was analyzed at the 0.05 probability level, the group for whom no bedtime sedative was ordered differed from both the group given a bedtime sedative and the group not given their PRN bedtime sedative. As Table 21.15 illustrates, the mean pain intensity score was higher for the group without an order for a bedtime sedative.

When analyzing the pain distress difference between groups at the 0.05 probability level, the group for whom no bedtime sedative was ordered differed from the group not given a PRN bedtime sedative but not from the group given a bedtime sedative. Table 21.15 shows that the group for whom

TABLE 21.15

MEANS AND STANDARD DEVIATIONS OF PAIN INTENSITY AND DISTRESS IN RELATION TO SEDATIVE USE

Sedative Use	Current (n = 40)		Worst (n = 40)		Average (n = 40)		Distress (n = 40)	
	$\overline{X}$	S.D.	$\overline{X}$	S.D.	$\overline{X}$	S.D.	$\overline{X}$	S.D.
Given	39.2	28.7	58.0	29.6	41.5	26.2	49.1	31.0
Not Given	34.1	24.4	56.2	26.7	42.0	21.5	39.3	25.6
Not Ordered	49.6*	28.4	70.3*	25.0	55.2**	24.0	52.8*	26.2

*Differs from both groups at 0.05 probability level
**Differs from "not given" group at 0.05 probability level

no bedtime sedative was ordered had the highest mean distress score too. However, the group who were given a bedtime sedative indicated a mean distress score just 4 points lower. Pain may have been interfering with sleep to create distress for those without a bedtime sedative order. It also may have been the reason that the other group took a bedtime sedative. Perhaps the group not given the bedtime sedative were less distressed because they decided not to take it but knew it was available if needed (see Table 21.16 for ANOVA results).

Discussion

Most of the cancer patients participating in this study described their pain on initial interview as moderate to very bad or very bad to excruciating. They continued to have pain intensity levels of 47.76 (mean average pain intensity) and 62.86 (mean worst pain intensity) on a 0 to 100 scale and a mean distress score of 50.49. For 76 percent of them, pain caused moderate to severe interference with living which was most apparent in irritability, decreasing mobility, and crying. When the medication regimes were evaluated, 70 percent of the patients reported that medication reduced the severity of the pain rather than completely relieving it, and 78 percent received pain relief for less than four hours. Since over half of the analgesic medications were ordered for four-hour intervals

TABLE 21.16

ANOVA Summary Table for Sedative Use By Pain Intensity and Distress

Source of Variation	D.F.	S.S.	M.S.	F Ratio	p
		Current (n = 40)			
Between Groups	2	14 410.6250	7205.3125	10.090	0.0001
Within Groups	337	240 642.1875	714.0715		
Total	339	255 052.8125			
		Worst (n = 40)			
Between Groups	2	12 797.0	6398.5000	8.778	0.0001
Within Groups	337	245 654.0	728.9436		
Total	339	258 451.0			
		Average (n = 40)			
Between Groups	2	12 385.8125	6192.9063	11.218	0.0001
Within Groups	337	186 045.8750	552.0647		
Total	339	198 431.6875			
		Distress (n = 31)			
Between Groups	2	7 980.7500	3990.3750	5.306	0.006
Within Groups	230	172 967.6250	752.0330		
Total	232	180 948.3750			

or longer, it appears that shorter intervals or larger doses were needed for better pain relief. Of special interest was the fact that 87 percent of the patients surveyed complained of moderate to excruciating pain, but 45 percent did not want their medication regimen changed. Understanding the patients' reasons for this might provide a better understanding of their fear system for better pain management.

Person correlations revealed that a relationship existed, at a statistically significant level, between patients' pain and their analgesic regime. Although this may simply indicate that patients' pain scores increased with their ARS, the fact that their pain and distress continued to be moderate, or above moderate for worst pain, with their current analgesics suggests that analgesic orders or administration schedules needed revising.

When comparing Demerol (meperidine) orders in this study with Marks and Sachar's (1973) study, the recommended therapeutic dose of Demerol (meperidine) 100 mg intramuscularly (I.M.) every three hours was never ordered. The most frequently ordered doses were 50 and 75 mg, and the prescribed administration intervals varied from two to six hours. It appears that these patients were also undermedicated with Demerol (meperidine). However, Kaiko, Foley, Grabinski, Heidrich, Rogers, Inturrisi, and Reidenberg's (1983) research indicates that long-time use of Demerol is not recommended because accumulation of normeperidine from meperidine breakdown causes toxic effects resulting in central nervous system (CNS) excitation.

Some interesting results concerning psychotropic drugs and bedtime sedatives were found during this study. Those patients in the group who did not receive any doses of PRN psychotropic drugs had statistically significant higher distress scores than the group for whom no psychotropic drugs were ordered. This suggests that patients for whom PRN psychotropic drugs were ordered might have benefited if nurses had given the medication. Perhaps greater emphasis on nursing assessment of pain distress is indicated. The group of patients who had no bedtime sedative ordered differed for pain intensity at a statistically significant level when compared with the other two groups. Also, the group who had no bedtime sedative order had a higher distress level at a statistically significant level than the group who did not receive any PRN doses but not the group who received a bedtime sedative. This suggests that patients who have a bedtime sedative order available if needed have less distress from their pain. Many patients commented about "never getting a good night's sleep" because of the pain, or, "If I could just get a good night's sleep, I could face the day." Bedtime sedatives may help patients sleep better, and just knowing that one is available if pain interferes with sleep may decrease distress. Further study is needed to clarify these results.

However, Bressler, Hange, and McGuire (1986) found that

pain routinely prevented 72 percent of a group of cancer outpatients from falling asleep and also awakened 66 percent from sleep. Furthermore, 28 percent of their sample suffered their worst pain between 10 P.M. and 4 A.M. while for another 26 percent worst pain occurred between 4 A.M. and 10 A.M. Therefore 54 percent indicated that pain during the night was a problem.

The following limitations exist in this study. (1) Not all subjects participated in all aspects of the study. On some days patients did not feel well enough to concentrate on pain scales and questionnaires. However, these problems are inherent in collecting data in any clinical setting. (2) Since this was an exploratory study, relationship between variables can only be noted because cause and effect cannot be determined. (3) The small sample size limits generalization of results. Nevertheless, the data suggest that these patients continued to have moderate levels of pain and distress in spite of their medication regimes and could have benefited from both revised analgesic orders from physicians and more perceptive administration of PRN medications by nurses.

Nurses' Perceptions of Cancer Patients' Pain

Purpose

The purpose of this second study was to assess nurses' perceptions of the pain suffered by cancer patients for whom they were caring, their beliefs and practices in managing these patients' pain with drugs, and their general concerns about using pain drugs for patients diagnosed with metastatic or terminal cancer. The questions investigated included:

1. Is there an association between the nurses' perception of the patients' pain level and their:
   a. Recommendation for frequency of administration of medication?
   b. Assessment of the adequacy of pain relief from the analgesic?
   c. Concern about addiction?

2. Is there an association between the nurses' concern with addiction for the patient and their:
   a. Recommendation about medication frequency?
   b. Perception of the duration of pain relief from analgesics?
   c. Assessment of the adequacy of the physicians' prescribed analgesic orders for relieving pain?
3. Are the nurses' years of clinical experience associated with their:
   a. Perception of the patients' pain intensity?
   b. Perception of the amount of pain relief obtained from the analgesic?
   c. Estimation of the duration of pain relief?
4. Is there an association between how often nurses recommend that patients should receive medication for pain and their belief about:
   a. Relieving or reducing pain for terminal cancer patients?
   b. Frequency of narcotic administration?
5. Is there an association between the nurses' perception of the adequacy of the analgesic for pain relief and their belief about:
   a. Relieving or reducing pain for terminal cancer patients?
   b. Frequency of narcotic administration? (Rankin and Snider, 1984, pp. 150–151)

Methodology

This descriptive study of nurses' perceptions of patients' pain from cancer was conducted at a midwestern university teaching hospital with a bed capacity of 1053.

Subjects. Fifty-two female nurses, who were caring for patients known to be suffering from terminal or metastatic cancer, consented to participate in this study during a thirty-three-week period. Their years of clinical experience ranged from less than six months to over ten years. As seen in Table 21.17, 57 percent of the nurses had less than three years clinical work experience.

TABLE 21.17

YEARS OF CLINICAL EXPERIENCE

Years in Clinical Nursing		n	%
Less than 6 months		9	17
6 months to 1 year		8	15
1 to 3 years		13	25
3 to 5 years		8	15
5 to 10 years		6	12
Over 10 years		2	4
No data		6	12
	Total	52	100

Instrument. A two-section questionnaire with previously established face and content validity was used to collect data from these nurses. The first section included nine items questioning the nurse about her perceptions of the pain of one specific cancer patient whose name was written in the space provided. The named patient was one for whom the nurse had been providing nursing care and who was known to be suffering from pain. Questions asked the nurse to estimate, from multiple options, the patient's pain intensity level, amount of pain relief obtained from analgesics, and duration of pain relief. Other items asked the nurse about her beliefs and practices concerning the adequacy of the prescribed analgesics in relieving pain, the dose interval required, the possibility of addiction for this patient, and any physical conditions or reasons for withholding or limiting analgesics.

The second section assessed the nurse's beliefs about use of analgesic drugs for patients in general who have metastatic or terminal cancer. These items asked about the purpose of narcotic administration in either reducing or relieving pain, the adequacy of the physicians' prescribed narcotic orders in relieving pain, the usual routine used when an order is written q3-4h, concern for drug addiction that limits the amount of analgesic medication given, and interpretation of PRN orders.

The last item asked if those from groups according to race, sex, weight, or pathology requested pain medication more frequently and consequently needed more critical evaluation before giving pain medication.

Procedure. To select nurses to participate in the study, day or evening charge nurses on hospital units were asked for the names of nurses who had been caring for specific patients who were known to have pain from cancer. It had been previously verified by the investigator that the selected patients were experiencing pain and were receiving analgesic medications for their pain. Those nurses confirming that they had been caring for the respective patients were asked to participate in the study by completing the questionnaire. Within the next two days, the completed questionnaire was collected from those nurses who consented to participate.

Results

Questionnaire Responses. As seen from Table 21.18, nurses perceived that 80.8 percent (42) of the patients experienced pain of moderate to extreme intensity. They estimated that 17.3 percent (9) of fifty-two patients received total relief from their pain, 67.3 percent (35) received moderate relief and were able to tolerate the pain, and only 13.4 percent (7) received little pain relief. As illustrated in Table 21.19, nurses assessed that 61.5 percent (32) received relief from their pain medications for four hours or less.

TABLE 21.18

NURSES' PERCEPTION OF PAIN INTENSITY

Pain Estimate		n	%
Don't Know		2	3.8
Mild		8	15.4
Moderate		13	25.0
Very Bad		19	36.6
Extreme		10	19.2
	Total	52	100.0

TABLE 21.19

NURSES' ASSESSMENT OF ANALGESIC DURATION

Analgesic Duration		n	%
Unable to Assess		4	7.7
Less than Two Hours		7	13.4
Two to Four Hours		25	48.1
More than Four Hours		16	30.8
	Total	52	100.0

The majority of these nurses (88.5%) indicated that the currently prescribed medications were adequate in spite of assessing that 61.5 percent of the patients received relief for four hours or less from their analgesic medications and only 17.3 percent received complete relief. In the first study which used the same patient population, 78 percent of the patients themselves reported receiving pain relief for less than four hours, and only 30 percent reported complete relief (Rankin, 1982). When responding to how often these patients should received medication for pain, 25 percent (13) of the nurses believed that the patients should received medications on a regular schedule rather than PRN, as demonstrated in Table 21.20. Within this group of thirteen, eight (15.4%) believed that these patients should receive pain medications as frequently as every one to two hours.

Although 84.6 percent (44) of this group of fifty-two

TABLE 21.20

INTERVALS NURSES RECOMMENDED FOR ANALGESIC ADMINISTRATION

Analgesic Interval		n	%
Unable to estimate		1	1.9
PRN at Infrequent Intervals		18	34.6
PRN q 3–4 h		20	38.5
Regular Schedule q 2–4 h		13	25.0
	Total	52	100.0

nurses denied being concerned about the possibility of addiction with the respective patients, 15.4 percent (8) identified that this was a concern. Most of these nurses (80.8%) denied that any physical condition existed for the patient that would contraindicate giving analgesic medication to the patient.

In responding to questions assessing their general beliefs about pain drugs for cancer patients with metastatic or terminal cancer, 42.3 percent (22) of the nurses noted that narcotics should be administered frequently enough to completely relieve pain, while 57.7 percent (30) indicated that narcotics should only reduce the pain. Fifty-eight percent (30) of the nurses believed that physicians generally order the "right amount" of narcotic for pain, but 27 percent (14) believed that too little is ordered or at too infrequent intervals. However, 10 percent (5) indicated that both too much and too little narcotic is generally ordered by physicians, and two chose not to answer this item.

When interpreting an order for an analgesic to be given PRN q3–4h, 44 percent (23) of the nurses would administer the medication every three hours PRN, while 42 percent (22) would administer it every four hours PRN. The remaining 14 percent (7) noted that their choice of which to administer would depend upon the specific patient.

When asked if general concern about drug addiction would cause them to restrict or limit the amount of analgesics given in a twenty-four-hour period to terminal cancer patients, only forty-five nurses responded. Of this group 82 percent (37) said "no" and 18 percent (8) said "yes." These responses were very similar to those given previously concerning drug addiction for specific patients wherein 84.6 percent of the nurses indicated that they were not concerned about addiction.

Analysis of items asking if those from groups according to race, sex, age, weight, or pathology requested pain medication more frequently revealed that most nurses believed that no differences existed between black and white people or between obese and thin people. However, adults were perceived as asking for more pain medication than the elderly, and females asking for more than males. Those patients with cancer were assessed as asking for more pain medication than those with kidney stones. Specific response frequencies for these items are presented in Table 21.21.

TABLE 21.21

PERCEIVED DIFFERENCES ACCORDING TO RACE, WEIGHT, SEX, AGE, AND PATHOLOGY IN REQUESTING ANALGESICS

Groups		n	%
Race			
White		4	8
Black		1	2
No Difference		43	90
	Total	48	100
Weight			
Obese		11	23
Thin		7	14.5
No Difference		30	62.5
	Total	48	100.0
Sex			
Female		30	65
Male		3	7
No Difference		13	28
	Total	46	100
Age			
Elderly (over 60)		5	10
Adult (20–60)		28	55
No Difference		18	35
	Total	51	100
Pathology			
Cancer		22	49
Kidney Stones		4	9
No Difference		19	42
	Total	45	100

Analysis of Questions. The statistical test chosen to analyze the data investigating the specific questions for this study was the chi-square test for independence. The level of significance selected was the 0.05 level of confidence.

In reviewing the data for the first question, a significant association was found to exist between nurses' perception of patients' pain levels and their recommendation for frequency of administration of medication. Nurses who assessed patients as suffering very bad or extreme pain recognized their need for analgesic medications at more frequent intervals as shown in Table 21.22. The nurses' perceptions of the patients' pain levels, however, appeared to be independent of their assessment of the adequacy of the analgesic in providing pain relief (X^2 = 0.418 with 2 d.f., p = 0.811). In addition, nurses' perception of patients' pain level appeared to be independent from their concern about addiction since the association between these variables did not reach the 0.05 level of significance.

TABLE 21.22

Association of Nurses' Perception of Patients' Pain Levels to Recommendation for Frequency of Medications

	Frequency Recommendation		
Pair Estimate	PRN at Infrequent Intervals	PRN q 3–4 h	Regular Schedule q 2–4 h
Moderate	12	5	4
Very Bad	2	10	6
Extreme	3	5	2

X^2 = 9.56323 (d.f. = 4); p = 0.0485.

Nurses' concern with addiction appeared independent from their recommendations about medication frequency when these data were analyzed for the second question. Also, the nurses' concern about addiction and their perception of the duration of pain relief from medications for these patients appeared to be independent observations. Furthermore, nurses' concern about addiction was independent from their assessment of the adequacy of physicians' prescribed analgesic orders because no significant association existed in this data either. It seems, then, that addiction was not a conscious factor in these nurses' assessment process.

For the third question, nurses' years of clinical experience did not have a significant association with perception of patients' pain intensity, assessment of obtained pain relief from medications, or estimation of duration of pain relief. Therefore, years of clinical experience also seemed to be independent from these nurses' assessment process.

Again, for the fourth question, no significant association was revealed between nurses' recommendation for the frequency of analgesic administration for specific patients and their general belief about the purpose of narcotics administration in completely relieving or simply reducing pain for terminal cancer patients, or with their general belief about the frequency of narcotic administration for cancer patients. Also, for the fifth question, no significant association was noted between nurses' perception of the adequacy of the analgesic for pain relief for specific patients and their general belief about the purpose of giving narcotics for relieving or reducing pain for terminal cancer patients, or with their general belief about the frequency of narcotic administration for cancer patients. Apparently, these nurses' beliefs about the nurses' goal for pain relief and beliefs about narcotic administration were independent from their assessment of the adequacy of the medication providing analgesia.

Additional Findings. Additional tests were done which also used the chi-square test for independence. One finding demonstrated an association at the 0.0088 level of probability between the nurses' estimate of the amount of relief obtained from the patients' analgesic medication and their assessment of the duration of that relief (Table 21.23). Interpretation of this result probably indicates that duration of analgesic relief is one variable among several used by nurses in assessing total relief obtained from analgesics.

Data pertaining to question 1 revealed that nurses' perception of patients' pain level and their assessment of the adequacy of obtained pain relief from analgesics appeared to be two independent observations. However, an association approaching significance was found $X^2 = 8.756$ with 4 d.f., $p = 0.0675$) between nurses' estimate of patients' pain intensity and their assessment of patients' relief obtained from ordered analgesics.

TABLE 21.23

ASSOCIATIONS OF NURSES' ESTIMATE OF OBTAINED RELIEF FROM MEDICATIONS TO DURATION OF RELIEF

	Relief Duration		
Obtained Relief	Less than 2 hrs	2–4 hrs	More than 4 hrs
Little	4	3	0
Moderate	3	18	11
Total	0	4	4

$X^2 = 13.56206$ (d.f. = 4); $p = 0.0088$;
Kendall's tau B = 0.39830; $p = 0.0017$.

As illustrated in Table 21.24, most patients were perceived as receiving moderate relief from pain regardless of pain intensity, but more patients with bad or extreme pain were perceived as receiving little pain relief than those with moderate pain. In addition, a significant association was noted between the nurses' perception of the adequacy of pain medication as ordered by physicians for the patients and the nurses' assessment of relief obtained from the ordered analgesics (Table 21.25). Nurses indicating that analgesics were inadequate in providing pain relief assessed that patients were receiving little or moderate pain relief, while some perceiving the medication as adequate noted that some patients received total relief from pain.

It would appear, then, that patients with bad or extreme pain were perceived by their nurses as receiving little pain relief, and those receiving little pain relief were then perceived as having inadequately ordered analgesics. However, simply suffering from bad or extreme pain did not necessarily indicate that pain relief was inadequate, and moderate relief of pain was often perceived as adequate.

Furthermore, a significant association was revealed between nurses' estimate of pain intensity and their general perception that physicians order appropriate amounts of analgesic medication for patients. As Table 21.26 indicates, more

TABLE 21.24

ASSOCIATION OF NURSES' PAIN ESTIMATE TO ESTIMATE OF OBTAINED RELIEF FROM MEDICATIONS

	Obtained Relief		
Pain Estimate	Little	Moderate	Total
Moderate	1	12	7
Very Bad	3	15	1
Extreme	3	6	1

X^2 = 8.75577 (d.f. =4); p = 0.0675.

TABLE 21.25

ASSOCIATION OF NURSES' PERCEPTION OF ADEQUACY OF PAIN MEDICATION TO ESTIMATE OF OBTAINED RELIEF FROM MEDICATIONS

	Medication Relief		
Medication Adequate	Little	Moderate	Total
Yes	4	32	9
No	3	3	0

X^2 = 8.06285 (d.f. = 2); p = 0.0177.

nurses believed inadequate amounts of analgesic medications were ordered by physicians for patients with extreme pain than for those with pain of lower intensities. In those cases, the majority of nurses believed that physicians ordered the right amount to control pain. It would seem that nurses perceive moderate pain as tolerable to patients.

Finally, an association at the 0.0998 probability level was noted between nurses' goals for narcotic administration and concern about addiction (Table 21.27). Apparently, more nurses who disclaim concern about addiction believe that narcotics should reduce rather than relieve pain. Although this does not reach the accepted 0.05 probability level, it identifies a trend consistent with the finding that moderate pain relief was perceived by nurses as being adequate.

TABLE 21.26

ASSOCIATION OF NURSES' PAIN ESTIMATE TO THEIR PERCEPTION OF PHYSICIANS' NARCOTIC ORDERS FOR CANCER PATIENTS IN GENERAL

	Physicians Orders	
Pain Estimate	Amount Right	Amount Not Right
Moderate	12	9
Very Bad	14	3
Extreme	3	7

$X^2 = 7.38334$ (d.f. = 2); $p = 0.0249$.

TABLE 21.27

ASSOCIATION OF NURSES' GOAL FOR NARCOTIC ADMINISTRATION TO CONCERN ABOUT ADDICTION

	Narcotic Administration Goal	
Addiction Concern	Relieve	Reduce
Yes	6	2
No	16	28

Corrected $X^2 = 2.70833$ (d.f. = 1); $p = 0.0998$;
Kendall's tau B = 0.28216; $p = 0.0220$.

Discussion

In this study, 89 percent of the participating nurses assessed that patients were receiving adequate medication for pain control, and yet 67 percent assessed that patients had moderate pain. This compares with data from the first study using the same patient population which documented that these patients suffered moderate pain in spite of their analgesic regimes so that 76 percent of them experienced moderate to severe interference with living because of the pain (Rankin, 1982). Although nurses and patients agreed that pain was of *moderate* intensity, the term itself may have different implications for each group. According to Melzack and Torgerson

(1971), when patients and physicians were asked to rank order pain descriptors according to a one to five pain scale, both groups agreed on rank order, but often patients attached a higher intensity to the words than physicians. Also, while 61.5 percent of the nurses evaluated that patients received pain relief for four hours or less, 78 percent of the patients in the first study indicated this (Rankin, 1982, p. 186).

For 57.7 percent of the nurses, the goal for narcotic administration was to reduce pain rather than relieve it, and this goal was apparently met since 70 percent of the patients in the first study indicated that their pain was reduced rather than completely relieved by their medication regimes (Rankin, 1982, p. 186). Complete relief of pain all the time may be unrealistic, but these data seem to indicate that these nurses often perceived moderate pain relief as an adequate goal.

Eighty-six percent of the nurses denied concern about addiction, and this appeared to be independent of their evaluation of duration of pain relief and recommendation for frequency of medication. Contrary to expectation, addiction was not a conscious factor associated with the pain assessment process for these nurses. A trend, however, was revealed between nurses' goals for narcotic administration and their concern about addiction.

From this second study, data appeared to indicate that these nurses recognized: (1) patients with bad or extreme pain needed their analgesics more often; (2) patients with bad or extreme pain received little pain relief; and (3) patients receiving little pain relief were receiving inadequate analgesic medication. However, assessment of bad or extreme pain for the patients did not indicate to these nurses that pain relief was inadequate.

Several limitations exist in this second study. First, not all factors influencing nurses' perceptions of pain were included on the questionnaire. Second, chi-square tests note association between variables, but cannot determine actual cause and effect. Third, responses on a questionnaire about beliefs and practices may not coincide with actual behavior. Nevertheless, when examining the results of the second study in terms of the first, nurses' perceptions of cancer patients' pain can be compared with the patients' own perceptions. Several implications were suggested: (1) Nurses need to concentrate upon evaluating analgesic relief and duration of that relief. Obtaining daily pain intensity scales from patients, asking patients about the amount of relief obtained in terms of percentages after giving pain medications, and noting the duration of analgesic effect each time would enable nurses to evaluate more objectively and accurately. (2) Goals for narcotic administration to patients with advanced and terminal cancer need to be discussed. Because quality of life is often equated with comfort, a goal to completely relieve pain when possible seems more appropriate than one to simply reduce it to moderate intensity. As Degner et al. (1982) noted, quality of life for cancer patients with pain improved when nurses became more knowledgeable about narcotics and accepted more responsibility for pain control. Grady (1986) emphasized that it is an ethical responsibility for nurses to be concerned with pain management to assure quality of life for these patients.

Quality of life for terminal cancer patients must be an ethical concern for physicians as well as nurses. Twycross (1982) stated that priorities should change from cure to "comfort care" when patients are expected to die within a few weeks or months. "The primary aim is then not to preserve life but to make the life that remains as comfortable and as meaningful as possible" (p. 84). This can be accomplished by appropriate use of analgesics and adjunct medications.

The WHO (1986), in a consensus statement, indicated that "pain relief was a realistic target for the majority of cancer patients throughout the world" (p. 5). Furthermore, the American College of Physicians (1983) has published position statements on drug therapy for patients in severe pain from terminal illness. Their goal for drug therapy is alleviation and suppression of existing pain, and prevention of recurring pain. They suggest that oral administration of a narcotic drug on a regular schedule will accomplish this. They believe that sufficient medication should be made available for treating these patients, and administration of narcotics in this way does not cause addiction, or psychological dependence, in the terminally ill.

Terminal cancer patients ask for or demand narcotics, not to experience their psychological effects but to obtain relief from pain for a few hours (Twycross, 1982). Those who seem to be "clock watchers" have either received inadequate pain control or have increased pain from progressive pathology. Clock watching will cease when memory and fear of pain is erased by adequate pain control (Twycross, 1974, 1982). According to Porter and Jick (1980), addiction is rare in hospitalized medical patients with no history of addiction. After examining the records of 11,882 patients receiving narcotics, they documented only four cases of addiction among them. Therefore addiction should not be considered an important problem for advanced cancer patients.

Recommendations for Using Drugs for Cancer Pain

According to Foley, pain can be adequately managed so that discomfort is controlled without functional impairment for 90 to 95 percent of the patients with cancer (Foley, 1979). This usually involves properly administering analgesic drugs. For instance, Bressler et al. (1986) found that the major factor cited for decreasing pain by 57 percent of their cancer outpatient group was use of analgesics. Narcotic analgesics have been especially effective in relieving severe pain in terminal illness for 97 percent of the patients (Foley, 1979). However, problems arise when narcotics and nonnarcotics are improperly prescribed or administered by health professionals (Bonica, 1984). Various principles and suggestions have been published to remedy this situation.

When pain occurs, the therapeutic strategy should be to (1) relieve pain at rest, on standing, and during activity, and (2) increase the hours of pain-free sleep (WHO, 1986). Analgesics should be given around the clock on a regular schedule so therapeutic blood levels remain constant, and the patient can remain free of pain. Also a sequential pattern for prescribing analgesics should be followed so nonnarcotic drugs are used first, weak narcotics next, and strong narcotics last. Thus, if pain persists or increases, drugs higher on the "ladder" sequence are used (WHO, 1986). For example, if aspirin around the clock is no longer effective, codeine can be added to the regime. If this ceases to be effective, morphine should be ordered instead. Aspirin, which acts peripherally, may be continued with the morphine, which acts centrally, because their additive therapeutic effect may provide the best pain relief.

Drugs used for cancer pain have been categorized as nonnarcotics, narcotics, and adjuvant analgesics (Foley, 1985). The most common drugs in each category will be listed along with a few comments about their use for cancer patients with pain.

Nonnarcotic Drugs

Nonnarcotic drugs include aspirin, Tylenol (acetaminophen), and nonsteroidal anti-inflammatory drugs such as Motrin or Advil (ibuprofen), and Naprosyn (naproxen) (Sellers, Mount, and Bethune, 1984). They are indicated for mild to moderate pain. Since these drugs inhibit prostaglandin synthesis, they are effective for metastatic bone pain and some soft tissue metastases which produce prostaglandins (Twycross and Lack, 1983). Their anti-inflammatory effect as well as additive effect when combined with narcotics make them useful for treating cancer pain (WHO, 1986). Although gastrointestinal side-effects are common, they may be controlled by administering the medications with milk, meals, or an antacid, or by using an enteric-coated form if available (Saunders, 1981). Because these drugs have ceiling effects, increasing the dose beyond its highest range does not produce additional analgesia (Foley, 1979). These medications do not cause tolerance or physical dependence.

Narcotic Drugs

Narcotic drugs include both weak and strong opioids, like codeine and morphine respectively. Generally, weak narcotics are indicated for moderate pain, while strong narcotics are required for severe pain (Sellers et al, 1984). Codeine, as the prototypic weak narcotic, is usually administered in doses of 30 to 60 mg. Besides providing analgesia, it is an effective cough suppressant. This effect can be doubly beneficial when coughing causes pain, as sometimes occurs with lung cancer. Because regular use of codeine causes severe constipation, laxatives need to be started concomitantly with the codeine to avoid the problem.

Drugs included in the strong narcotic category include morphine, Dilaudid (hydromorphone), and Dolophine (methadone). Morphine, the most commonly used, is the prototype against which the others are compared in determining equianalgesic doses. Brompton's cocktail and heroin (diamorphine) are no longer recommended because studies have demonstrated that the same effects can be achieved by morphine alone (Twycross, 1974; Twycross and Lack, 1983; Twycross and Lack, 1984).

These drugs are associated with the development of physical dependence and tolerance. Physical dependence is that physiological adaptation of the tissues to repeated administration of a drug so that without it, withdrawal symptoms occur. Tolerance is defined as the gradual development of resistance to the effects of a repeatedly administered drug which requires that the dose be increased to maintain the same effect. Thus, the interval between doses must be shortened or the size of the dose must be increased to maintain the same effect from the medication. Physical dependence and tolerance seem to occur concurrently (Jaffe 1980).

Morphine is available in oral as well as injectable forms. Oral forms include concentrated solutions as well as controlled-release tablets. Morphine does not have a dose-related ceiling effect. Therefore doses may vary considerably among patients since each patient's dose must be titrated to completely relieve his or her pain. Also, as tolerance develops or pain increases, doses must be increased to maintain the pain-free state. Specific directions for titrating doses have been published (Wright, 1981; Twycross and Lack, 1983; Twycross and Lack, 1984; Portenoy, Moulin, Rogers, Inturrisi, and Foley, 1986).

The following guidelines, which were synthesized from

several sources, are suggested for using narcotic analgesics in pain management:

1. Start with a specific drug appropriate for the type of pain (Foley, 1985).
2. Know the duration, pharmacokinetic properties, equianalgesic doses, and oral: parenteral ratio for the prescribed drug (Foley, 1985).
3. Adjust the route of administration to the patient's needs (Foley, 1985).
   A. Use oral medications if possible (Twycross and Lack, 1984).
   B. Use parenteral routes which are the most convenient and comfortable for the patient.
      i. Use intravenous lines already in place for:
         a. a narcotic bolus by intravenous (I.V.) drip over fifteen to thirty minutes;
         b. continuous narcotic by I.V. drip via an infusion pump (Fraser, 1980);
         c. a patient controlled analgesia pump (Keeri-Szanto, 1976; Graves, Foster, Batenhorst, Bennett, and Baumann, 1983).
      ii. Use patient controlled analgesia (PCA) subcutaneously (Campbell, Mason, and Weiler, 1983; Coyle, Mauskop, Maggard, and Foley, 1986).
      iii. Rotate injection sites systematically when giving I.M. or subcutaneous injections:
         a. use ventrogluteal sites for I.M. injections because they cause the least pain for patients (Eland, 1983);
         b. use Z-track technique because site discomfort the day following injection is less than when standard technique is used (Keen, 1986).
   C. Use rectal suppositories if patients have difficulty taking oral narcotics (Rogers, 1986).
   D. Use oral morphine solution sublingually to avoid first pass effect in the liver, and provide analgesia for patients with gastrointestinal obstruction, lim-

ited venous access, or reduced muscle mass for parenteral administration (Hirsch, 1984; Foley, 1984).

4. Administer medications every four hours around the clock after initial titration of the dose (Twycross and Lack, 1984; Foley, 1985).
5. Allow patients' wishes to determine the balance between level of pain relief and obtunding effects of high doses of analgesics (Cleeland, Rotondi, Brechner, Levin, MacDonald, Portenoy, Schutta, and McEniry, 1986).
6. Monitor the response carefully (Twycross and Lack, 1984).
7. Combine drugs to provide additive analgesia and reduce side-effects (Foley, 1985).
8. Anticipate side-effects, like constipation, drowsiness, nausea, and vomiting, and treat them preventively with laxatives, amphetamines, and antiemetics (Foley, 1985).
9. Watch for tolerance so analgesic doses or schedules can be adjusted or a stronger, more effective drug ordered (Foley, 1985).
10. Prevent insomnia by using a larger dose of morphine at bedtime for more prolonged pain relief and better sleep (WHO, 1986). Awaken patients to give regularly scheduled analgesics to prevent pain from recurring if a larger dose is not given (Twycross and Lack, 1984; WHO, 1986).
11. Write a PRN analgesic order along with an around-the-clock analgesic so that the nurses have something to alleviate pain if the regularly scheduled regimen does not work (Spross, 1985).
12. Avoid meperipine because repeated doses may cause (a) hyperirritability of the CNS resulting in shakiness, irritability, tremors, twitches, muscle jerking, and generalized motor seizures (Foley, 1979; Kaiko et al. 1983); (b) mood changes (Kaiko et al., 1983); and (c) painful tissue damage from muscle fibrosis when given intramuscularly (McCaffery, 1987).

Adjuvant Analgesics

Adjuvant analgesics include medications such as the steroids, tranquilizers, antidepressants, and antianxiety agents, which in themselves do not produce analgesia but with other analgesics promote better pain control. This probably occurs because they enhance analgesia, ameliorate symptoms, or treat side-effects (WHO, 1986). Steroids, which decrease inflammation and edema, have been useful for relieving pain associated with nerve compression, spinal cord compression, and headache from increased intracranial pressure (Sellers et al., 1984; WHO, 1986). Tranquilizers, like Compazine (prochlorperazine) and Thorazine (chlorpromazine), act as antiemetics and antipsychotics. They are most helpful when the psychological distress component of pain is high but are also indicated for rectal or bladder spasms (Sellers et al., 1984). Elavil (amitriptyline), the antidepressant most commonly used for cancer patients, relieves the dysesthetic pain of deafferentation and postherpetic neuralgia. Since it also produces a hypnotic effect, it is often prescribed at bedtime to improve patients' sleep patterns (Sellers et al., 1984; WHO, 1986). Antianxiety agents, like Valium (diazepam) and Vistaril or Atarax (hydroxyzine), are used to treat pain caused by muscle spasm (WHO, 1986).

In summary, both nurses and physicians have an ethical responsibility to see that quality of life is maintained for cancer patients with severe pain. This can be achieved by appropriate prescription, administration, and evaluation of analgesic drugs. If doses of analgesic medications are individually adjusted, without unnecessary concern for addiction, patients should remain free of pain. Perhaps, then, pain will no longer be automatically associated with cancer.

References

American College of Physicians, Health and Public Policy Committee. (1983), Drug therapy for severe, chronic pain in terminal illness. *Ann. Intern. Med.*, 99/6:870–873.

Bolund, C. (1982), Pain relief through radiotherapy and chemotherapy. *Acta Anaesthes. Scand., Suppl.*, 74, 26:114–116.

Bonica, J.J. (1953), *The Management of Pain*. Philadelphia: Lea & Febiger.

———(1978), Cancer pain: A major national health problem. *Cancer Nurs.*, 1/4:313–316.

———(1982), Management of cancer pain. *Acta Anaesthes. Scand. Suppl.*, 74, 26:75–82.

———(1984), Treatment of cancer pain: Current status and future needs. *Pain*, Suppl., 2:196.

Bressler, L.R., Hange, P.A., & McGuire, D.B. (1986), Characterization of the pain experience in a sample of cancer outpatients. *Oncol. Nurs. Forum*, 13/6:51–55.

Campbell, C.F., Mason, J.B., & Weiler, J.M. (1983), Continuous subcutaneous infusion of morphine for the pain of terminal malignancy. *Ann. Intern. Med.*, 98/1:51–52.

Cassell, E.J. (1983), The relief of suffering. *Arch. Intern. Med.*, 143/3:522–523.

Charap, A.D. (1978), The knowledge, attitudes, and experience of medical personnel treating pain in the terminally ill. *Mt. Sinai. J. Med.*, 45/4:561–580.

Charkes, N.D., Durant, J., & Barry, W.E. (1972), Bone pain in multiple myeloma. *Arch. Intern. Med.*, 130/1:53–58.

Cleeland, C.S. (1984a), Assessing pain in cancer: The patient's role. In: *Symposium on the Management of Cancer Pain*, ed. *Hospital Practice*. New York: HP Publishing, pp. 17–21.

———(1984b), The impact of pain on the patient with cancer. *Cancer*, 54:2635–2641.

———Rotondi, A., Brechner, T., Levin, A., MacDonald, N., Portenoy, R., Schutta, H., & McEniry, M. (1986), A model for the treatment of cancer pain. *J. Pain & Symp. Management*, 1/4:209–215.

Cohen, F.L. (1980), Postsurgical pain relief: patients' status and nurses' medication choices. *Pain*, 9/2:265–274.

Cohen, R.S., Ferrer-Brechner, T., Pavlov, A., & Reading, A.E. (1985), Prospective evaluation of treatment outcome in patients referred to a cancer pain center. *Clin. J. Pain*, 1/2:105–109.

Coyle, N., Mauskop, A., Maggard, J., & Foley, K.M. (1986), Continuous subcutaneous infusions of opiates in cancer patients with pain. *Oncol. Nurs. Forum*, 13/4:53–57.

Daut, R.L., & Cleeland, C.S. (1982), The prevalence and severity of pain in cancer. *Cancer*, 50/9:1913–1918.

Davitz, L.L., & Davitz, J.R. (1980), *Nurses' Responses to Patients' Suffering*. New York: Springer.

Degner, L.F., Fujii, S.H., & Levitt, M. (1982), Implementing a program to control chronic pain of malignant disease for patients in an extended care facility. *Cancer Nurs.*, 5/4:263–268.

Derrick, W. (1972), Management of pain. *Cancer Bull.*, 24/3:46–48.

Eland, J. (1983), Children's pain: Developmentally appropriate efforts to improve identification of source, intensity, and relevant intervening variables. In: *Nursing Research: A Monograph for Non-Nurse Researchers*, eds. G. Felton & M. Albert. New York: McGraw-Hill, pp. 64–79.

Engel, G.L. (1962), *Psychosocial Development in Health and Disease*. Philadelphia: W.B. Saunders.

Foley, K.M. (1979), The management of pain of malignant origin. In:*Current Neurology*, Vol. 2, eds. H.R. Tyler & D.M. Dawson. Boston: Houghton Mifflin, pp. 279–302.

———(1981), *The Management of Cancer Pain*, Vol. 1. Nutley, NJ: Hoffmann La Roche.

———(1982), Clinical assessment of cancer pain. *Acta Anaesthes. Scand. Suppl.*, 74, 26:91–96.

———(1984), A review of pain syndromes in patients with cancer. In: *Symposium on the Management of Cancer Pain*, ed. *Hospital Practice*. New York: HP Publishing, pp. 7–16.

———(1985), The treatment of cancer pain. *New Eng. J. Med.*, 313/2:84–95.

Fox, L.S. (1982), Pain management in the terminally ill cancer patient: An investigation of nurses' attitudes, knowledge, and clinical practice. *Milit. Med.*, 147/6:455–460.

Fraser, D.G. (1980), Intravenous morphine infusion for chronic pain. *Ann. Intern. Med.*, 93/5:781–784.

Grady, M.W. (1986), Pain management for the terminally ill patient. *Nurs. Admin. Quart.*, 10/3:38–44.

Graves, D.A., Foster, T.S., Batenhorst, R.L., Bennett, R.L., & Baumann, T.J. (1983), Patient-controlled analgesia. *Ann. Intern. Med.*, 99/3:360–366.

Grier, M.R., Howard, M., & Cohen, F. (1979), Beliefs and values associated with administering narcotic analgesics to terminally ill patients. In: *Clinical and Scientific Sessions.* Washington, DC: American Nurses Association, pp. 211–222.

Hackett, T.P. (1971), Pain and Prejudice. *Med. Times*, 99/2:130–146.

Hirsch, J.D. (1984), Sublingual morphine sulfate in chronic pain management. *Clin. Pharm.*, 3/6:585–586.

Hunt, J.M., Stollar, T.D., Littlejohns, D.W., Twycross, R.G., & Vere, D.W. (1977), Patients with protracted pain: A survey conducted at the London Hospital. *J. Med. Ethics,* 3/2:61–73.

International Association for the Study of Pain (IASP), Subcommittee on Taxonomy (1979), Pain terms: A list with definitions and notes on usage. *Pain*, 6/3:249–252.

Inturrisi, C.E. (1984), Pharmacology of narcotic analgesics. In: *Symposium on the Management of Cancer Pain*, ed. *Hospital Practice*. New York: HP Publishing, pp. 22–29.

Jacox, A., Pain Alleviation through Nursing Intervention. Unpublished Final Report. Federal Grant NU00467–3.

———(1979), Assessing pain. *Amer. J. Nurs.*, 79/5:895–900.

———Stewart, M. (1973), *Psychosocial Contingencies of the Pain experience.* Iowa City: University of Iowa.

———Rogers, A.G. (1981), The nursing management of pain. In: *Cancer Nursing*, ed. L.B. Marino. St. Louis: C.V. Mosby, pp. 381–404.

Jaffe, J.H. (1980), Drug addiction and drug abuse. In: *The Pharmacological Basis of Therapeutics*, eds. A.G. Gilman, L.S. Goodman, & A. Gilman. New York: Macmillan, pp. 535–584.

Johnson, J.E. (1973), Effects of accurate expectations about sensations on the sensory and distress components of pain. *J. Pers. Soc. Psychol.*, 26:261–275.

———Rice, V.H. (1974), Sensory and distress components of pain. *Nurs. Res.*, 23/3:203–209.

Kaiko, R.F., Foley, K.M., Grabinski, P.Y., Heidrich, G., Rogers, A.G., Inturrisi, C.E., & Reidenberg, M.M. (1983), Central nervous system excitatory effects of meperidine in cancer patients. *Ann. Neurol.*, 13/2:180–185.

Keen, M.F. (1986), Comparison of intramuscular injection techniques to reduce site discomfort and lesions. *Nurs. Res.*, 35/4:207–210.

Keeri-Szanto, M. (1976), Demand analgesia for the relief of pain problems in "terminal" illness. *Anesthes. Rev.*, 3/2:19–21.

Lamerton, R. (1973), The pains of death. *Nurs. Times,* 69/2:56–57.

Lazarus, R.S. (1966), *Psychological Stress and the Coping Process.* New York: McGraw-Hill.

———Folkman, S. (1984), *Stress, Appraisal, and Coping.* New York: Springer.

Lucas, V., & Huang, A. (1977), Letter: Vinblastine-related pain in tumors. *Cancer Treat. Rep.*, 61/9:1735–1736.

Marks, R.M., & Sachar, M.D. (1973), Undertreatment of medical inpatients with narcotic analgesics. *Ann. Intern. Med.*, 78/2:173–181.

Mathews, G.J., Zarro, V., & Osterholm, J.L. (1973), Cancer pain and its treatment. *Sem. Drug Treat.*, 3/1:45–53.

McCaffery, M. (1979), *Nursing Management of the Patient with Pain*, 2nd ed. Philadelphia: J.B. Lippincott.

———(1987), Giving meperidine for pain: Should it be so mechanical. *Nurs.*, 87, 17/4:61–64.

Melzack, R. (1975), The McGill Pain Questionnaire: Major properties and scoring methods. *Pain*, 1/3:277–300.

———Torgerson, W.S. (1971), On the language of pain. *Anesthes.*, 34:50–59.

Murphy, T.M. (1973), Cancer pain. *Postgrad. Med.*, 53/6:187–194.

Oster, M.W., Vizel, M., & Turgeon, L.R. (1978), Pain of terminal cancer patients. *Arch. Intern. Med.*, 138/12:1801–1802.

Parker, R.G. (1974), Selective use of radiation therapy for the cancer patient with pain. In: *Advances in Neurology*, Vol. 4, ed. J.J. Bonica. New York: Raven Press, pp. 491–493.

Pilowsky, M.D., & Bond, M.R. (1969), Pain and its management in malignant disease. *Psychosom. Med.*, 31/5:400–404.

Portenoy, R.K., Moulin, D.E., Rogers, A., Inturrisi, C.E., & Foley, K.M. (1986), IV infusion of opioids for cancer pain: Clinical review and guidelines for use. *Cancer Treat. Rep.*, 70/5:575–581.

Porter, J., & Jick, H. (1980), Addiction rare in patients treated with narcotics. *New Eng. J. Med.*, 302/2:123.

Rankin, M.A. (1980), The progressive pain of cancer. *Topics in Clin. Nurs.*, 2/1:57–73.

———(1982), Use of drugs for pain with cancer patients. *Cancer Nurs.*, 5/3:181–190.

———Snider, B. (1984), Nurses' perceptions of cancer patients' pain. *Cancer Nurs.*, 7/2:149–155.

Rogers, A., (1977), Drugs for pain. In: *Proceedings of the Second National Conference on Cancer Nursing*. New York: American Cancer Society, pp. 39–43.

———(1986), The use and availability of rectal narcotics. *J. Pain & Symp. Management*, 1/4:229–230.

Roller, A.C., ed. (1986), WHO outlines global cancer pain relief program. *Oncol. News/Update* 1/6:11.

Sanford, R.A., & Patrick, B.S. (1977), Management of pain of malignancy. *J. Miss. State Med. Assn.*, 28/9:230–232.

Saunders, C. (1976), Control of pain in terminal cancer. *Nurs. Times*, 72/29:1133–1135.

———(1981), Current views on pain relief and terminal care. In: *The Therapy of Pain*, ed. M. Swerdlow. Philadelphia: J.B. Lippincott, pp. 215–241.

Sellers, E.M., Mount, B.M., & Bethune, G.W. (1984), *Cancer Pain: A Monograph on the Management of Cancer Pain*. Ottawa: Minister of Supply and Services, Canada.

Senescu, R.A. (1963), The development of emotional complications in the patient with cancer. *J. Chronic Dis.*, 16:813–832.

Shawver, M.M. (1977), Pain associated with cancer. In: *Pain: A Source Book For Nurses and Other Health Professionals*, ed. A.K. Jacox. Boston: Little, Brown, pp. 373–389.

Spross, J.A. (1985), Cancer pain and suffering: clinical lessons from life, literature, and legend. *Oncol. Nurs. Forum*, 12/4:23–31.

Sternbach, R.A. (1968), *Pain: A Psychophysiological Analysis*. New York: Academic Press.

Stewart, M.L. (1977), Measurement of clinical pain. In: *Pain: A Source Book for Nurses and Other Health Professionals*, ed. A.K. Jacox. Boston: Little, Brown, pp. 107–137.

Twycross, R.G. (1974), Clinical experience with diamorphine in advanced malignant disease. *Internat. J. Clin. Pharmacol.*, 9/3:184–198.

———(1975), Diseases of the central nervous system: Relief of terminal cancer. *Brit. Med. J.*, 4/5990:212–214.

———(1978), The target is a pain-free patient. *Nurs. Mirror*, 147/24:38–39.

———(1982), Ethical and clinical aspects of pain treatment in cancer patients. *Acta Anaesthes. Scand. Suppl.*, 74, 26:83–90.

———(1984), Cancer pain management. *Iss. Oncol.*, 1/4:3–5.

———Fairfield, S. (1982), Pain in far-advanced cancer. *Pain*, 14/3:303–310.

———Lack, S.A. (1983), *Symptom Control in Far Advanced Cancer: Pain Relief.* London: Pitman Limited.

——— ———(1984), *Oral Morphine in Advanced Cancer.* Beaconsfield, Bucks, U.K.: Beaconsfield.

Volicer, B., & Bohannon, M. (1975), A hospital stress rating scale. *Nurs. Res.*, 24/5:352–359.

World Health Organization. (1986), *Cancer Pain Relief.* Geneva: World Health Organization.

Wright, Z. (1981), From I.V. to P.O: titrating your patient's pain medication. *Nursing*, 81, 11/7:39–43.

22

Counseling the Chronic Pain Patient

RICHARD J. BECK, PH.D., C.R.C., N.C.C.
AND PAUL LUSTIG, PH.D.

INTRODUCTION

The effects of chronic pain are an enormous burden to any society. For those suffering with chronic low back pain alone the costs are $23 billion annually in Workers' Compensation and Social Security payments, long-term disability payments, and legal fees. This malady accounts for 24 percent of all time lost from work; 30 percent of all compensation claims are due to low back injuries. Research has shown that the problem leads to chronic unemployment: Conley and Noble (1978) cited research on Workers' Compensation claims in five states and concluded that unemployment among those with permanent, but only partial disabilities (i.e., the physician in the case believed that the individual was able to return to some form of employment, albeit with limitations), was rife, ranging from 22 to 49 percent depending on the state.

More recent research has produced similar results. Beck (1987) studied nonscheduled permanent partial cases in Wisconsin (82 percent back injured) and found that 36 percent of workers returned to their former employers and were still with them after three years. However, of the remainder, more than two out of three were unemployed. The factors associated with unemployment were primarily length of convalescence, age, and external locus of control; also, the most difficult cases seemed to be referred to rehabilitation workers. There was an association between rehabilitation services being involved, and poor outcome, just as there was between being referred for rehabilitation and having a longer period of convalescence. In addition, chronic pain literature defines the length of convalescence as one factor in chronicity of pain; another is the presence of profound emotional consequences of the pain, mainly depression and anxiety (Sternbach, 1974; Bergman and Werblun, 1978).

Eaton (1979) has succinctly and comprehensively described the major obstacles to rehabilitating the chronic pain patient who is receiving Workers' Compensation. He cited nine major obstacles: (1) a protracted period of recuperation; (2) the receipt of Workers' Compensation benefits; (3) employer rejection of the injured worker; (4) worker personality factors (e.g., low self-esteem, external locus of control, and poor adjustment to disability); (5) family reinforcement of the patient's sick role status; (6) dependence on drugs; (7) insensitive tactics by claims adjusters; (8) attorney reinforcement of the invalid role and blocking of rehabilitation efforts; and (9) union contracts imposing limitations on lighter work entry.

Hanson-Mayer (1984) and others have focused on the concept of secondary gain as an explanatory phenomenon in chronic low back pain. These authors have argued that the maintenance of chronic pain has as much to do with the expectation by the patient of some kind of reinforcement for having the pain, as it has to do with tissue damage. Moreover, these authors ascribe pain which occurs in the absence of explanatory organic factors, to the expectation of reinforcement, or secondary gain. Tuck (1983) takes the concept of "gain" a step further, and describes "tertiary gain" as those gains made by significant parties involved with the injured worker; for example, the fact that the fee for the attorney's services is commensurate with the size of the disability award, and that the referrals to a rehabilitation specialist are partly based on the specialist's ability to attenuate the compensation paid to the injured worker. It seems clear that psychologists and other rehabilitation workers must be prepared to deal with both intrinsic factors (i.e., depression, anxiety, and others) and extrinsic or environmental factors when attempting to assist the chronic pain patient. However, as Tuck (1983) illustrated, since the service provider does not work in a vacuum, and is susceptible to the pressures of various forces (especially financial reward), it is critical for that provider to understand the chronic pain patient, and the emotional and environmental consequences of that patient's pain, not only for the patient, but for all parties involved with the patient. This chapter will attempt to analyze these factors, as well as provide some discussion on counseling strategies which may be helpful in returning the patient to as productive a life-style as possible, as well as appropriate roles which can be assumed by service providers. Since the majority of those who assist chronic pain patients (at least in the low back pain area) are rehabilitation counselors and affiliated occupations, the theoretical underpinnings of these professional approaches will be emphasized here. The question of service provision and alternative roles also impinges on questions of ethics, especially in view of tertiary gain considerations. Therefore, some discussion of ethical conduct will be part of this analysis.

Patient and Situational Variables

Patient Variables

Chronic pain is a dichotomous phenomenon, one side belonging to the domain of musculoskeletal and tissue damage, and the other to the psychological, which includes perceptual, behavioral, emotional, demographic, and cognitive factors. The way that chronic pain patients are described depends in part upon the factors which are emphasized.

Fordyce (1976) has developed a way of looking at pain behavior and treating it with applied learning theory, and his model is in use at many pain clinics and treatment centers. He believes that pain can only be identified through the verbal and nonverbal communication of patients, and that it is this communication, not the pain itself, which should be treated. He further believes that much of pain behavior (complaining, limping, etc.) is not only physiological, but operant as well, designed to elicit certain "rewards" from the environment, such as attention from significant others, compensation, and other forms of secondary gain.

Sternbach (1974) has described the emotional component of chronic pain. He emphasize the interpersonal manipulativeness of many pain patients. Sternbach believes that pain is central to the identity of the chronic pain patient since painful illness or injury plus unmet emotional needs leads to behavior resulting in the meeting of those needs through chronic pain. He also differentiated chronic pain patients from acute patients, in that the former patients cannot ascribe a sense of meaning to the pain; the pain is, therefore, difficult to treat and becomes associated with confusion, anxiety, bitterness against others who are enjoying life without pain, despair, a sense of injustice and indignation, and hopelessness. The chronic pain patient becomes locked in a vicious cycle of anxiety, worry, and sleepless nights. However, the cycle of misery cited above is sometimes an inevitable response to the way some individuals cope with disability, combined with the response of significant others to their prolongation in the sick role.

Berven, Habeck, and Malec (1985) used a cluster analysis procedure in analyzing the Minnesota Multiphasic Personality Inventory (MMPI-168) profiles of 120 rehabilitation medicine inpatients, and identified four patient clusters characterized as the following: (1) no clinical elevations (about half the sample); (2) depression (significantly female); (3) somatic focusing; and (4) personality disorganization. Further discriminative analysis revealed that ruminative worry and openness to identifying problems accounted for the majority of the differentiation.

Pilling, Brannick, and Swenson (1967) concluded after reviewing the MMPI profiles of pain patients and interviews with them that pain may be substituted for feelings of anxiety and depression.

Engel (1959) characterized pain-prone patients as having excessive conscious or unconscious guilt feelings, which the experience of pain serves to relieve. For him, chronic pain patients are often intolerant of success.

Beutler, Engle, Oro'-Beutler, Daldrup, and Meredith (1986) proposed that difficulty expressing anger and controlling intense emotions are predisposing factors linking both depression and chronic pain. They believe that chronic pain and depression may be disturbances in processing intensely emotional information, which then affects both the immune system and interpersonal relationships.

Various authors have emphasized the perceptual elements of chronic pain, such as those who describe the relationship between temperament and arousal (Eysenck and Eysenck, 1968; Johnson, 1982). According to this theory, introversion and extraversion are representations of the interaction between the environment and the organism's underlying endogenous arousal level. Extraverts are thought to be less likely to identify nociceptive stimuli as painful and have a higher tolerance for both intensity and duration of pain, then introverts. Johnson (1982) found in a study of eighty-five chronic low back pain patients hospitalized for treatment, that this group was significantly more introverted than college students or patients with spinal cord injuries.

The cognitive aspects of chronic pain have been described by several authors (Melzack, 1973; and Turk, Meichenbaum, and Genest, 1983). They propose that cognitions are primary in the experience of pain: cognitions precede and direct emotional responses. They offer much research to show that pain patients who receive cognitive reorientation show an increase in their ability to cope with pain, and a reduction in their experience of pain.

Still other authors espouse psychophysiological concepts of chronic pain. Flor, Turk, and Birbaumer (1985) and other researchers have demonstrated the link between stress and pain, which is in turn exacerbated by emotional reactions to pain such as anxiety, depression, or somatization. Another concept in this area is that of the pain–muscle spasm–pain cycle (Keefe, Block, Williams, and Surwit, 1981). In this view, an initial event such as an accident triggers reflexive muscle spasms, accompanied by vasoconstriction, the release of pain-producing substances, and pain. With time, an attempt is made to minimize additional muscle spasm and pain by restricting movement. When this occurs, muscle shortening may bring on fatigue, which predisposes muscles to more spasm and increased pain. If this cycle continues, periods of pain become more frequent, and the pain can become chronic and last for years.

A third approach in the psychophysiological area is that of the neuromuscular pain model (Dolce and Raczynski, 1985). These researchers point out that many pain patients have muscular asymmetries and abnormally low levels of paraspinal muscle activity which produce instability in the spine, and irritation and impingement of spinal nerves, thereby inducing pain.

In addition to the models presented above, there are various other factors which have been mentioned in the literature as correlates of chronic pain. One element which seems critical in chronic pain is that of time. With its passage, pain goes from the acute stage to a chronic stage. With the development of chronicity, personality changes occur in the individual which may affect the person's very identity (Sternbach, 1974). Lynch (1979) reviewed the chronic pain literature and noted that pain patients seem to be initially severely depressed, mildly hypochondriachal, and mildly hysterical; in time they become progressively less depressed (perhaps pain becomes a "mask" for the less acceptable depression), but more severely hypochondriachal and hysterical. He noted that the probability of successful rehabilitation decreases with time.

Another element which seems to be associated with chronic pain is that of poor premorbid adjustment. Various researchers have found chronic pain patients to have a substantially greater history of depression (Schaffer, Donlon, and Bittle, 1980), and poorer premorbid adjustment and social maturity (Kalla, 1977).

Finally, some researchers have cited various demographic correlates of chronic pain. Melzack (1973) reported that reactivity and tolerance of pain is related to cultural and socioeconomic status. Low back pain is clearly related to the strength factors in occupations. Other researchers have pointed out that chronic pain may be a symptom of a dysfunctional marriage (Delvey and Hopkins, 1982).

Situational Variables

The chronic pain patient often receives some form of disability compensation (Beck, [1987], found that 40 percent of unemployed injured workers cited this as their primary source of income). Turpin (1987) also demonstrated, through his research on pain patients evaluated at a hospital pain center, the association between the disincentive influence of compensation, and chronic pain and unemployment.

Several factors inherent in Workers' Compensation, the primary disability compensation system, contribute to "pain games" which are played by the injured worker and by others in the process. One of these factors is the basis for making compensation payments. Wage replacement (usually two-thirds to three-fourths of preinjury wage up to a maximum) is paid to the injured worker until a physician (either the patient's own or one who examines the patient at the request of the insurance carrier or employer) states that the worker has reached a "healing plateau" which indicates that maximum healing has probably been achieved, even though some residual disability may remain. Since this compensation may represent more security to a patient (who fears further injury) than an attempt to return to employment, the individual may resist making positive reports to the doctor.

Another factor is the way in which states pay compensation to workers for permanent disability after the healing period has ended, and with it, wage replacement. Some states pay workers on the basis of functional, or medical, factors; others pay on the basis of lost earning capacity; and some states do both. Regardless of the basis for payment, there is an incentive for some workers to attempt to increase their monetary settlements through maximizing their disability. Attorneys may consciously or unconsciously aid this attempt since their fees are based on the size of the disability award.

Physicians can become obstacles in the process of rehabilitating the chronic pain patient. Hackett (1971) surveyed the attitudes of health care providers toward chronic pain patients and concluded that: (1) health care providers disbelieve that patients have pain in the absence of demonstrable chronicity; (2) they treat chronic pain from an acute pain model; (3) they tend to undermedicate patients and overestimate the seriousness of iatrogenic drug addition; (4) they use placebos incorrectly; and (5) they do not refer patients to psychological or psychiatric services until other treatment strategies fail. These attitudes can result in patient confusion, frustration, and hopelessness. They can also induce a certain amount of defensiveness in a physician who can feel that he or she is not getting anywhere with a patient. The physician may not actively cooperate with rehabilitation professionals who query the physician regarding the patient's progress, and otherwise seek guidance regarding the patient's vocational rehabilitation and other matters.

Insensitive claims adjusters and rejecting employers can also increase hostility in the injured worker which can be displaced toward rehabilitation workers who attempt to help the injured person return to a job, or try to help him or her to achieve a more positive adjustment to the disability. Often, these workers perceive collection of their wage replacement benefit, or increasing the size of their disability award, as ways of vindicating themselves or "getting revenge" against those who they believe are treating them unfairly. Litigation to determine the extent of permanent partial disability occurs in 40 to 50 percent of cases in many states (Conley and Noble, 1978; Beck, 1987).

Secondary Gain

This area was chosen for examination as a separate topic, because it is, in the opinion of the authors, the most misunderstood concept in the area of chronic pain, and one that contributes to more rehabilitation failure and counselor bias than any other. As a concept, it is an important ingredient in the understanding of chronic pain, but like the concept of "motivation," it can either add to, or present an obstacle to, effective counseling practice.

The concept of secondary gain is a fairly frequent explanation of the lack of rehabilitation movement of many of our clients. It is even more frequently used in workers' compensation cases, legal situations, and in private rehabilitation agencies. In addition, we have given additional names to the same or similar concepts. Among them are disincentives and the "worker's disability syndrome" (Hanson-Mayer, 1984).

The concept of secondary gain tends to mean that the patient holds on to a disabling or nonvalid symptom, because the person gets greater benefits by holding on to the symptom, than by discarding it. It also implies that the symptoms which the person holds are minor or less important. Although sometimes unconscious, it implies a conscious control in which the person weighs the benefits and discomforts on both sides of the ledger or balance sheet. In using secondary gain as a basis for decision making, the client goes against what society would consider beneficial to the person and to others.

The concept of secondary gain was introduced by Freud (1936). Freud made the distinction between the primary process in symptom formation and secondary gain. The primary process in the formation of symptoms is a neurotic process, which is developed because of a breakdown of one's protective capabilities. The primary process controls anxiety. Secondary gain has no part in the production of symptoms. The person does not develop symptoms in order to enjoy some advantages. Freud remarked that "one does not cut one's leg off for the purpose of such gains as living in indolence on his pension" (p.33).

In today's use of secondary gain in rehabilitation, there tends to be an omission of the emotional consequences of a disability. Among the emotional concomitants of a disability may be an attack upon the person's self-esteem and role in society. In other words, the person may see him or herself as less competent, desirable, and respected than was the case before the disability. The person may believe that their salary will be drastically reduced, thus reducing how society values the person. The person may believe that they are not the man or woman they were before.

A second concomitant of a disability is often the need to have others see the disability as catastrophic, dire, and tragic. Thus, others will appreciate the physical and psychological suffering and fright that the person is going through.

Most of us tend to need acceptance by others. If there is a test of the degree of acceptance, it occurs when we do poorly, fail, or become less than we have been. The need for others to understand and accept the disabling condition as dire and tragic is related to our need for social acceptance.

Another emotional concomitant of disability is that for many it results in seeing oneself as less competent than others (who seem to expect that the disabled person can perform at a similar level). In this additional aspect of the disability, the less one thinks of oneself, the less one is ready to take on new tasks. Since the person has been seriously hurt once, there tends to be a desire to prevent further injury and failure. The consequence is that often the person avoids doing what could be done before, because failure would be extremely painful. Doing a new task is also fraught with danger. The person might fail and thereby expose to himself and to others the degree of incompetence the injury has caused. The end result of this anxiety is that the person often doesn't try to do much because he or she needs to avoid failure.

The following case is an example of this avoidance principle:

> A woman, aged forty-five, is a single parent. She has raised a child, who was born out of wedlock, to adolescence. She has worked and supported the child. She is faced with two strong forces or pushes. She works in a hospital–institution for the severely and profoundly retarded, who also have medical–physiologic problems in addition to the mental retardation. She is an attendant, and dislikes her job intensely. On the other hand, she needs to work in order to show her strength and independence. The image which she has and wants to portray is that of a hard-working, serious minded person. She would have great difficulty accepting welfare assistance. She cannot stop working because of what it might do to her child's attitude toward her. So,

> on the one hand, she needs to work, while on the other hand, she can't stand the job. She can't even quit her job and look for another. She doesn't have enough savings to tide her over. In addition, she has grave doubts that she can get another job of at least equal pay. She is trapped in her present situation, and if she continues in it, there will be some serious deterioration. So her psyche or ego does a creative thing. While still expressing a very strong desire to continue working, she develops a back problem as a result of lifting the children. Whether it is medially supported or psychologically caused is immaterial. She can't lift. She cannot continue to do what she has been doing. She receives workers' compensation and immediately makes preparation for developing a new occupational skill by registering in the local vocational–technical school. By doing so, she has proven to everyone that she can no longer work in her former employment.

If there was a Machiavelli in this situation it was her unconscious psyche, which selected a method that was acceptable to her and others of getting away from what was disliked and moving toward what was wanted. There is always a danger that the person may be shifting the arena of difficulty because of another, as yet undetected conflict, or the new occupation is not a really desirable one.

The misuse of secondary gain as a concept in counseling the chronic pain patient is precisely that it prevents any possible progress the patient might make. It is a dangerous interpretive concept. It tends to interfere or even destroy a helping relationship. It may give us a reason for ridding ourselves of a difficult case, but too often the difficulty in case handling has resulted not from secondary gain, but from concerns inappropriate to case handling.

First, what does the concept do to our service relationship? If the client has a need for acceptance, to be seen as having suffered a dire insult, implying that the client's behavior is the result of some economic benefit that will result from not doing anything about employment, tells the client that we see him or her as a conniving, dishonest, materialistic, lying, malingering, deceptive person. Even if this is not actually stated, many clients have a tremendous need to know that others accept the tragic consequences of the disability, and they are extremely sensitive to the failure to communicate this. The result is to force the client to resist this negative conception, to protect himself by an increasing tenaciousness, and eventually to become angry with the counselor who does not accept the fear and the uncertainty resulting from the disability. Most of all it reflects a lack of respect for the client's failings and humanity.

Finally, the label of secondary gain is often applied to clients who are above all ambivalent in their attitude toward their disability. To a certain degree, ambivalence is a typical reaction to chronic pain. In fact, the lack of ambivalence is arguably descriptive of malingerers. It is the hallmark of successful counseling to help the client become aware of ambivalent attitudes and feelings and to help resolve that ambivalence, in favor of making choices which are consistent with the client's values, interests, abilities, aptitudes, and needs.

Counseling Approaches

Counseling models and techniques can be either unidimensional or multidimensional, and interpersonal or intrapersonal in dealing with the psychosocial problems of chronic pain patients. In unidimensional approaches, such as learning theory, the focus is on one aspect of the patient's condition; for example, behavior. In multidimensional approaches, such as cognitive counseling strategies, the focus of counseling switches between the cognitive–evaluative motivational–affective, and the sensory–discriminative components. For example, the patient learns that he or she can exert some control over the sensory–discriminative component of pain through relaxation techniques and controlled breathing. The patient learns that he or she can exert control in the motivational–affective component by acquiring skills in attention–diversion and imagery manipulations, in order to counteract feelings of helplessness and absence of control. And finally, the patient can learn to deal with the cognitive–evaluative component through learning how to reconceptualize the pain experience, identifying painful stressors, and learning how to prepare for them and handle them, and by learning new coping skills to handle pain, and self-reinforcement techniques to reward successful coping (Meichenbaum 1977).

Counseling approaches can be interpersonal in the sense that they may focus on the person's behavior, or communication of pain experience, to others. Thus, learning theory approaches focus on the patient's communication of perceived pain, and reality therapy (Glasser, 1965) focuses on accomplishing objectives in order to learn responsibility for the satisfaction of one's own needs.

Intrapersonal approaches include those which focus on the person's evaluation of the total pain experience, and their feelings, attitudes, and reactions to that experience. Commonly, counseling the intrapersonal condition involves a series of stages. The first stage is one of acceptance of the person's perception by the counselor, who communicates a recognition that there is good reason for supporting the existence of pain. The second stage is one of empathy and value. This underlies a recognition that the person has been suffering and as such has manifested human strength far beyond what the average person is asked to do. The third stage is one of examining the choices. It involves selection or method of coping with the pain. If the person chooses not to succumb to the pain, this is the "action stage" in which pain rehabilitation takes place.

The level of counseling skill of the professional working with the patient is a consideration in the choice of counseling approaches. But anyone who seeks to counsel the chronic pain patient should be aware of the varying treatment approaches, so that he or she may either practice them with pain patients, or refer the pain patient to another professional for that service.

Also, the professional working with the chronic pain patient should be aware of the correlates of chronic pain, and disability in general, in order to have the capability of forming working hypotheses and choosing counseling practices with which to test these hypotheses. For example, knowing that a client is extraverted may lead to utilizing counseling approaches which are less intrapersonal and more experiental, as suggested by Malec (1985).

Behavior Management

A unidimensional approach that is frequently employed by pain clinics and treatment centers is that developed by Fordyce (1976) and others (Rachlin, 1985). Fordyce applies learning theory principles developed by Skinner and other learning-behavioral proponents, to the chronic pain problem. He views chronic pain symptomatology as developing independently following its acute stage, and as being directly related to both pathological and operant components. The latter include social reinforcement, financial remuneration, and avoidance of fear. Since this symptomatology can only be assessed via communication from the patient (both verbal and nonverbal), these pain behaviors should be the targets of treatment, using operant conditioning principles. Keefe and Gil (1986) have described criticisms and limitations with this model: it is expensive, usually requiring inpatient hospitalization; important contingencies are difficult or impossible to control (e.g., patient family members, attorneys); the actual reduction of pain may not occur, resulting in frustration by both patient and referring physician; and many patients may not be appropriate candidates for referral (those whose organicity is commensurate with stated pain, and so on).

Psychodynamically Oriented Therapies

Another unidimensional approach with chronic pain patients is the application of psychodynamic theories (Freud, 1915; Rogers, 1951; Szasz, 1955) in therapy or counseling, where the intervention consists of a sharing of inner worlds. Bellisimo and Tunks (1984) point out that an objective for psychodynamic therapy with pain patients is to "promote the patient's understanding of the manner in which the pain evolved and the function that it served; this involves its role in the basic emotional economy of the patient as 'primary gain' and its secondary entrenchment as part of the patient's style of operating because of the addition of 'secondary gain'" (p. 102).

These authors provide a very useful and compelling view of the effect of a painful event on the life of the patient:

> Should a problem of chronic pain arise, a number of events and changes may follow. Events such as work and participation in family affairs may be curtailed; the sense of security, self-efficacy, and sameness that flows from these activities may be impaired. The results of loss of function may indeed be serious or even catastrophic, with loss of income and house, damaging the family's future. If so, the importance of the injury event and the changes occasioned, is heightened in proportion to the perceived threat to the self. It is an easy step from here to the development of the fantasy that if only the pain could be taken away, all of the other unpleasant consequences would also be reversed. In this way, the "problem" is, in the eyes of the sufferer, reduced to a solitary cause and solution—one, however, that is forever elusive. This fantasy is furthered by regression, which invests the therapist in the role of parental omnipotence, viewed ambivalently, however, as potentially withholding from the clamoring needy self. The sense of being changed may be further accentuated over time by the forgetting and blurring of the details, more and more emphasis being given to the pain and loss. The search for the former self is likely a fantasy in major part, because one finds an almost universal tendency among chronic pain patients to speak in glowing terms of their premorbid selves, whereas on careful inquiry of the patient and other family members, one often finds that premorbid function was less than ideal [p. 116–117].

Psychodynamic therapy or counseling offers the pain patient the opportunity to gain insight into the relationship between his pain and personality, and to facilitate corrective emotional experience. It is also an opportunity for the patient to rebuild needed self-confidence, improve self-concept, increase responsibility taking, and decrease dependency.

The limitations of this technique have to do with time and efficiency, as well as patient need. First, psychodynamically oriented counseling or therapy is oftentimes intensive, with commensurately high cost, which many patients can ill-afford, and many sources of third-party funding (e.g., insurers, employers) may resist underwriting. The objectives of this therapy are often quite subjective, with therapists and patients often disputing counseling outcomes.

Along with the ambiguity of outcomes, psychodynamic approaches often do not deal with the complex issues having to do with the demands of insurers, employers, attorneys, physicians, and other parties. Psychodynamically oriented therapy is not primarily interested in holding a patient to a certain value system, and therefore it may ignore the hidden values which are communicated to the patient: that medical progress is good and lack of it implies malingering on the part of the patient; that a specific disability should only require a given amount of time to heal (which the United States government has recently embodied in paying for certain medical services according to criteria established for diagnostic related groups [DRG's]; that a patient should be interested in, and should do everything possible, to try to get back to work; and that psychotherapy itself amounts to "hand-holding" and does not deal with the hard issues involved with return to work.

Finally, patient needs often extend beyond those related to the objectives of psychotherapy. They may have more to do with other more practical matters, such as occupational change, job finding, clearing up ambiguous medical problems, and so on. The following case history will illustrate the point:

> One of the authors had received a referral for counseling, Mrs. M., who had a shoulder and arm disability in which she had severe limitation in range of motion and severe pain when she moved her affected arm. On the first visit with the client, she wept upon relating the details of her accident and her disability, and how it affected her daily life. The only relief that she could obtain from her constant pain were brief episodes after she visited her chiropractor, who had treated her for over a year. She seemed fearful of doing any kind of job and reported other negative effects of the injury—interference with her role as a grandmother and wife, sleepless nights, loss of appetite. The counselor's first hypothesis was that she had chronic pain syndrome which included a heavy depressive component, but decided to refer her to an excellent orthopedist for a definitive diagnosis. He reported that she had a frozen shoulder, a

complication of her original tissue damage, and he recommended further treatment including surgery and physical therapy. With time and treatment, her pain became better and she was able to resolve problems of occupation and to resume a satisfying family life.

This vignette illustrates that had the counselor pursued his original hypothesis of a depressive reaction associated with chronic pain, the counseling therapy chosen might not have been an effective treatment due to the acuteness of the medical problem. The counselor took it upon himself to provide medical management coordination and obtain a definitive medical diagnosis before proceeding with a counseling approach to depressive symptoms, which ultimately succeeded in making the entire process more effective. In addition, the counselor became more potent in the eyes of the client, because he was addressing the matter of the client's first concern, her pain, as the first step in helping her.

Cognitive–Behavioral Therapy

Cognitive approaches are based upon the belief that patient cognitions, or perspectives, of their experiences are primary and precede and condition their emotional reactions (e.g., depression and anxiety), affect their sensory pain perception, cause hyperactivity in affected muscles and provoke spasm, and direct their behavioral responses (for a thorough discussion of these themes, see Melzack and Wall [1965]; Melzack and Casey [1968]; Beck [1987]; Flor and Turk [1984]). Because the cognitive model incorporates sensory, psychological, affective, and behavioral coping factors, it is a multidimensional approach.

Although a wide variety of therapeutic procedures fall in the category of cognitive "reorientation" (education, relaxation, desensitization, reduction of medications), perhaps the most widely recognized cognitive approach is that of Turk (1978) which is based on Meichenbaum's theory of behavior change (1977). Applied to chronic pain, Meichenbaum's approach has three phases: (1) education of the patient regarding his pain and how intervention will benefit him; (2) training the patient in the use of a variety of coping techniques to be used in the various aspects of the pain problem; and (3) the implementation of the learned coping skills. The skills in phase 2 include the use of relaxation techniques, self-directed strategies in dealing with attention (directed imagery) and noxious stimulation, and reorienting cognitions involving attributions, labeling, and self-statements.

Biofeedback is another mode of therapy which is closely allied with the cognitive and operant-conditioning behavioral schools. In this therapy, the patient is hooked up by a network of leads to an electronic system which is capable of measuring otherwise involuntary bodily responses, such as blood pressure, muscle tension, brain waves, and so on. These responses are amplified and converted into signals which the patient may readily identify, such as the movement of the needle in a meter, varied audible tones, or flashing lights. The objectives of this therapy are to allow the patient to gain an awareness of physiological states which may affect his or her pain, learn how to exert some control over these states, and to then generalize these newly acquired skills outside the laboratory (Budzynski, 1973).

Other psychological interventions used in the treatment of chronic pain include hypnosis and family counseling (discussed in detail in Bellisimo and Tunks [1984]).

Rehabilitation Counseling

Rehabilitation counselors who work with chronic pain clients often differ from other professionals (e.g., psychologists) with regard to counseling objectives (adjustment to disability versus fundamental changes in personality or behavior), the setting in which they work, referral sources, and the variables to which they pay attention. For example, rehabilitation psychologists and other psychologists often work in hospitals or clinic settings, in which they use the counseling and therapeutic approaches outlined above. However, most rehabilitation counselors who work with chronic pain patients are employed in other settings which are not conducive to using some of the therapies that have been described above (especially the unidimensional approaches). These counselors work in proprietary rehabilitation offices primarily, with another large group working for state institutions, and still others working directly for insurance companies or employers.

The fact that rehabilitation psychologists and other psychologists are often licensed, and are graduates of the American Psychological Association's approved graduate programs, makes them eligible for third-party payments (i.e., medical and other insurance plans) while rehabilitation counselors often are not. Therefore, rehabilitation counselors, especially those who work in the proprietary rehabilitation sector, receive their referrals from insurance companies or employers who pay Workers' Compensation benefits and who would like to limit their exposure, or total liability for indemnity payments and medical costs, through helping the injured worker to return to work as soon as possible. The rehabilitation counselor is thus under a set of expectations from the referral source to provide the most cost-effective services possible in order to realize the goal of helping the client achieve a productive life-style. That is not to say that psychologists do not have some of these same expectations placed upon them, but their referrals do not totally depend upon satisfying the expectations of insurers and employers such as is the case with those counselors who work in the private, proprietary rehabilitation sector. Many of the referrals to psychologists come from physicians and other medical professionals whose expectations may differ from those of insurance companies as to length and cost of treatment, focus on work, and attention to issues of exposure.

Rehabilitation counseling as a profession also differs from psychology in its concept of the roles and functions of the counselor. In rehabilitation, for example, the case manager role is seen as just as important as the "self-actualizer" role (Cassell and Mulkey, 1985). As a manager, the functions of the counselor include planning, organizing, directing, coordinating, and controlling. In working with chronic pain patients where many parties are involved (lawyers, physicians, physical therapists, employers, psychologists, and insurance companies, etc.) the manager role often leads the rehabilitation counselor to becoming the de facto team leader, whose functions are to coordinate communication between all parties, act as a negotiator (Beck, 1985) and clarifier, and to ultimately come up with a rehabilitation plan or program which is built on the consensual agreement of all parties.[1] In fact, one of the managing roles of the rehabilitation counselor may be to refer a client in need of in-depth pain therapy to a pain clinic, which employs rehabilitation or other psychologists (e.g., in the case of the client with severe depressive characteristics).

Rehabilitation counseling itself differs somewhat from psychology in that it has more of a systems view of treating the disabled individual than the closely related professions of clinical or counseling psychology (see Cottone [1987], for a complete description of this point of view). In this view, the client and his or her disability interact in reciprocation with environmental factors including the referral source, employer, client's family, and all other factors in the environment.[2]

Thomas, Butler, and Parker (1987) state that the client's achievement of rehabilitation goals is predicated upon counseling, especially *psychosocial counseling*, which they define thus:

> The term psychosocial counseling comes from the concept that a handicap is the cumulative result of society's imposition of psychosocial barriers (e.g., negative attitudes) on persons with disabilities. The internalization of demeaning psychological and sociological influences may lead to a negative self-image and other psychosocial difficulties. Consequently, effective rehabilitation counselors typically focus their efforts on the amelioration or removal of psychosocial problems and on the resultant personal adjustment problems faced by their clients [p. 65–66].

Rehabilitation counseling as a profession has its basis in various theories of adjustment to disability, including attitudes

[1]As a negotiator, the counselor must be careful not to represent the interests of either party, and must strive to assume the role of an authoritative, neutral third party.

[2]The use of pain as a secondary gain is a result of this reciprocal process, when a need for succorance and support are not met, and the person is forced into creating a chronic pain situation as a means of communicating the extent of the disability's devastation.

of others toward the disabled, and of disabled people toward themselves and their own disabilities. Cook (1987) cited Lewin's (1935, 1936) field theory and the somatopsychologists (Barker, Wright, Meyerson and Gonick, 1953; Dembo, Leviton, and Wright, 1956) who incorporated his theory into broader theories of adjustment to disability. He also cited the work of researchers who have studied the problems of society's attitudes in relation to disabled individuals (English, 1971; Siller, 1976; Livneh, 1986) in his discussion of the experiences which disabled people confront and their possible range of responses to them. In his review, disabled people face being relegated to a minority group status with much stigma being associated with that new status, and he pointed out that they can respond to this status, and to their impairment, with a range of reactions from succumbing to overcoming.

The authors' view of the stages that an individual with chronic pain may experience is a modification of that described by Livneh (1986) and include: (1) shock; (2) awareness of vulnerability (both physical and financial); (3) depression; and (4) establishment of defenses which can include confusion, selective attention, unnecessary risk taking, denial, repression, withdrawal, regression, displacement, projection, substitution–compensation, and sublimation. The social response to a disability (or, how others respond) involves: (1) anguish and upset because it affects them; (2) identification with the sufferer; (3) awe at the heroics of the suffer; and (4) rejection. The sequence of personal response depends upon the reciprocal behavior of how others have responded and the typical way by which the person responds to adversity. The person's choices involve: (1) focus, either on the disabling condition itself or ignoring or minimizing it; (2) coping, or, one's attitude toward the disability, which may vary from acquiescence, to succumbing, exploiting, rejecting, or overcoming; and (3) blaming, which may be directed at the person, at others, or at the situation or disabling condition.

In an illustration of research conducted on response patterns to disability of a population of chronic pain patients specifically, Johnson (1982) studied fifty subjects with chronic back pain to determine if personality traits as measured by the

Millon Clinical Multiaxial Inventory (MCMI) predicted life activities by these patients after treatment, using the Activity Pattern Indicator (API) as a measure of the criterion variables. He found that subjects grouped themselves into three clusters: (1) those who were working and/or meeting household responsibilities, but reported having little joy in life; (2) those who met household responsibilities, were actively involved in social and recreational activities, and pleased with the quality of their lives, despite continuing vocal complaints of pain; (3) those who were inactive, depressed, socially isolated, and dissatisfied with their lives. No significant relationship was found between personality traits and outcome, however.

Rehabilitation counselors usually hold an eclectic approach to counseling the physically disabled, including chronic pain patients. In addition, they typically use work itself as a therapeutic tool with chronic pain patients (Catchlove and Cohen, 1982), which differentiates them from some psychologists in clinic and hospital settings. For example, rehabilitation counselors often use a gradualized return to work, wherein the injured worker starts a few hours per day and gradually increases hours with the support of medical and psychological intervention. This approach is intended to help the client overcome fear of work, secure the client's compensation until he feels comfortable in taking on the demands of a permanent job, and to help him recondition physically. Besides educating the client as to the nature of chronic pain (e.g., using descriptions borrowed from such theories as Melzack and Wall's gate control theory) the counselor can train the client to use cognitive techniques in gradualized return to work or "work hardening" programs, in which the client can utilize various coping techniques, such as self-talk strategies (Turk, 1978), relaxation, and attention diverting.

Other techniques from which the eclectic counselor can borrow include the psychodynamic, in order to communicate acceptance and approval to the client, deal with intense feelings (e.g., anger, depression, hostility, and blaming), and resolve a certain amount of ambivalence; behavioral, in order to effectively use contingencies and reinforcements in helping the client make decisions and deal with phobic situations involving pain and reintegrating into society or the workforce; and reality therapy, which is actually a blend of a variety of approaches, although it is more closely aligned with the behavioral approach than any other.

Rehabilitation counseling involves more roles than the profession of psychology, and is oftentimes more art than science. Part of that art is the counselor's knowing his or her own limitations in skill, limitations in time with which to practice counseling skills, and the circumstances surrounding the referral of the client (e.g., if the client is referred by an insurer, the counselor must be aware that the establishment of an implicit "counseling contract" between counselor and client may be problematic). The counselor also must have a feel for when to refer the client to another professional, such as a psychologist or psychiatrist who has an awareness of chronic pain conditions.

Reality Therapy Applied to Chronic Pain Counseling

Beck (1985), and Lynch and Beck (1987) defined the problem of chronic pain, and reviewed counseling theories for their appropriateness in conforming to the needs of this patient population. He concluded that reality therapy was an ideal model for working with chronic pain clients. This approach has many advantages for the rehabilitation counselor. First, it facilitates accountability (since this is what referral sources demand) by documenting client achievements, which have been expressed in operational and objective terms. It seems to fit very well with maladjusted clients who have responded to their disabilities by blaming others and the situation, succumbing to their pain, and have become overly dependent and irresponsible regarding their own recovery. This approach's inventor, William Glasser (1965, 1972) described those in therapy in similar terms to those applied to many chronic pain patients served by rehabilitation counselors: (1) they deny the reality of the world around them; (2) they have taken on a "failure" identity; and (3) they retreat into unreality through their pain and use of pain narcotics.

Glasser also suggested that these individuals, in order to

improve, need to be involved with another individual who is truly "involved" with life, and that this is the appropriate role of the counselor. Beside being truly involved with the client, the counselor must guide the client back to a productive life-style through the use of behavioral contracting and focusing on what the client *does* rather than what the client says. This approach seems most appropriate during that stage of the rehabilitation process when the client feels a degree of safety, acceptance, and trust with the counselor, and when it seems apparent that the client is ready to work on a plan to reintegrate back into productive activity.

Beck (1985) cited a list of suggestions which were made for the reality therapist by Bassin (1976), and which seem particularly appropriate with regard to counseling the chronic pain client.:

1. Be warm, friendly and honest. It is essential to avoid false promises and to openly describe the limits of the relationship.
2. Reveal yourself to the client. Do not present the facade of the aloof professional.
3. Concentrate on the here and now. Clients should not be allowed to dwell on the perceived origins of their problems.
4. Use the first-person pronouns "I" and "me" as much as possible. The client wants personal, human contact.
5. Concentrate on behaviors rather than feelings.
6. Ask "what" rather than "Why" questions; the latter engender excuses.
7. Insist that clients evaluate their own behavior. Transmit the message that the client is responsible for his or her behavior, and that viewing behavior in relation to goals is a way of assuming responsibility.
8. Help the client formulate a plan. The plan should specify the client's goals, proceed in easily attainable steps, be specific in planning (e.g., "How many employers will you call for appointments this week?"). The plan should be written to provide objective guidelines and time frames.

9. Do not acknowledge client excuses.
10. Move the client into a group as soon as possible. For the chronic pain client, consider YMCA membership, volunteer work, return to former employment, and so on. Group involvement helps wean the client from the counselor; the client begins to satisfy needs with group members.[3]
11. Use praise, encouragement, and other social rewards. Verbal reinforcement, as well as a pat on the shoulder, handshake, and other similar gestures convey the notion "I like you, I care for you, you're doing well."
12. Do not "press" the client too hard; do not be pushy. Confront the client when appropriate, but attempt to increase client involvement through being open to discussion on a wide range of topics of interest to the client.
13. Never give up. The client will often test the rehabilitation counselor, especially when the counselor is being effective. Paradoxically, chronic pain clients frequently demonstrate increased pain as their life situation grows better.

To summarize the context in which the rehabilitation counselor provides services, especially in the private sector, the following description is offered.

The chronic pain patient may come to the counseling relationship with a complex of attributes which can pose obstacles to the counseling process. Such a patient has probably spent several months to several years unemployed and receiving disability compensation. Depression or anxiety, or both, may be present, as well as hypochondriasis, hysteria, confusion, hostility, and the identity of an invalid. The patient may also have a desperate need for the counselor to acknowledge his or her pain. The patient will usually have a degree of ambivalence toward the issue of adjustment to disability and return to employment.

[3]When considering helping the client move into a group-oriented activity, it is well to remember that one of the client's main problems may be physical deconditioning, and that a reconditioning program may promote many of the client's physical needs as well as emotional and social ones through modeling and vicarious learning.

The patient's environment is likely to contain elements which facilitate, and some which frustrate, counseling efforts. The Workers' Compensation system is likely to have set up expectations in the patient's mind of a financial reward which is contingent upon the maintenance of the patient's pain. There may have been role changes in the patient's family which encourage the patient's pain identity, or loss of family support which has affected his or her coping ability.

The source of the referral of the patient may present the counselor with an ethical dilemma: who is the client? The counselor risks violating ethical principles if he or she attempts to represent the interests of the disability compensation referrer at the expense of the patient. Cottone (1982) cited instances where counselors "set up" their clients for litigation in view of the difficulty of making progress with these clients, and in view of the fact that these counselors are rewarded by the referring insurance carrier for helping to minimize the insurer's liability for benefits by making additional referrals. In too many instances, "medical management" is a euphemism for glorified claims adjusting by tricking the physician into making an "end of healing" statement, or a statement as to the patient's residual disability percentage.

The proprietary rehabilitation counselor may have the backing of the insurance carrier to follow the patient as long as necessary to produce results, as well as the ability to coordinate the activities of a wide range of professionals involved with the patient. The hospital counselor or psychologist might have to end their involvement when the period of hospitalization ends. Also, the psychologist's time may be expensive to the point that an insurance carrier may prefer to purchase the services of other professionals, and the psychologist may not be interested in the role of coordinator or job developer, which many pain patients need.

Finally, the level of ability of the individual counselor is a consideration in the counseling process. Bozarth, Rubin, Krauft, Richardson, and Bolton (1974) studied rehabilitation counselors over a five-year period and concluded that three interaction styles of counselors could be identified: information providers, therapeutic counselors, and information exchangers, and that higher levels of interpersonal skills tended to be related to higher vocational gain at closure, higher monthly earnings at follow-up, positive psychological change ten months or more following intake, and greater job satisfaction at follow-up. The implication for rehabilitation counseling of chronic pain clients is that this group requires counseling services from the most skilled group of counselors in view of all the psychosocial difficulties associated with chronic pain, but it remains to be seen whether they are receiving the highest level of services. Matkin (1982) surveyed rehabilitation counselors in the private sector regarding areas which they believed to be the most important in terms of serving their clients (largely chronic pain clients), and they rated psychological evaluation and counseling, group counseling, and work adjustment services as less important because of the extended nature of these services.

Rehabilitation counselors are not trained to provide in-depth psychotherapy, as a rule. They use counseling methods to provide clients with help in adjusting to their disability (helping the client to prevent the disability from overwhelming him or her, clarifying values, resolving ambivalence, learning new coping and vocational skills, ameliorating financial difficulties, learning more responsible and effective behaviors, and so on). The counselor does not aim for fundamental personality change on the part of the client, unless that counselor has received specialized training beyond the graduate program. However, the counselor must be able to identify when the client needs more in-depth therapy than the counselor can deliver, and to recommend referral either to an individual psychologist or other psychotherapist, or to a hospital pain center, depending on the nature of the problem.[4]

SUMMARY

This chapter has endeavored to discuss counseling of the chronic pain patient in view of the multiplicity of characteristics

[4]For example, unresponsive depression or severe phobic reactions may signal a need for referral to a therapist. Constant pain complaints and lack of progress due to such may suggest a formal pain clinic program to instigate movement in the direction of productive activities.

that are ascribed to this category of patient, the variety of counseling strategies that are in common use, and the professional roles of those who do the counseling. It has attempted to make the point that all approaches, and all roles have merit as well as limitations, and that it is important for all professionals to know when to refer a patient to another professional who may have more capabilities in certain areas (this is part of the team approach which is ideal with this and other groups of disabled individuals).

Ethical considerations were discussed also, particularly knowing who the client is (the patient, or the insurer), and not using interpretive concepts such as "secondary gain" as an excuse to label a client and curtail further services.

The chapter elaborated rehabilitation counseling as applied to chronic pain patients, since rehabilitation counselors take a somewhat different approach to the psychosocial problems of chronic pain patients than do more traditional professions such as psychology, psychiatry, and nursing.

References

Barker, R.G., Wright, B.A., Meyerson, L. & Gonick, M.R. (1953), *Adjustment to Physical Handicap. A Survey of the Social Psychology of Physique and Disability*, 2nd ed. New York: Social Science Research Council, Bulletin 55.

Bassin, A. (1976), The reality therapy paradigm. In: *The Reality Therapy Reader*, eds. A. Bassin, T. Bratter, and R. Rachin. New York: Harper & Row, pp. 265–280.

Beck, R. (1985), Understanding and counseling the chronic pain patient in proprietary rehabilitation. *J. Rehab.*, 51/3:51–55.

———(1987), *A Survey of Rehabilitation Outcomes of Wisconsin Injured Workers with Non-scheduled Disabilities.* Unpublished doctoral dissertation, University of Wisconsin, Madison.

Bellissimo, A., & Tunks, E. (1984), *Chronic Pain: The Psychotherapeutic Spectrum.* New York: Praeger.

Bergman, J., & Werblun, M. (1978), Chronic pain: A review for the family physician. *J. Fam. Pract.*, 7:685–693.

Berven, N., Habeck, R., & Malec, J. (1985). Predominant MMPI-168 profile clusters in a rehabilitation medicine sample. *Rehab. Psychol.*, 30/4:209–219.

Beutler, L.E., Engle, D., Oro'-Beutler, M.E., Daldrup, R., & Meredith, K. (1986), Inability to express intense affect: A common link between depression and pain? *J. Consult. Clin. Psychol.*, 54/6:752–759.

Bozarth, J.D., Rubin, S.E., Krauft, C.C., Richardson, B.K., & Bolton, B. (1974), Client counselor interaction, patterns of service, and client outcome: Overview of project, conclusions, and implications. *Arkansas Studies in Vocational Rehabilitation*, No. 19. Fayetteville: Arkansas Rehabilitation Research and Training Center.

Budzynski, T.H. (1973), Biofeedback procedures in the clinic. *Sem. Psychiat.*, 5:537–546.

Cassell, J., & Mulkey, S.W. (1985), *Rehabilitation Caseload Management: Concepts and Practice*. Austin, TX: Pro-Ed.

Catchlove, R., & Cohen, K. (1982), Effects of a directive return to work approach in the treatment of workman's compensation patients with chronic pain. *Pain*, 14:181–191.

Conley, R., & Noble, J. Jr. (1978), Workers' compensation reform: Challenge for the 80's. *Amer. Rehab.*, 3/3:19–28.

Cook, D. (1987), Psychosocial impact of disability. In: *Rehabilitation Counseling: Basics and Beyond*, ed. R. Parker. Austin, TX: Pro-Ed.

Cottone, R. (1982), Ethical issues in private-for-profit rehabilitation. *J. Appl. Rehab. Counsel.*, 13/3:14–17.

———(1987), A systemic theory of vocational rehabilitation. *Rehab. Counsel. Bull.* 30 3:167–176.

Delvey, J., & Hopkins, L. (1982), Pain patients and their partners: The role of collusion in chronic pain. *J. Marit. & Fam. Ther.*, 8/1:135–142.

Dembo, T., Leviton, G.L., & Wright, B.A. (1956), Adjustment to misfortune: A problem of social-psychological rehabilitation. *Artif. Limbs*, 3:4–62.

Dolce, J.J., & Raczynski, J.M. (1985), Neuromuscular activity and electromyography in painful backs. Psychological and biomechanical models in assessment and treatment. *Psycholog. Bull.*, 97:502–520.

Eaton, M. (1979), Obstacles to the vocational rehabilitation of individuals receiving Worker's Compensation. *J. Rehab.*, 45/2:59–63.

Engel, G.L. (1959), Psychogenic pain and the pain-prone patient. *Amer. J. Med.*, 26:899–918.

English, R.W. (1971), Correlates of stigma towards physically disabled persons. *Rehab. Res. & Pract. Rev.*, 2:1–18.

Eysenck, H.J., & Eysenck, S.B.G. (1968), *Personality Structure and Measurement*. San Diego: Knapp.

Flor, H., & Turk, D.C. (1984), Etiological theories and treatments for chronic back pain: I. Somatic factors. *Pain*, 19:105–121.

——— ———Birbaumer, N. (1985), Assessment of stress-related psychophysiological reactions in chronic back pain patients. *J. Consult. & Clin. Psychol.*, 53:354–364.

Fordyce, B. (1976), *Behavioral Methods in Chronic Pain and Illness*. St. Louis: C.V. Mosby.

Freud, S. (1915), The dynamic of transference. *Collected Papers*, Vol. 2. New York: Basic Books, 1959, pp. 99–108.

———(1936), *The Problem of Anxiety*. New York: W.W. Horton.

Glasser, W. (1965). *Reality Therapy: A New Approach to Psychiatry*. New York: Harper & Row.

———(1972), *The Identity Society*. New York: Harper & Row.

Hackett, T.P. (1971), Pain and prejudice: Why do we doubt that the patient is in pain? *Med. Times*, 99:130–132.

Hanson-Mayer, T. (1984), The worker's disability syndrome. *J. Rehab.*, 50/3:50–54.

Johnson, K. (1982), Introversion and chronic pain, 1982 (unpublished). (Available from the Department of Rehabilitation Medicine, University Hospital and Clinics, University of Wisconsin—Madison).

Kalla, J.N. (1977), The effects of premorbid adjustment upon treatment outcome of chronic pain patients. *Diss. Abstr. Intern.*, 50:5025B–5026B. (University Microfilms no. 7802832.)

Keefe, F.J., Block, A.R., Williams, R.B., & Surwit, R.S. (1981), Behavioral treatment of chronic pain: Clinical outcome and individual differences in pain relief. *Pain*, 11:221–231.

———Gill, K.M. (1986), Behavioral concepts in the analysis of chronic pain syndrome. *J. Consult. & Clin. Psychol.*, 54/6:776–783.

Lewin, K. (1935), *A Dynamic Theory of Personality.* New York: McGraw-Hill.

——— (1936), *Principles of Topological Psychology.* New York: McGraw-Hill.

Livneh, H. (1986), A unified approach to existing models of adaptation to disability. Part II. Intervention Strategies. *J. Appl. Rehab. Counsel.*, 17/2:6–10.

Lynch, R. (1979), Vocational rehabilitation of workers' compensation clients. *J. Appl. Rehab. Counsel.*, 9/4:164–167.

———Beck, R. (1987), Rehabilitation counseling in the private sector. In: *Rehabilitation Counseling: Basics and Beyond*, ed. R. Parker. Austin, TX: Pro-Ed.

Malec, J. (1985), Personality factors associated with severe traumatic disability. *Rehab. Psychol.*, 30/3:165–172.

Matkin, R. (1982), Rehabilitation services offered in the private sector: A pilot investigation. *J. Rehab.*, 48/4:31–33.

Meichenbaum, D.H. (1977), *Cognitive-Behaviour Modification: An Integrative Approach.* New York: Plenum Press.

Melzack, R. (1973), *The Puzzle of Pain.* New York: Basic Books.

———Casey, K.L. (1968), Sensory, motivational and central control determinants of pain: A new conceptual model. In: *The Skin Senses*, ed. D. Kenshalo. Springfield, IL: Charles C. Thomas.

———Wall, P.D. (1965), Pain mechanisms: A new theory. *Science*, 50:971–979.

Pilling, L.F., Brannick, T.L., & Swenson, W.M. (1967), Psychological characteristics of psychiatric patients having pain as a presenting symptom. *Can. Med. Assn. J.*, 97:387–394.

Rachlin, H. (1985), Pain and behavior. *Behav. & Brain Sci.*, 8:43–53.

Rogers, C.R. (1951), *Client-centered Therapy: Its Current Practice, Implications and Theory.* Boston: Houghton Mifflin.

Schaffer, C.B., Donlon, P.T., & Bittle, R.M. (1980), Chronic pain and depression: A clinical and family history survey. *Amer. J. Psychiat.*, 137/1:118–120.

Siller, J. (1976), Attitudes toward disability. In: *Contemporary Vocational Rehabilitation*, eds. H. Rusalem & D. Malikin. New York: New York University Press, pp. 67–69.

Sternbach, R.A. (1974), *Pain Patients: Traits and Treatments.* New York: Academic Press.

Szasz, T. (1955), The nature of pain. *Arch. Neurolog. Psychiat.*, 74:174–181.

Thomas, K., Butler, A., & Parker, R. (1987), Psychosocial counseling. In: *Rehabilitation Counseling: Basics and Beyond*, ed. R. Parker. Austin, TX: Pro-Ed.

Tuck, M. (1983), Psychological and sociological aspects of industrial injury. *J. Rehabilitation*, 49/3:20–25.

Turk, D.C. (1978), Cognitive-behavioural techniques in the management of pain. In: *Cognitive Behaviour Therapy: Research and Applications*, eds. J.P. Foreyt & D.P. Rathjen. New York: Plenum Press.

———Meichenbaum, D., & Genest, M. (1983), *Pain and Behavioral Medicine: A Cognitive-Behavioral Perspective.* New York: Guilford Press.

———Rudy, T.E. (1986), Assessment of cognitive factors in chronic pain: A worthwhile enterprise? *J. Consult. & Clin. Psychol.*, 54/6:760–768.

Turpin, J. (1987), The relationship of self-efficacy variables to work status among workers' compensation claimants. *Diss. Abstr, Internat.*, 47/9:4010B.

23

Understanding Pediatric Pain: A Developmental Perspective

JOSEPH P. BUSH, PH.D.

The most common types of chronic pediatric pain are associated with renal infections, Crohn's disease, vertebral disease and intraspinal tumor (Apley, 1976), hemophilia (Nossel, 1980), sickle-cell anemia (Bunn, 1980), and cancer, the second leading cause of death in one- to fourteen-year-olds (O'Malley, Koocher, Foster, and Slavin, 1979). The most common types of recurrent pediatric pain are probably headache and intermittent abdominal pain with no identifiable organic etiology. There is evidence that recurrent abdominal pain is the most commonly encountered pain complaint in children between six and fifteen years of age, occurring in about 10 percent of school-aged children to an extent sufficient to disrupt academic functioning (Astrada, Licamele, Walsh, and Kessler, 1981). A number of research studies have indicated that an organic lesion is identified in less than 10 percent of these children (Green, 1967; Stone and Barbero, 1970). As many as 13 percent of children from ten to twelve years old

Acknowledgments. Preparation of this manuscript was supported by a Biomedical Grant from the Virginia Commonwealth University College of Humanities and Sciences. The author gratefully acknowledges the assistance of Carolyn Cockrell, B. S., Stephen Harkins, Ph.D., and Catherine Radecki, Ph.D.

suffer frequent nonmigrainous, and another 5 percent suffer from migraine, headaches (Tomasi, 1979). Procedural pain also affects a substantial number of children. Some of the more common types are bone marrow aspiration and lumbar puncture, burn debridement, chemotherapy, surgery, and orthodontia.

A Developmental Perspective

Physical Development

There is some disagreement as to when children begin to feel pain and whether they feel as much pain as adults under similar conditions. McGraw (1963) evaluated the responses of seventy-five infants to pinprick. A few hours after birth, infants showed no apparent response, but by one week they responded with diffuse body movements, crying, and local reflex withdrawal. At one month, infants showed increasing organization and response specificity, including localization of response, deliberate withdrawal of the stimulated area, and more anticipatory avoidant behaviors when exposed to visual stimuli associated with pinprick. These results strongly suggest that nociception, if not pain perception per se, is present at least from birth.

The main arguments that infants feel less pain are based upon cortical immaturity and incomplete myelination. Studies have in fact shown that higher levels of electric shock are needed to elicit pain responses on the first day after birth than at three months (Gildea and Quirk, 1977). Recent research on infant vocalizations, however, have provided evidence that even neonates experience pain. Porter, Miller and Marshall (1986) recorded and analyzed the cries of thirty infants during circumcision. They found distinctive acoustical features (longer crying, shorter quiet intervals, higher peak frequencies, etc.) to be consistently associated with the more invasive phases of the surgical procedure. Furthermore, these cries were later judged by adults to be the most "urgent" of the recorded vocalizations. Beyond infancy, moreover, empirical and clinical evidence indicate that pain thresholds tend to increase over the course of childhood (Lollar, Smits, and Patterson, 1982).

Cognitive Development

McGraw's (1963) pinprick studies suggest that infants' pain behaviors appear in a fixed developmental sequence (deliberate responses to painful stimulation, followed by anticipatory fear and avoidance behaviors), and are well formed by the age of two years. This progression parallels Piaget's sensorimotor stage of cognitive development, culminating in the ability to form and maintain mental representations of objects. This theory explains why young infants emit pain responses only during aversive stimulation, but not before or for long after. The lack of well-developed cognitive representations implies an absence of memory for painful events.

Piaget's theory has also been used to construct a developmental model of children's concepts of illness. Interviews with twenty-four normal children at three age levels corresponding to stages at which children, according to Piaget's theory, think in qualitatively different ways, revealed that children's illness concepts conform to Piaget's model (Bibace and Walsh, 1980). These authors describe a detailed developmental formulation of children's illness concepts with categories of illness explanations corresponding to specific Piagetian cognitive developmental stages (Bibace and Walsh, 1981). More recently, similar work has been reported concerning children's concepts of pain. Gaffney and Dunne (1986) evaluated verbal definitions of pain obtained from 680 Irish five- to fourteen-year-olds. They report deriving their scoring categories from content analysis of the children's protocols, rather than imposing them upon the data. Children in three age groups corresponding to Piagetian cognitive developmental levels differed significantly in use of definitions falling into twelve scoring categories. With increasing age, children's pain definitions were increasingly abstract and general, and are interpreted by the authors as consonant with Piaget's theory. Five- to seven-year-old children manifested the cognitive characteristics described by Piaget's preoperational stage: centering on perceptually salient features and juxtaposing elements (e.g., pain and injury) without demonstrating any understanding of the relationship between them. An example of a preoperational response might refer to: ". . . when it hurts in your head . . . you can get it when you bump your head on something." Eight- to ten-year-olds used definitions typical of Piaget's concrete operational stage, showing the advent of relatively more abstract thinking and awareness of the psychological concomitants of pain: ". . . pain is something that hurts you, you feel miserable and . . . you start crying. . . " (p. 114). Finally, the eleven- to fourteen-year-olds used the most abstract and introspectively sophisticated definitions, consistent with Piaget's notion of formal operational thought: "Pain is the total opposite of joy. It can be mental or physical and varies with the intensity of the injury . . ." (p. 112). These children also were likely to report more accurate and useful physiological details in their verbalizations. The authors caution that there was considerable overlap between stages, consistent with Piaget's notion of decalage (Ginsburg and Opper, 1969) which states that qualitative developmental changes in cognition are gradual and partial in nature, rather than sudden, complete, and final.

The importance of qualitative developmental differences in children's conceptualizations of illness lies in several areas: (1) the impact of cognition on children's subjective pain experiences; (2) the adaptation of verbal and nonverbal techniques for communicating information and advice to help children in pain; (3) the assessment of children's pain; (4) the design and delivery of pain management interventions; (5) the ability of children to communicate about their pain; and (6) the residual learning children will accrue as a result of the pain experience. It has also been found that illness concepts tend to lag behind overall cognitive development, and that there appear to be no sex or socioeconomic differences (Perrin and Gerrity, 1981).

Research has also shown that attribution of self-blame for illness decreases with age, and that adultlike (abstract and complex) understanding of illness usually awaits adolescence (Perrin and Gerrity, 1981). Conflicting evidence has been reported by researchers looking more specifically at pain, however. Interviews with 994 five- to twelve-year-olds revealed uniformly unsophisticated conceptualizations of pain with no evidence for Piagetian developmental trends (Ross and Ross, 1984). Clearly, more direct investigation of developmental trends in children's pain-related cognitions is needed. It does appear evident, however, that children's pain concepts are qualitatively different from those of adults.

Cognitive distortions about pain and illness in children associated with unsophisticated conceptualizations may result in heightened emotional reactions and fear (Whitt, 1982; Beales, 1983). Some children seem to believe that painful medical procedures, illness, and hospitalization represent punishment for wrongdoing (Perrin and Gerrity, 1981) or aggressive intentions on the part of the health professional (Farley, 1981). Furthermore, research investigating children's understanding of the physician's behaviors and social role has yielded findings consistent with this explanation. Haight, Black, and DiMatteo (1985) evaluated four- and five-year-olds' understanding of the social roles of doctor and patient. They reported that these children demonstrated having considerable detailed information about social roles and behaviors, but that their understanding of the reasons for the physicians' behaviors was quite limited. Clearly, this lack of understanding leaves the child susceptible to cognitive distortion when subjected to painful medical procedures. This distortion may be explained by the Piagetian notions of imminent causality and animism, which characterize the preschool child's egocentric reasoning. Older children who are very upset and frightened about pain may regress to this more primitive level of reasoning, making such distortions difficult to identify and correct. Thus, pain management techniques addressing cognitive factors are likely to be more effective if timed to precede mobilization of intense anxiety (Armstrong, Gil, Dahlquist, Ginsburg, and Jones, 1983). Additionally, induction of positive affective responses to the person of the physician (or other caregiver) may inhibit development of dysfunctional cognitions regarding punishment and aggressive intent. Consistent with this, Bush and Holmbeck's (1987) study of 286 children revealed that children's ratings of their liking for medical personnel were inversely correlated with their ratings of how much they would try to avoid contact with those personnel.

Cognitive changes in childhood also render different sorts of stimuli threatening to different children. One study found that preschool children were most threatened by medical instruments, school-aged children by aspects of their interactions with medical personnel, and adolescents by implications for their health and physical integrity (Steward and Steward, 1981). Separation and stranger anxiety are often more significant than physical factors in preschool children, whereas for older children learned anxiety resulting from previous medical experiences is more likely to be a problem.

Likewise, cognitive coping strategies employed by children in painful and other stressful situations also appear to undergo developmental change. Brown, O'Keefe, Sanders, and Baker (1986) examined age trends in children's cognitions in response to two stressful situations, one of which involved receiving an injection in a dentist's office. The proportion of children reporting cognitive coping strategies, and the variety of these strategies, increased with age. Positive self-talk was the most commonly used strategy, followed by attention diversion. Coping cognitions were associated with lower levels of trait anxiety. On the other hand, the investigators reported that catastrophizing cognitions were more frequent than coping cognitions in all age groups. These results, consistent with Ross and Ross (1984), suggest the existence of developmental trends in cognitive coping ability which may be necessary but not sufficient for actual utilization of these abilities when dealing with pain. A recent study of pediatric oncology patients by Worchel, Copeland, and Barker (1987) replicated the finding that cognitive coping is utilized more by older (in this case adolescent) than younger children. Similarly, information seeking was found to increase markedly with age in five- to eleven-year-olds studied prior to elective surgery (Peterson and Toler, 1986).

Psychosocial Development

Pain behaviors serve a communication function in the patient's interpersonal relationships. An example of this is the child whose pain behaviors elicit parental attention and concern. Many young children have learned that crying in a frightening situation is likely to lead to maternal comfort-giving behaviors. More crying was observed in four- to ten-years-olds with their mothers present during venipuncture than in those whose mothers remained in the waiting room (Gross, Stern, Levin, Dale, and Wojnilower, 1983). Parent–child interaction may also exacerbate pain responses through emotional contagion (Escalona, 1953), by which parental anxiety is communicated directly to the child, as well as by disinhibition of child fear behaviors (Shaw and Routh, 1982). Conversely, parental presence may provide a discriminative stimulus for relaxation and other coping behaviors. Among 994 five- to twelve-year-olds interviewed about pain, 99 percent reported parental presence as the most helpful factor (Ross and Ross, 1984). There does not appear to be a consensus on the desirability of parental presence during painful procedures. Rather, such a determination seems to require consideration of what the parent actually does while interacting with the frightened child (Bush, Melamed, and Cockrell, in press). Research suggests that parent–child interaction in stressful medical situations varies as a function of the child's age and that children are helped more by parents with whom they have better relationships, and whose own anxiety does not interfere with capable parental functioning (Bush, Melamed, Sheras, and Greenbaum, 1986).

Children's psychosocial developmental status also affects their interactions with health professionals. Inefficient and at times iatrogenic behaviors may be engaged in by physicians, nurses, and others whose emotional responses and lack of knowledge about child development reduce their objectivity and effectiveness. Examples include the well-meaning physician whose "need to help" leads to unnecessary and invasive diagnostic procedures with the recurrent abdominal pain child (Barr and Feuerstein, 1983), or the nurse for whom the aversiveness of witnessing intense pain in the child undergoing burn treatment leads to insensitivity and attribution of pain complaints to the child's oppositionality. Psychosocial development influences how children handle pain, how they communicate about it, and what effects it has on future development. Clinical descriptions of characteristic pain manifestations in children of different ages have been provided by several authors (e.g., Stoddard, 1982). Interviews with 264 six- to twelve-year-old short-term inpatients indicated that as children grow older their pain behaviors increasingly conform to their perceptions of a socially defined illness role (Campbell, 1975). This social learning might be expected to be strongly influenced by exposure to familial pain and illness models. Children's coping abilities also develop as children grow older. Bush and his colleagues (Bush et al., 1986), observing fifty mother–child dyads awaiting outpatient pediatric examination, reported negative correlations between children's behavioral distress and both prosocial and exploratory coping behaviors. Older children were found to engage more frequently in exploration independent of parental facilitation, suggesting more self-sufficient coping repertoires.

The Clinical Significance of Pain in Children

Medical Care

Quality, location, temporal patterning, and environmental responsiveness of pain are important in differential diagnosis (Apley, 1976) and treatment. Differential diagnosis of migraine and psychomotor seizure, for example, requires information about the prodrome and degree of impairment of consciousness (Tomasi, 1979). Questioning a child about this in a manner he or she can understand and obtaining a valid and interpretable response is likely to be difficult. The potential for inaccurate assessment by clinicians unsophisticated in child development is significant (this will be discussed more fully later in this chapter). Better data about children's pain could preclude the need for expensive and often dangerous and painful diagnostic procedures. These data might also be useful in evaluating the affective component in children's pain responses as well as in assessing the effectiveness of analgesics.

The strict dichotomizing of psychogenic and somatogenic

pain has been justifiably disputed (Barr and Feuerstein, 1983). Differential diagnosis of psychogenic pain is likely to become a red flag in the child's medical record, and is typically made solely on the basis of clinical judgment (Painter, Morrison, and Evens, 1965). Diagnosing psychogenicity on the basis of an absence of physical findings alone is poor practice. Such diagnosis minimally requires identification of positive findings of individual psychopathology or dysfunctional family interaction patterns, together with a rationale linking these underlying problems with the presenting symptom. Possible consequences of an incorrect diagnosis of psychogenicity include inappropriate treatment, damage to the credibility of the physician in the eyes of the child and his or her family, and leading some to the erroneous conclusion that a child with psychogenic pain does not have "real" pain. Such a diagnosis should be specific, as well justified as an "organic" diagnosis, should access more appropriate treatment rather than merely providing an excuse for failure to find an organic diagnosis, and should be made only by a qualified professional.

Impact on the Child

The state of knowledge relating to sequelae of children's pain experiences is woefully inadequate. Studies have shown that a high proportion of children with recurrent abdominal pain either maintain their symptoms or develop other pain complaints (reviewed in Barr and Feuerstein [1983]). Retrospective studies have suggested that adults with chronic pain had more childhood pain than adults without chronic pain (Varni, Bessman, Russo, and Cataldo, 1980). It has also been observed that children in chronic pain who cope inadequately are at risk for depression (Masek, Russo, and Varni, 1984). On the other hand, successfully handling pain in childhood may result in positive learning, for example acquisition of coping skills, enhanced self-esteem, or desensitization of previously feared medical stimuli. Little research has investigated this possibility (but see Parmelee, [1986], for a discussion of the potentially beneficial developmental effects of childhood illness).

The operant learning model suggests that children's pain behaviors, complaints, and even the subjective experience of pain may be maintained beyond the point of recovery from the original physical cause by contingent reinforcement. Such reinforcement may be positive (e.g., attention and comfort-giving behaviors by parents) or negative (e.g., avoidance of chores). Reinforcing consequences of pain complaints were cited by one-third of 994 five- to twelve years olds interviewed (Ross and Ross, 1984). Operant learning of pain behaviors often underlies school phobia. The "school phobic" child presents pain complaints in the morning and is allowed to remain at home. Research suggests that avoiding separation from mother, rather than avoiding school, is the effective reinforcer.

The respondent learning model suggests that stimuli which children encounter together with pain-inducing stimuli acquire the capacity to elicit pain-associated responses (fear, anxiety, avoidance, pain complaints, subjective experience of pain). Thus, for example, the personnel, equipment, and setting associated with debridement may come to elicit the same responses as debridement itself (Kelley, Jarvie, Middlebrooke, McNeer, and Drabman, 1984). Anticipatory fear is related to degree of pain reported during medical procedures, just as previous traumatic medical experience has a negative effect on children's handling of subsequent procedures. A study of nine two- to twelve-year-olds undergoing burn dressing changes documented a tendency toward decremented discrimination between painful and nonpainful events (Kavanaugh, 1983).

At least three family interaction patterns have been noted as contributing to dysfunctional learning about pain. The first of these is modeling and reinforcement. A child exposed to a pain model may imitatively acquire a repertoire of pain behaviors as a means of coping with stress. If these behaviors elicit parental reinforcement the child may fail to develop other more adaptive coping strategies. While some researchers have questioned whether any relationship exists between psychogenic pain in children and exposure to familial pain models (Barr and Feuerstein, 1983; McGrath, Goodman, Firestone, Shipman, and Peters, 1983), others have reported higher incidence rates of somatization disorder in relatives of children with "functional" than "organic" pain (Routh and Ernst, 1984), as well as higher numbers of chronic pain patients in the families of children with chronic pain than in children with relatively pain-free chronic diseases (Violon and Giurgea, 1984). A recent study by Bennett, Hatcher, Richstmeier, and Conrad (1987) replicated this finding and provided further evidence for a modeling explanation of this coincidence. In this study, children with unexplained abdominal pain identified more familial pain models than did children suffering from pain attributable to a diagnosed condition (sickle-cell anemia); reported more positive consequences following pain; and rated their pain as similar to that of the models. Studies of adults with chronic pain syndromes have also revealed high concordance rates, relative to healthy individuals, with parental illness behavior models (Turkat and Rock, 1984).

Another family factor influencing children's learning about pain is described by the emotional contagion hypothesis (Escalona, 1953). According to this model, maternal anxiety is communicated directly to the child, primarily by nonverbal means. Thus, exposure to an anxious parent is likely to disrupt positive coping, inhibit relaxation, and in general exacerbate the negative affect accompanying a painful experience. This model has received broad empirical support in research showing substantial correlations between parental and child dental anxiety (reviewed in Melamed and Bush [1985]).

Finally, pain complaints may be supported by family system psychopathology. Minuchin's work with psychosomatic families (Minuchin and Fishman, 1979) has illustrated several family interaction patterns in which the child's symptom functions to diffuse marital conflict, maintain inappropriate intergenerational relationships, or to "express" the psychopathology of one of the parents. Research on children with recurrent abdominal pain with no identified organic etiology has shown that, while these children do not differ from their healthy or behaviorally disordered peers, their mothers had significantly higher Beck Depression Inventory scores (Hodges, Kline, Barbero, and Flanery, 1985). Minuchin emphasizes that family system variables are more clearly implicated in the maintenance, rather than the etiology, of the child's symptoms.

Symptoms associated with organic lesions may be maintained by their acquired function in maintaining family system homeostasis.

Effects of Pediatric Pain on Others

Significant others are liable to experience a child's pain as highly stressful. Effects on parent–child interactions may include enhanced parental functioning (Stoddard, 1982) or parental withdrawal, reinforcement of overdependent child behaviors, and exacerbation of spousal conflict. A survey of 181 staff respondents in ninety-three burn units revealed a tendency to engage in cognitive distortion in order to avoid awareness of causing pain to children (i.e., as a result of treatment procedures) (Perry and Heidrich, 1982). Several typical distortions have been described in the nursing literature (Eland and Anderson, 1977).

Assessment of Pediatric Pain

Factors to Consider

Assessment should always include cognitive developmental status, especially level of sophistication of illness concepts and pain-related beliefs. Children may generate grotesque fantasies when their information is incomplete or when the explanations with which they are provided are developmentally inappropriate. Developmental change is extensive within childhood, and so different assessment techniques are likely to be needed with preschoolers, school-age children, and adolescents. Whereas a school-aged child can provide a reasonably sophisticated description of his or her pain, younger children cannot be relied upon to describe accurately the time patterns or other subtle state changes associated with painful conditions.

Assessment of pain associated with medical procedures should include a focus on anticipatory anxiety (Beales, 1983). Much of the anxiety exacerbating children's pain may be related to the stress of hospitalization (Gildea and Quirk, 1977), with its imposition of separation from parents, unfamiliar routines, and exposure to other sick or injured patients. Developmental trends are to be expected in terms of which aspects of hospitalization are experienced as stressful. Stress from normal as well as traumatic events may also underlie chronic intractable pain complaints (Barr and Feuerstein, 1983).

A number of child personality characteristics have been suggested as playing a significant role in pain responses. Coping style is probably the most well-documented factor. Information-seeking behavior has been found, by naturalistic research in the outpatient pediatric clinic, to be correlated with lower levels of child distress during medical procedures (Bush et al., 1986). Peterson and Toler (1986) investigated this coping disposition in children more directly. They administered the Coping Strategies Interview to fifty-nine five- to eleven-year-olds prior to minor elective surgery. Information-seeking scores on this measure were validated by parents' ratings of children's typical coping behaviors in other situations and preference for information acquisition as well as by observer, nurse, and parent ratings of the child's actual information-seeking behaviors during blood tests, anesthesia induction, and postsurgical recovery. These scores were significantly predictive of parents' ratings of the child's having coped well with aversive medical procedures in the past, and of better adaptation and less distress before as well as after surgery. Other child coping behaviors include self-distraction, withdrawal, "playing doctor" (desensitization), and clinging to mother. It is important to recognize that coping processes or defenses which would normally be considered pathognomic may be adaptive in children coping with intense pain.

The only other personality variable for which adequate evidence exists to support its routine assessment is health locus of control (Whitt, 1982; Masek et al., 1984; Perrin and Shapiro, 1985). However, the child's cognitions about the meaning of the pain (Beales, 1983; Beales, Keen, and Lennox Holt, 1983) have been shown to be related to perceived pain intensity and emotionality of response, and should also be assessed. In addition, of course, it is important to screen for more severe psychopathology. While diagnosis of child somatization disorder is complicated by contradictory literature and difficulties in assessment, recent work by Ernst, Routh, and Harper (1984) has contributed to the clarification of symptomatic patterns present in children with chronic functional abdominal pain. Their findings may help to facilitate the development of a more well-defined and empirically based taxonomy of childhood psychosomatic disorders.

A particularly critical factor in the assessment of pediatric pain involves the functional relationships between pain behaviors and environmental consequences. Particularly in cases of recurrent pain, the clinician should look for both operant and respondent patterns maintaining the symptoms, though these may be important in procedural pain as well (Brunnquell and Hall, 1982). Related to the question of respondent learning is the influence of children's past medical and pain experiences. Emotional responses to a traumatic previous experience may be elicited by environmental cues perceived by the child as signaling a similar experience.

Parental attitudes toward medical care and the quality of their relationships with the child are further factors likely to be of importance (Melamed and Bush, 1985). Assessment should include the child's exposure to "pain models," as well as the anxiety and coping responses (including beliefs about the cause and expected cure of the child's pain) of both parents (Varni, 1984). It is also important to evaluate the impact of the child's pain and associated symptomatology on the family system (Minuchin and Fishman, 1979), including the question of what would change in the family if the child's pain disappeared.

Some studies have identified apparent gender differences in children's pain responses. Greater anxiety was found in girls than boys among four- to seven-year-olds following elective surgery (Melamed and Siegel, 1975). It has also been found by several researchers (Lollar et al., 1982; Bush and Holmbeck, 1987) that girls report more pain when directly questioned about medical events, and that they are likely to engage in more emotional expression and other-directed comfort-seeking than boys (Katz, Kellerman, and Siegel, 1980). These differences may be associated with cultural norms discouraging expression of fear and dependency in males.

Existing Assessment Techniques

Interviews and Observation. Since all psychometric assessment instruments for pediatric pain are currently in an experimental stage, the clinician must rely heavily on interview and observation. Child interviewing demands sophistication in the area of child development and general interviewing skills. Child as well as parent interview data are likely to be heavily confounded by demand characteristics and other sources of response bias. Research has suggested that children and their parents overestimate headache activity, and that trends in degree and type of response bias appear to vary as a function of child age (Burke, Andrasik, Blanchard, and Attanasio, 1984). Parental interview may be facilitated by employment of objective ratings with which parents can describe their children's pain behaviors. For example, Budd and Kedesdy (1987) have developed a scale for rating situations and events surrounding the occurrence of child headaches, reporting that scores on the scale's Attention Consequences factor were significantly related to treatment outcome.

Particularly with younger children, observation of behavior is probably the most valuable source of information. Its advantages include its applicability during actual pain experiences, its lack of reactivity if conducted unobtrusively, and the possibility of using trained nonprofessionals. Observational data have been found to be sensitive to children's responses to pain management interventions (Kelley et al., 1984). Several structured observational schedules are reviewed by Varni (1984) who has also reported good results using child self-observation by means of a pain diary (Masek et al., 1984). Most research studies using trained observers have established adequate interrater reliability. Research on children's responses during painful medical procedures has, however, been encumbered by a lack of consistency and demonstrated validity in observational measures (Katz, Kellerman, and Siegel, 1980). Jay and Elliot's (1984) Observational Scale of Behavioral Distress is a promising tool which may help to meet this need. It has been shown to be valid and reliable for use during bone marrow aspirations, and incorporates intensity weights as well as quantifying variety and duration of child distress behaviors.

Self-Report Measures. Several questionnaires have been developed, but none has undergone extensive validation nor attained widespread use. An adjective checklist has been developed (Savedra, Gibbons, Tesler, Ward, and Wegner, 1982; Tesler, Ward, Savedra, Wegner, and Gibbons, 1983) which may be useful with children over nine years old, but its psychometric properties are largely undefined and it should be considered at this time as a promising research tool. Of related interest is the Illness Impact Inventory (Zeltzer, Kellerman, Ellenberg, Dash, and Rigler, 1980), which has been used with adolescents to obtain ratings of areas in which an illness is perceived as having the greatest impact on one's life.

Probably the most promising format for assessment of young children's pain, however, is the visual analog scale (Bradley, Prokop, Gentry, VanDerHeide, and Prieto, 1981). For example, a 10 cm scale representing pain severity has been demonstrated to yield scores which correlate significantly with observer-rated postsurgical pain behaviors in a small sample of nine- to fifteen-year-olds (Abu-Saad and Holzemer, 1981). A five-point scale drawn into a picture of a thermometer has been used to assess fear of medical stimuli (Melamed and Siegel, 1975), as well as pain. Bush and Holmbeck (1987), found that children's responses on this instrument differentiated painful from nonpainful stimuli, showed the expected age-related decreases in painfulness ratings, and correlated with self-reported tendencies to avoid contact with health care professionals. Another, very different type of analog scale is the pressure algometer (Lollar et al., 1982), with which children indicate when pain from physical pressure equals the pain they are describing, or when it reaches various tolerance thresholds. Yet another type of analog scale is the body chart, consisting of front- and rearview human body outlines, with which children have been shown to be able accurately to indicate pain locations (Eland and Anderson, 1977).

Another approach to obtaining self-report data from children while avoiding some of the problems associated with questionnaires involves the use of structured interviews. A particularly promising instrument of this type, the Coping Strategies Interview, was developed by Siegel (1981) to evaluate methods children use for coping with distress. The child is asked to talk about how he or she copes in medical settings in general and during a recent specific stressful medical procedure, and then to give relevant coping advice to a best friend.

Projective instruments have also been used to evaluate pediatric pain. The Pediatric Pain Inventory (Lollar et al., 1982) consists of twenty-four drawings of pain-evoking events about which children respond to a series of questions concerning their beliefs, attitudes, and estimated pain magnitude. The authors report adequate internal consistency, convergent and discriminant validity based on administration to 240 four- to nineteen-year-olds. Unruh, McGrath, Cunningham, and Humphreys (1983) analyzed 109 drawings by five- to eighteen-year-olds suffering from migraine or musculoskeletal pain. Several drawings were obtained from each child, and adequate reliability was established for classification of the drawings' contents. These and other authors (Scott, 1978) have reported consistent color associations with pain.

Physiological Measures. Assessment of autonomic arousal may be used for evaluating the distress–anxiety component of pain in children (Gildea and Quirk, 1977). Jay and her colleagues (Jay, Elliot, and Varni, 1986), for example, found that heart rate and diastolic blood pressure prior to pediatric bone marrow aspirations were predictive of observed and self-rated distress during the procedure.

Clinical Management of Pediatric Pain

Techniques for managing pediatric pain may be broadly grouped into pharmacological and psychosituational approaches. Regarding both of these approaches, child developmental factors must be carefully considered in individualizing the regimen, and multiple approaches must usually be used. Further research is clearly needed on interactions among behavioral and pharmacological interventions (Houpt, Moore, and Weinstein, 1986).

Pharmacological Approaches

Anesthesia. While techniques for inducing and maintaining general anesthesia in children are beyond the scope of this review, two problematic issues will be raised. The first of these involves traumatic reactions to induction. Advantages of adequate psychological preparation have been known to anesthesiologists for years, including need for less premedication and less anesthetic agent, more rapid induction, shortened excitement state, and less disruption of the operating room (Jackson, 1951). Steward (1980) recommends using intravenous administration with older children, letting younger children hold the mask, and allowing parental presence during induction. A second problematic area involves the practice of not anesthetizing infants in surgery, including circumcision. This practice has come under severe criticism by authors who note that these infants require physical restraint, show autonomic and endocrinal responses strongly suggestive of pain, and have a right to anesthesia (Swafford and Allan, 1968; Gross and Gardner, 1980).

Caudal blocks were utilized following genital surgery in twenty-two children and found to be easily administered as well as more effective than intramuscular injections of morphine, while producing fewer side-effects (Lunn, 1979). Penile nerve blocks have also been found to be effective in infants undergoing circumcision, but are rarely used (Jensen, 1981). Dixon, Snyder, Holve, and Bromberger (1984), comparing full-term infants undergoing circumcision with and without lidocaine nerve block, found that the unanesthetized infants received scores on the Brazelton Neonatal Assessment Scale indicating significantly more behavioral difficulties following surgery and on the following day. Little or no research has been done in evaluating combinations of nerve blocking and behavioral techniques.

Analgesics. A number of carefully controlled studies have documented the apparently prevalent practice of undermedicating children in pain (Perry and Heidrich, 1982; Mather and Mackie, 1983). One study compared analgesics prescribed and administered to fifty children and fifty matched adults following open heart surgery (Beyer, DeGood, Ashley, and Russell, 1983). Children were more often administered doses of analgesics below recommended ranges, and medication was discontinued sooner than with adults. Surprisingly, little if any empirical research has investigated the consequences of adequate compared to inadequate analgesic medication in pediatric patient populations. Speculations regarding the reasons underlying these medication practices are unsubstantiated by empirical data, and include a number of possible factors (Eland and Anderson, 1977; Beyer et al., 1983). These include beliefs that children feel less pain and that pediatric pain cannot be evaluated, reluctance to give narcotics to children, the belief that children require less analgesia, the fact that children may avoid expressing pain in order to avoid injections, and the aversive consequences children may provide to those who inject them with analgesics. In addition, some undermedication may be due to prevalent misinformation regarding the analgesic potency of commonly used drug combinations. One particularly popular category of such medications includes combinations of antipyretics with opioids, such as combining acetaminophen with codeine. The widespread belief that this drug combination acts synergistically has not been demonstrated to be true, and in fact numerous studies have consistently established that an additive effect is achieved (reviewed in Beaver [1984]). This is not surprising, since opioids act centrally while acetaminophen and other pyretics exert their effects on the peripheral nervous system. While research has indicated that these combinations are effective and efficient in their additive analgesic effects (i.e., the combination is superior to doubling the dose of either drug alone), prescriptions written upon the assumption of a synergistic effect will overestimate the analgesic potency of the medication. On the other hand, potential negative effects of analgesic medication should not be ignored. Aside from the well-known risks of respiratory depression with anesthesia and addiction to narcotics, these include possible interference with production and release or metabolism of endorphins (Kavanaugh, 1983), reinforcement of pain complaints, leading to acquisition of maladaptive coping patterns (Olness and MacDonald, 1981), excessive sedation (Wakeman and Kaplan, 1978), and possible adverse reactions to large narcotic doses (Moore and Goodson, 1985).

Undermedication may erode the patient's trust and risk acceleration of symptomatic behavior as a plea for more help, and violates the right to adequate control of pain and suffering which is one of the most fundamental responsibilities of the health care professional. PRN orders are strongly cautioned against in cases of chronic pain, because providing relief (negative reinforcement) contingent on pain complaints may increase sick-role behaviors (McGrath and Vair, 1984). Scheduled painful procedures should be postponed when premedication has not yet taken effect (Gross and Gardner, 1980), and adjunctive psychological techniques such as relaxation and distraction should be used to enhance analgesia (Wakeman and Kaplan, 1978; Kavanaugh, 1983). Several researchers have recommended administering analgesics orally (Schultz, 1971), or intravenously (Mather and Mackie, 1983) whenever children are already on intravenous tubes, and have suggested a number of other techniques of potential value with children which merit further investigation. These include preparing injection sites with aerosol cooling agents or applying small quantities of liquid topical anesthetics to lacerations, followed by slow injection of local anesthetic, prior to suturing (Beyer and Byers, 1985). When a child is found to be excessively anxious in anticipation of a medical procedure, anxiolytic medications may be helpful (Stoddard, 1982), though a number of nonpharmacological techniques are available which are probably more effective and have positive (skill enhancement) rather than potentially iatrogenic side-effects.

Psychological Interventions

Hypnosis, Distraction, and Relaxation. A wide variety of therapeutic approaches are subsumed under the category of hypnosis, and the distinctions among these, distraction, and relaxation techniques are even more uncertain where young children are concerned. Hypnosis has been utilized most extensively with children undergoing painful procedures in which anxious anticipation is significant (Zeltzer and LeBaron, 1982). Wakeman and Kaplan (1978) noted that children make better hypnotic subjects than adults. It has also been shown that children are capable of mastering self-hypnotic techniques and using these effectively to control recurrent pain due to migraine (Olness and MacDonald, 1981). As with hypnotic induction, specific techniques for distracting children in pain must be geared to the child's developmental level. Distraction should engage all of the major sensory modalities, and imagery and rhythmic breathing should be employed. Particularly promising results have been found in several single case studies of the effectiveness of distraction techniques employing video technology with children undergoing painful medical procedures (Kelley et al., 1984; Kolko and Rickard-Figueroa, 1985).

Relaxation training has been used with children to help reduce anxiety and may therefore enable the child to benefit from other interventions, such as preparatory information. In fact, relaxation may be the effective component in biofeedback (Labbé and Williamson, 1983) and hypnosis. Relaxation training was found significantly to reduce migraine activity in six seven- to twelve-year-olds, as compared to EMG biofeedback and waiting-list controls (Masek et al., 1984). Applications of relaxation training to children with chronic disease pain (hemophilia) and procedural pain (burn treatment) have been reviewed by Varni (1984). McGrath and Vair (1984) recommend that relaxation training in young children is facilitated by use of a "comfort object" (e.g., a teddy bear) along with gentle touching and soothing talk, while older children benefit more from pleasant conversation and individually selected imagery as adjuncts to traditional breathing and muscle relaxation instructions.

Biofeedback. Most of the published research evaluating the effectiveness of biofeedback in pediatric pain management has focused on migraine. Studies utilizing frontalis electromyograph (EMG) biofeedback with child migraineurs are reviewed by Varni (1984), who concludes that such treatment has not been shown to be more effective than progressive muscle relaxation training. In one randomized treatment study of eighteen eight- to twelve-year-old migraineurs, relaxation training and pain behavior management, with and without EMG biofeedback, were equally efficacious (and superior to waiting list controls) in reducing headache activity following treatment and at one-year follow-up (Fentress, Masek, Mehegan and Benson, 1986). Finger temperature biofeedback with autogenic training was used in the treatment of migraine in three nine- to thirteen-year-olds (Labbé and Williamson, 1983). All subjects showed decreased finger temperature as well as posttreatment and follow-up decreases in headache frequency, intensity, duration, and medication usage. The authors later replicated these results, using autogenic feedback training, in an experimental design utilizing a waiting list control group. At end of treatment and at one-month follow-up, 93 percent of the treatment group children showed at least 50 percent reductions in headache activity, as opposed to no improvement in control group children. Six-month follow-up of eight of the thirteen treated children indicated consistent maintenance of gains (Labbé and Williamson, 1984).

Family Therapy. Family therapy is increasingly recognized as the treatment of choice with children in whom family factors appear to be prominent, such as is often the case with recurrent abdominal pain. Family therapy may be conducted from a number of orientations, though the cognitive–behavioral and structural–systems approaches appear to be most effective. Behavioral approaches emphasize altering contingencies in the familial environment so as to extinguish pain complaints and reinforce healthy coping, as well as teaching family members adaptive strategies for managing stress. Minuchin and his colleagues (Minuchin and Fishman, 1979; White, 1979) have reported particular success using the latter approach with "psychosomatic families" by focusing therapeutic efforts on altering the interactive patterns which maintain pain symptoms, rather than dealing with presumed etiological factors.

Management and Preparation Techniques. These approaches typically employ interventions based on social learning principles, and have been shown by empirical research to be highly effective in a number of applications, particularly when behavioral regulation and anxiety reduction are major goals (reviewed in Melamed and Bush, 1985). Preparatory techniques utilizing modeling, often presented via videotape, have been found to be particularly useful with children hospitalized for elective surgery (Melamed and Siegel, 1975), leading to reductions in both pre- and postoperative anxiety. Research has also demonstrated the effectiveness of contingency management in improving children's handling of medical procedures. Varni et al. (1980) employed contingent attention for well behaviors and ignored pain behaviors in a three-year-old burn patient. They found their treatment to be effective, reporting in addition increased cooperativeness and positive self-statements relating to rehabilitation. Positive results were also reported with children in burn treatment (Kavanaugh, 1983), utilizing an intervention designed to maximize predictability and control. Children in the treatment group were given cues signaling "safe time" and times when a potentially painful procedure was imminent; they also were encouraged to participate in treatment; for example, helping remove splints and bandages.

Several authors have utilized Piaget's theory of cognitive development as a basis for recommended approaches to communicating medical information to children of different ages (Perrin and Gerrity, 1981; Beales, 1983; McGrath and Vair, 1984). The need for specialized training in developmentally appropriate communication skills is underscored by a study in which pediatricians, nurses, and child development students were asked to estimate the ages at which children made various responses to questions about illness (Perrin and Perrin, 1983). Physicians and nurses tended to approach all children as if they were in middle childhood, overestimating young children's conceptual sophistication and underestimating that of older children. Two common types of miscommunication illustrating these errors are, respectively, telling preschool children that their pain is time-limited or that it denotes healing, and talking to school-aged children as if they were much younger.

Preparation for stressful medical procedures, usually involving some combination of information and suggestions for coping with pain and anxiety, is one of the most clearly indicated interventions with child patients. Preparatory intervention has been described and found effective for anesthesia induction (Jackson, 1951), postoperative pain management (Mather and Mackie, 1983), and painful treatment and diagnostic procedures (Beales, 1983; Varni, 1984; Fassler, 1985). Researchers have also reported successful results following preparatory programs directed to child inpatients together with their parents (Campbell, Clark, and Kirkpatrick, 1986). Preprocedural preparation may be difficult with very young children (Steward and Steward, 1981), however, and should be tailored to the individual child (Gross and Gardner, 1980; Melamed and Bush, 1985). Preparatory programs are not inevitably benign in their effects. Indiscriminant, inexpert, or ill-timed exposure of children to informational or modeling presentations may cause sensitization and induction of excessive anxiety (Wilson, 1981; Faust and Melamed, 1984). Perhaps most dangerous, however, is providing the child with inaccurate information such as describing an upcoming painful procedure as nonpainful (McGrath and Vair, 1984). This erodes the child's belief that the adults responsible for his or her care can be trusted, and is likely to make the child anticipate pain in other, truly nonpainful procedures.

Individual Psychotherapy. Though traditional forms of individual psychotherapy have been used with pediatric pain patients, particularly when a psychogenic component has been diagnosed, there is a paucity of evaluation research in this area (Barr and Feuerstein, 1983). Follow-up of seventy-four children with abdominal or headache pain diagnosed as at least partly psychogenic revealed that those receiving psychotherapy showed no more improvement than those not in treatment (Friedman, 1972). In addition, it has been argued (Varni et al., 1980) that psychotherapy employing empathy as a major component may exacerbate pain by positively reinforcing pain complaints.

Other Interventions. Counterirritation is a method of pain management in which cutaneous stimulation, such as rubbing or transcutaneous nerve stimulation, is used to reduce the perceived intensity of localized pain. Few studies have empirically evaluated the effectiveness of systematic counterirritant techniques in pediatric applications, though a few authors have reported favorable results (reviewed in Beyer and Byers [1985]).

CONCLUSION

Among the clinical recommendations which may be made on the basis of available evidence, one must be particularly emphasized. This is the importance of taking developmental factors into consideration. The child's developmental status carries implications for interpretation of clinical symptomatology, design and interpretation of assessment, communication with the child, and intervention. Furthermore, the complexity of taking developmental factors into account must be appreciated. Physical, cognitive, and psychosocial development are all of importance. Expertise in child development and in communicating with children must not be regarded as incidentally acquired. The state of the art in pediatric pain assessment is such that interviewing and behavioral observation must be heavily relied upon, because applicable psychometric instruments are at an experimental stage. Programmatic curricula and supervised experience are essential to the acquisition of these competencies. Consultation with a pediatric psychologist or other qualified professional should be frequently utilized by clinicians working with children in pain. The need for an interdisciplinary approach cannot be overemphasized with this highly vulnerable population.

Areas in which further research is needed include: (1) development and validation of assessment techniques for pediatric pain; (2) investigation of short and long-term effects of "inadequate" analgesic medication for children with moderate to severe acute pain; (3) empirical evaluation of intervention techniques addressing "psychogenic pain" syndromes, preparing children for painful medical procedures and managing pain in chronic conditions; (4) further research into relatively unexamined techniques such as counterirritation; and (5) evaluation of training for physicians and nurses in developmentally appropriate communication and management approaches.

REFERENCES

Abu-Saad, H., & Holzemer, W. (1981), Measuring children's self-assessment of pain. *Iss. Comprehen. Pediat. Nurs.*, 5:337–349.

Apley, J. (1976), Pain in childhood. *J. Psychosom. Res.*, 20:383–389.

Armstrong, F., Gil, K., Dahlquist, L., Ginsburg, A., & Jones, B. (1983), Behavioral intervention to facilitate coping with chemotherapy in pediatric cancer patients. Paper presented to the Association for Advancement of Behavior Therapies, Washington, DC. October.

Astrada, C., Licamele, W., Walsh, T., & Kessler, E. (1981), Recurrent abdominal pain in children and associated DSM-III diagnoses. *Amer. J. Psychiat.*, 138:687–688.

Barr, R., & Feuerstein, M. (1983), Recurrent abdominal pain syndrome: How appropriate are our basic clinical assumptions? In: *Pediatric and Adolescent Behavioral Medicine: Issues in Treatment*, ed. P. McGrath. New York: Springer, pp. 13–27.

Beales, J. (1983), Factors influencing the expectation of pain among patients in a children's burn unit. *Burns*, 9:187–192.

——— Keen, J., & Lennox Holt, P. (1983), The child's perception of the disease and the experience of pain in juvenile chronic arthritis. *J. Rheumatol.* 10:61–65.

Beaver, W. (1984). Combination analgesics. *Amer. J. Med.*, 77:38–53.

Bennett, R., Hatcher, J., Richstmeier, A., & Conrad, H. (1987), Social modeling and unexplained pediatric pain. *Eighth Annual Proceedings, Society of Behavioral Medicine*, 5A:43–56.

Beyer, J., & Byers, M. (1985), Knowledge of pediatric pain: The state of the art. *Child. Health Care*, 13:150–159.

——— DeGood, D., Ashley, L., & Russell, G. (1983), Patterns of postoperative analgesic use with adults and children following cardiac surgery. *Pain*, 17:71–81.

Bibace, R., & Walsh, M. (1980), Development of children's concepts of illness. *Pediatr.*, 66:912–917.

——— ——— (1981), Children's conceptions of illness. In: *Children's Conceptions of Health, Illness and Bodily Functions*, eds. R. Bibace & M. Walsh. Washington: Jossey-Bass, pp. 31–48.

Bradley, L., Prokop, C., Gentry, W., VanDerHeide, L., & Prieto, E. (1981), Assessment of chronic pain. In: *Medical Psychology: Contributions to Behavioral Medicine*, eds. C. Prokop & L. Bradley. New York: Academic Press, pp. 91–117.

Brown, J., O'Keefe, J., Sanders, S., & Baker, B. (1986), Developmental changes in children's cognition to stressful and painful situations. *J. Pediat. Psychol.*, 11:343–357.

Brunnquell, D., & Hall, M. (1982), Issues in the psychological care of pediatric oncology patients. *Amer. J. Orthopsychiat.*, 52:32–44.

Budd, K., & Kedesdy, J. (1987), Investigation of environmental factors in pediatric headache: The Children's Headache Assessment Scale. *Eighth Annual Proceedings, Society of Behavioral Medicine*, A3:67–68.

Bunn, H. (1980), Disorders of hemoglobin structure, function, and synthesis. In:

Harrison's Principles of Internal Medicine, eds. K. Isselbacher, R. Adams, E. Braunwald, R. Peterson, & J. Wilson. New York: McGraw-Hill, pp. 1560–1562.

Burke, E., Andrasik, F., Blanchard, E., & Attanasio, V. (1984), Correspondence between parent and child report of headache: Interview versus diary data. *Society of Behavioral Medicine Proceedings, Fifth Annual Scientific Session*, p. 9.

Bush, J., & Holmbeck, G. (1987), Children's attitudes about health care: Initial development of a questionnaire. *J. Pediatr. Psychol.*, 12:429–443.

——— Melamed, B., & Cockrell, C. (1989), Parenting children in a stressful medical situation. In: *Stressful Life Events*, ed. T. Miller. Madison,CT: International Universities Press, pp. 643–657.

——— Melamed, B., Sheras, P., & Greenbaum, P. (1986), Mother–child patterns of coping with anticipatory medical stress. *Health Psychol.*, 5:137–157.

Campbell, J. (1975), Illness is a point of view: The development of children's concepts of illness. *Child Develop.*, 46:92–100.

Campbell, L., Clark, M., & Kirkpatrick, S. (1986), Stress management training for parents and their children undergoing cardiac catheterization. *Amer. J. Orthopsychiat.*, 56:234–243.

Dixon, S., Snyder, J., Holve, R., & Bromberger, P. (1984), Behavioral effects of circumcision with and without anesthesia. *J. Development. & Behav. Pediatr.*, 5:246–250.

Eland, J., & Anderson, J. (1977), The experience of pain in children. In: *Pain: A Sourcebook For Nurses and Other Health Professionals*, ed. A. Jacox. Boston: Little, Brown, pp. 453–473.

Ernst, A., Routh, D., & Harper, D. (1984), Abdominal pain in children and symptoms of somatization disorder. *J. Pediatr. Psychol.*, 9:77–86.

Escalona, S. (1953). Emotional development in the first year of life. In: *Problems of Infancy and Childhood*, ed. M. Senn. California: Science and Behavior Books.

Farley, G. (1981). Cognitive development. In: *Understanding Human Behavior in Health and Illness*, eds. R. Simons & H. Pardes. Philadelphia: Williams & Wilkins.

Fassler, D. (1985), The fear of needles in children. *Amer. J. Orthopsychiat.*, 55:371–377.

Faust, J., & Melamed, B. (1984), Influence of arousal, previous experience, and age on surgery preparation of same day of surgery and in-hospital pediatric patients. *J. Consult. & Clin. Psychol.*, 52:359–365.

Fentress, D., Masek, B., Mehegan, J., & Benson, H. (1986), Biofeedback and relaxation response training in the treatment of pediatric migraine. *Development. Med. & Child Neurol.*, 28:139–146.

Friedman, R. (1972), Some characteristics of children with "psychogenic" pain. *Clin. Pediatr.*, 11:331–333.

Gaffney, A., & Dunne, E. (1986), Developmental aspects of children's definitions of pain. *Pain*, 26:105–117.

Gildea, J., & Quirk, T. (1977), Assessing the pain experience in children. *Nurs. Clin. N. Amer.*, 12:631–637.

Ginsburg, H., & Opper, S. (1969), *Piaget's Theory of Intellectual Development*. Englewood Cliffs, NJ: Prentice-Hall.

Green, M. (1967), Diagnosis and treatment: Psychogenic, recurrent abdominal pain. *Pediatr.*, 40:84–89.

Gross, A., Stern, R., Levin, R., Dale, J., & Wojnilower, D. (1983), The effect of mother–child separation on the behavior of children experiencing a diagnostic medical procedure. *J. Consult. Clin. Psychol.*, 51:783–785.

Gross, S., & Gardner, G. (1980), Child pain: Treatment approaches. In: *Pain: Meaning and Management*, eds. W. Smith, H. Merskey, & S. Gross. New York: Spectrum, pp. 127–142.

Haight, W., Black, J., & DiMatteo, M. (1985), Young children's understanding of the social roles of physician and patient. *J. Pediat. Psychol.*, 10:31–43.

Hodges, K., Kline, J., Barbero, G., & Flanery, R. (1985), Depressive symptoms in children with recurrent abdominal pain and in their families. *J. Pediatr.*, 107:622–626.

Houpt, M., Moore, P., & Weinstein, P., eds. (1986), Progress in pain and anxiety control #1: Integrating pharmacological and behavioral therapeutic modalities and research methodologies. In: *Proceedings of a Research Workshop on Dental Anxiety Sponsored by the National Institute of Dental Research*, September 12–13, 1985, Bethesda, MD. *Anesthesia Progress*, p. 33.

Jackson, K. (1951), Psychological preparations as a method of reducing the emotional trauma of anesthesia in children. *Anesthesiol.*, 12:293–300.

Jay, S., & Elliot, C. (1984), Behavioral observation scales for measuring children's distress: The effects of increased methodological rigor. *J. Consult. & Clin. Psychol.*, 52:1106–1107.

——— ——— Varni, J. (1986), Acute and chronic pain in adults and children with cancer. *J. Consult. & Clin. Psychol.*, 54:601–607.

Jensen, B. (1981), Caudal block for postoperative pain relief in children after genital operations: A comparison of bupivicaine and morphine. *Acta Anaesthes. Scand.*, 25:373–375.

Katz, E., Kellerman, J., & Siegel, S. (1980), Behavioral distress in children with cancer undergoing medical procedures: Developmental considerations. *J. Consult. & Clin. Psychol.*, 48:356–365.

Kavanaugh, C. (1983), Psychological intervention with the severely burned child: Report on an experimental comparison of two approaches and their effects on psychosocial sequelae. *J. Child Psychiat.*, 22:145–156.

Kelley, M., Jarvie, G., Middlebrooke, J., McNeer, M., & Drabman, R. (1984), Decreasing burned children's pain behavior: Impacting the trauma of hydrotherapy. *J. Appl. Behav. Anal.*, 17:147–158.

Kolko, D., & Rickard-Figueroa, J. (1985), Effects of video games on the adverse corollaries of chemotherapy in pediatric oncology patients: A single-case analysis. *J. Consult. & Clin. Psychol.*, 53:223–228.

Labbé, E., & Williamson, D. (1983), Temperature biofeedback in the treatment of children with migraine headache. *J. Pediat. Psychol.*, 8:317–326.

——— ——— (1984), Treatment of childhood migraine using autogenic feedback training. *J. Consult. & Clin. Psychol.*, 52:968–976.

Lollar, D., Smits, S., & Patterson, D. (1982), Assessment of pediatric pain: An empirical perspective. *J. Pediat. Psychol.*, 7:267–277.

Lunn, J. (1979), Postoperative analgesia after circumcision. *Aneathes.*, 34:525–555.

Masek, B., Russo, D., & Varni, J. (1984), Behavioral approaches to the management of chronic pain in children. *Pediatr. Clin. N. Amer.*, 31:1113–1131.

Mather, L., & Mackie, J. (1983), The incidence of postoperative pain in children. *Pain*, 15:271–282.

McGrath, P., Goodman, J., Firestone, P., Shipman, R., & Peters, S. (1983), Recurrent abdominal pain: A psychogenic disorder? *Arch. Dis. Childhood*, 58:888–890.

——— Vair, C. (1984), Psychological aspects of pain management of the burned child. *Children's Health Care*, 13:15–19.

McGraw, M. (1963), *The Neuromuscular Maturation of the Human Infant.* New York: Harper.

Melamed, B., & Bush, J. (1985), Family factors in children with acute illness. In: *Health, Illness, and Families: A Life-span Perspective,* eds. D. C. Turk & R. D. Kerns. New York: Wiley, pp. 183–219.

——— & Siegel, L. (1975), Reduction of anxiety in children facing hospitalization and surgery by use of filmed modeling. *J. Consult. & Clin. Psychol.,* 43:511–521.

Minuchin, S., & Fishman, H. (1979), The psychosomatic family in child psychiatry. *Annu. Amer. Acad. Child Psychiat.,* 18:76–90.

Moore, P., & Goodson, J. (1985), Risk appraisal of narcotic sedation for children. *Anesthes. Progr.,* 32:129–139.

Nossel, H. (1980), Disorders of blood coagulation factors. In: *Harrison's Principles of Internal Medicine,* eds. K. Isselbacher, R. Adams, E. Braunwald, R. Petersdorf, & J. Wilson. New York: McGraw-Hill, pp. 1560–1562.

Olness, K., & MacDonald, J. (1981), Self-hypnosis and biofeedback in the management of juvenile migraine. *Developmen. & Behav. Pediatr.,* 2:168–170.

O'Malley, J., Koocher, G., Foster, D., & Slavin, L. (1979), Psychiatric sequelae of surviving childhood cancer. *Amer. J. Orthopsychiat.,* 49:608–616.

Painter, P. Morrison, J., & Evens, R. (1965), Galvanic skin response: Differences in organic and psychogenic pain of children. *Amer. J. Dis. Child.,* 110:265–269.

Parmelee, A. (1986). Children's illnesses: Their beneficial effects on behavioral development. *Child Develop.,* 57:1–10.

Perrin, E., & Gerrity, S. (1981), There's a demon in your belly: Children's understanding of illness. *Pediatr.,* 67:841–849.

——— Perrin, J. (1983), Clinicians' assessment of childrens' understanding of illness. *Amer. J. Dis. Child.,* 137:874–878.

——— Shapiro, E. (1985), Health locus of control beliefs of healthy children, children with a chronic physical illness, and their mothers. *J. Pediatr.,* 107:627–633.

Perry, S., & Heidrich, G. (1982), Management of pain during debridement: A survey of U.S. burn units. *Pain,* 13:267–280.

Peterson, L., & Toler, S. (1986), An information seeking disposition in child surgery patients. *Health Psychol.,* 5:343–358.

Porter, F., Miller, R. & Marshall, R. (1986), Neonatal pain cries: Effect of circumcision on acoustic features and perceived urgency. *Child Develop.,* 57:790–802.

Ross, D., & Ross, S. (1984), Childhood pain: The school-aged child's viewpoint. *Pain,* 20:179–191.

Routh, D., & Ernst, A. (1984), Somatization disorder in relatives of children and adolescents with functional abdominal pain. *J. Pediat. Psychol.,* 9:427–437.

Savedra, M., Gibbons, P., Tesler, M., Ward, J., & Wegner, C. (1982), How do children describe pain? A tentative assessment. *Pain,* 14:95–104.

Schultz, N. (1971), How children perceive pain. *Nurs. Outlook,* 19:670–673.

Scott, R. (1978), "It hurts red:" A preliminary study of children's perception of pain. *Percept. & Motor Skills,* 47:787–791.

Shaw, E., & Routh, D. (1982), Effect of mother presence on children's reactions to aversive procedures. *J. Pediat. Psychol.,* 7:33–42.

Siegel, L. (1981), Naturalistic study of coping strategies in children facing medical procedures. Paper presented at the meeting of the Southeastern Psychological Association, Atlanta.

Steward, D. (1980), Anesthesia for pediatric outpatients. *Can. Anesthes. Soc. J.,* 27:412–416.

Steward, M., & Steward, D. (1981), Children's conceptions of medical procedures. In: *New directions for child development: Children's conceptions of health, illness, and bodily functions,* eds. R. Bibace & M. Walsh. San Francisco: Jossey-Bass, pp. 67–83.

Stoddard, F. (1982), Coping with pain: A developmental approach to the treatment of burned children. *Amer. J. Psychiat.*, 139:736–740.

Stone, R., & Barbero, G. (1970), Recurrent abdominal pain in childhood. *Pediatr.*, 45:732–738.

Swafford, L., & Allan, D. (1968), Pain relief in the pediatric patient. *Med. Clin. N. Amer.*, 52:131–136.

Tesler, M., Ward, J., Savedra, M., Wegner, C., & Gibbons, P. (1983), Developing an instrument for eliciting children's descriptions of pain. *Percept. & Motor Skills*, 56:315–321.

Tomasi, L. (1979). Headaches in children. *Pediatr.*, 5:13–19.

Turkat, I., & Rock, D. (1984), Parental influences on illness behavior development in chronic pain and healthy individuals. *Pain*, Supplement 2: Fourth World Congress on Pain of the International Association for the Study of Pain, S15.

Unruh, A., McGrath, P., Cunningham, S., & Humphreys, P. (1983), Children's drawings of their pain. *Pain*, 17:385–392.

Varni, J. (1984), Pediatric pain: A biobehavioral perspective. *Behav. Therap.*, 7:23–25.

——— Bessman, C., Russo, D., & Cataldo, M. (1980), Behavioral management of chronic pain in children: A case study. *Arch. Physical Med. & Rehab.*, 61:375–378.

Violon, A., & Giurgea, D. (1984), Familial models for chronic pain. *Pain*, 18:199–203.

Wakeman, R., & Kaplan, J. (1978), An experimental study of hypnosis in painful burns. *Amer. J. Clin. Hypnos.*, 21:3–12.

White, M. (1979), Structural and strategic approaches to psychosomatic families. *Fam. Proc.*, 18:303–314.

Whitt, J. (1982), Children's understanding of illness: Developmental considerations and pediatric intervention. In: *Advances in Developmental and Behavioral Pediatrics: A Research Annual*, Vol. 3, eds. M. Woolraich & D. Routh. Greenwich, CT: JAI Press, pp. 163–201.

Wilson, J. (1981), Behavioral preparation for surgery: Benefit or harm? *J. Behav. Med.*, 4:79–102.

Worchel, F., Copeland, D., & Barker, D. (1987), Control-related coping strategies in pediatric oncology patients. *J. Pediatr. Psychol.*, 12:25–38.

Zeltzer, L., Kellerman, J., Ellenberg, L., Dash, J., & Rigler, D. (1980), Psychological effects of illness in adolescence. II. Impact of illness in adolescents: Crucial issues and coping styles. *J. Pediatr.*, 97:1032–1035.

———LeBaron, S. (1982), Hypnotic and nonhypnotic techniques for reduction of pain and anxiety during painful procedures in children and adolescents with cancer. *J. Pediatr.*, 101:1032–1035.

24

Chronic Pain and the Role of the Clinical Social Worker

RANJAN ROY, ADV. DIP. S.W.

INTRODUCTION

Social work appears to be a relative latecomer to the field of chronic pain (Roy, 1981, 1987a), and social work literature on chronic pain is virtually nonexistent. Nevertheless, in view of the complexity of the psychosocial problems related to chronic pain, the necessity of social work involvement with the chronic pain patient cannot be left to chance.

THE PATIENT AS A PERSON

From the pioneering work of a number of researchers such as Sternbach (1974) it has been clearly demonstrated that persons with chronic pain consistently present a cohesive set of personality characteristics. This has been evident in the profile of these individuals on the Minnesota Multiple Personality Inventory (MMPI). On the MMPI the chronic pain patients demonstrate an elevation on the hypochrondriasis, hysteria,

Acknowledgments. I am deeply indebted to Mrs. June Clarke for her assistance in the preparation of this chapter.

and the depression scales, which is commonly known as conversion V. There has been much debate in the literature about the value of this MMPI finding, but arguably the finding has been able to establish beyond any serious doubt that chronic pain sufferers as a group tend to demonstrate psychological distress of a similar nature. Pilowsky (1969) and Pilowsky, Murrell, and Gordon (1976) have developed the Illness Behavior Questionnaire (IBQ) to delineate the patient's reaction to illness. The IBQ has seven scales: general hypochrondriasis, disease conviction, somatic versus psychological perception of illness, affective inhibition, affective disturbance, denial, and irritability. Pilowsky and Spence (1976) compared 100 patients with pain that had not responded to conventional treatment with a comparison group of 40 patients attending rheumatology, radiotherapy, pulmonary, and physiotherapy clinics. They found a significant difference on the scale of disease conviction, suggesting that patients with intractable pain tended to be more convinced as to the presence of disease, were somatically preoccupied, and seemingly were unable to accept reassurance from their physician. They concluded that "this response pattern [was] maybe most usefully conceptualized as a form of abnormal illness behaviour" (p. 66). The purpose of this brief excursion into the psychological profile of chronic pain patients and their reaction to illness is to establish that psychological and social factors are clearly implicated in what is commonly called the chronic benign pain syndrome.

From a psychodynamic perspective, it has been suggested that early childhood experiences may very well play a significant role in the etiology of chronic pain disorders (Roy, 1984). The primary proponent of this proposition is Engel (1959), who, in his seminal paper entitled "Psychogenic Pain and the Pain Prone Patient," clinically demonstrated that child abuse and neglect predisposed the victims to the development of "pain prone disorders." Generally speaking, as indicated earlier, a pain-prone patient demonstrates a history of a harsh and punitive childhood; prominence of guilt, and use of pain to expiate guilt; an inability to express anger directly, and turning in of anger on the self; a personal history characterized by suffering and a defeatist attitude, and an inability to tolerate success; strong, unusually unconscious, conflictual sexual impulses, which appear symbolically as pain; pain developed to reflect the loss or potential loss of another person. In short, for these individuals pain becomes a way of life and almost a reason for living. While theoretically Engel's proposition is an attractive one, it has failed to receive empirical validation to date (Roy, 1985a). Nevertheless, in clinical practice chronic pain patients with a past history of child abuse are certainly not uncommon (Roy, 1982). This particular perspective is important, as will become evident in one of the case discussions later in this section.

In sum, it is quite clear that chronic pain sufferers are psychologically vulnerable, tend to demonstrate a similar pattern of reaction to illness, and may indeed have a very damaged sense of self as a consequence of child abuse and deprivation.

Despite measurable progress in new treatment for chronic pain, the most critical factor that has implication for all health care professionals as well as social work is the chronic pain patients' relative unresponsiveness to traditional medical interventions (Holzman and Turk, 1986). Arguably, some of their problems are iatrogenic. Generally, as a group they are subject to mixed medical messages which range from "there is something wrong with you, but I don't know what it is" to "perhaps your problem is all in your head." Chronic pain sufferers are frequently sad, dependent on drugs, socially withdrawn, subject to multiple surgeries, and mentally and physically disabled. Of course it would be incorrect to suggest that all chronic pain patients demonstrate all the characteristics, but quite surprisingly many of the characteristics are frequently present. Drug dependency, and central nervous system (CNS) side effects due to a multitude of pharmacological treatments are presumably interrelated in some ways and are not uncommon among chronic pain sufferers. Multiple surgeries may be common among certain groups but not among others. For example, it is totally unlikely that chronic headache patients experience any surgical interventions, whereas it is certainly not uncommon among chronic back pain sufferers. Some of the other characteristics, such as the dysphoric mood and depression associated with loss of self-esteem, and psychosocial withdrawal and physical incapacity, have been the source of considerable debate in the pain-depression literature. A central question of this debate has been whether or not chronic pain sufferers, or more accurately the problem of chronic pain itself, is not some form of mood disorder. Consensus at this point in history appears to be that a percentage of chronic pain patients are indeed clinically depressed (Roy, Thomas, and Matas, 1984; Romano and Turner, 1985). Perhaps the debate about the presence of depression in chronic pain sufferers has been to a certain extent at the expense of ignoring the vast changes of fortune that many of these patients experience. Those changes are bound to cause a considerable amount of grief. In short, the relationship between social factors and dysphoric mood in these patients remains an underresearched area.

Therefore, it is quite imperative that the influence of social factors on the chronic pain patient should be examined in some depth. Sternbach, Murphy, Akeson, and Wolf (1973) observed that "typically he (chronic pain patients) has given up employment and subsists on welfare, social security, and disability income. He does little, if anything, in the home, spends only three or four hours a day on his feet, and frequents clinics and doctor's offices. In terms of self-concept, he is an invalid". Embedded in that statement are the most devastating consequences of chronic pain, namely, the traumatic nature of the role changes for these individuals. In many instances, a reasonably well-functioning human being following the onset of the pain problem and over a period of time undergoes a complete metamorphosis as far as his identity is concerned. From being a breadwinner, parent, lover, friend, and many other roles, the only identity that remains meaningful is that of a chronic patient. The Parsonian concept of the sick role, which implies that the sick person ultimately recovers and resumes normal living, is rendered ineffectual in the context of chronic pain sufferers (Gallagher and Wrobel, 1982).

Chronic pain patient often suffers from a sense of alienation from the society. His normal sources of succor and self-esteem magically melt away leaving the patient in a state a social limbo. He is jobless, friendless, no longer an effective provider for his family, a caring, loving parent or spouse. In that situation he has no choice but to assume the identity of a chronic patient. As Sternbach et al. (1973) pointed out, by this time the chronic pain patient indeed is an invalid.

Given the magnitude of social and emotional changes in these patients, the role of a clinical social worker may indeed be self-evident. But it is not always so. Perhaps an effective way of delineating social work activities in relation to this person would be by presenting three cases with overlapping, but at the same time, unique problems. This will also provide an opportunity for demonstrating what Germain (1980) has described as the social context for social work practice. Mr. L. was fifty-four years old when he was involved in a car crash causing injury to his right leg and fracturing it in several places. His past history of pain and accident was quite remarkable. Over a period of some sixteen years he had sustained four falls prior to the auto accident. Since the initial accident, until his inception into the pain clinic, he had nine surgeries, but in spite of his health problems he continued to work, with only minor lapses, until the final accident. Following that he decompensated rather rapidly to a point where he felt utterly helpless and was unable to return to his job. He also became severely hypertensive and was referred to the pain clinic by his family physician.

His premorbid history was quiet unremarkable. He was born in a French-speaking working-class family. His family moved to an English-speaking part of Canada where he encountered serious problems in English-speaking schools. He fell back steadily and only obtained an eighth grade education. He could barely read and write. His father was alive and lived with him, and his mother had died a year earlier. His three siblings were in excellent health. As a young man, he was heavily involved in sports and maintained his sporting activities until his last accident in his midfifties. Mr. L. was married with five children, two of whom had left home. His wife was in poor health and suffered from migraine and low back pain. She also had knee surgery for reasons that remained unclear to him. His eighteen-year-old daughter had a problem with vertigo and migraine. She was not receiving any active treatment. The family situation was vastly complicated by the fact that one of his sons was living with a woman, which was against the dictates of Mr. L.'s Roman Catholic religion, and there was a child by this marriage who had not been baptized. There was considerable family dissension over this matter, and Mr. L. was acutely affected by his son's "misconduct." The family picture that emerged was one of great deal of tension and unhappiness characterized by a lot of pain, financial difficulties, and interpersonal wrangles.

Mr. L.'s relationship with his wife and children had deteriorated to a point that they avoided him as much as possible. Prior to his last accident he was rather an easygoing man, but now he was mostly irritable and very critical of his family members. He also developed a habit of flying into inexplicable rage. This kind of behavior in Mr. L. resulted in avoidance by other members of his family which further added to his sense of loneliness and rejection. Review of his daily activities revealed that he was far from bedridden or housebound. He got up early every morning, had his breakfast, and went out for walks. He met with his pals everyday at a local hotel. Until about two years prior to the accident, Mr. L. had a serious drinking problem, but was not drinking anymore. Instead he was taking in an inordinate amount of medication, which was a combination of narcotics, plain analgesics, and Diazepam. The day he came to the pain clinic, he had taken ten Percodan and three Valium.

During the course of the interview he expressed his fear of "cracking up." He was also having nightmares, which involved losing his right leg. He demonstrated a tremendous amount of preoccupation with his pain problem and he was very sad. He cried on several occasions during the preliminary interview and described himself as an invalid. He had lost his sexual urges, and in fact could no longer get an erection. This, combined with his loss of occupational role, in his mind, totally emasculated him. He was very preoccupied with this last point. He expressed some vague suicidal thoughts. He was very adamant, however, that suicide was forbidden by his religion and he would never do it. There were times when he wondered what his life was all about, and, indeed, if it was worth continuing. He complained that his sense of loss and depression had been further accentuated by his mother's death. However, his main problem was still his pain. He was bitter about all the surgeries he had been subjected to, and was openly hostile toward the medical profession. He was convinced in his own mind that all those past surgeries had played a part in his ongoing pain problem and he was deeply disappointed that no one had been able to help him since his last accident.

Formulation was that this rather simple and nice man, with an unusual history of accidents and surgeries, became a victim of his own pain and was showing many signs of psychological disintegration and social alienation. He was sad and depressed, although perhaps not clinically, and his central sense of identity as a man and a provider was under serious challenge. With his past problem with alcohol, it was not surprising that he was overly dependent on drugs. Although he described himself as an invalid, a review of his daily living did not indicate that he had been immobilized by his illness or that he was totally dependent. At the point of his inception into the pain clinic, he was without a definite purpose and therefore quite unable to reflect on any kind of a plan to pull himself out of the doldrums.

Social Work Intervention. It must be noted at the outset that this man categorically refused to involve his family in the treatment. He regarded his problem as his own, and he felt very strongly that involving his family would be a further sign of his inability to deal with his own problems. In any event, he failed to understand how his family could be of any help since the problem was one of pain. He was also very skeptical about involvement with a social worker, but he acquiesced by simply stating that he was willing to try anything.

The first task was to help Mr. L. to establish more realistic goals for himself. He was very committed to returning to his job as a truck driver, which seemed highly unlikely to happen. This is not an unusual problem, because returning to work is almost universally seen as a realistic measure of success. This man literally had no control over his own life and felt victimized by the legal system, the Workmen's Compensation Board (WCB), the health care professionals, and so on. It was quiet imperative to give this man a sense of control over his own life. To that end a task-centered approach which has been enunciated by Reid and Epstein (1978), was adopted. This approach is predicated on behavioral principles and it is of a short-term nature. It assumes that people are by and large motivated to find solutions to painful situations so long as they play a part in determining the solutions that are designed to give them a sense of mastery over themselves.

As a starting point, discussion with Mr. L. centered on prioritizing his problems. It must be recognized that all this had been done in close collaboration with the other members of the pain clinic, including a physician and a physiotherapist. The goals were first and foremost to bring the patient's medication under control; a systematic exploration to find tasks that would be meaningful and gratifying to the patient; the exploration of solutions for his problems with his son, and improving relationship with his wife. He was advised by a urologist that his sexual dysfunctioning had been caused by his low mood, that there was no organic basis for it. Mr. L. found this to be very reassuring.

To begin with, Mr. L. was seen once a week for the first six weeks, and then at greater and greater intervals. The entire therapeutic alliance lasted for just over a year. During this time he became a volunteer in an old peoples' home. He was persuaded by his family and friends, and through lengthy discussion with the social worker, that the enjoyment he derived from his grandchild outweighed the fact that his son was not married. In any event the son had given every indication that he was planning to marry in the near future. In the sphere of his social activities, Mr. L. became somewhat better organized. Prior to the last accident, he had been very interested in hockey and curling, and while he could no longer participate in these activities he resumed his association with his old friends, and began to take a renewed interest in sports again. At home there was a remarkable change in his relationship with his wife. He generally became quite concerned about her well-being, and she in turn took his side more and more in family conflicts and helped him to reestablish his role as head of the household. They took a short holiday during which Mr. L. discovered that he was still capable of sexual activities, which restored his self-confidence in large measure.

It would be wrong to assume that Mr. L. was "cured" of his pain problem in any sense. He continued to complain about his pain, and his overdependency on drugs, while vastly improved, was still a problem. Social work intervention enabled this individual to regain his position within the family, improve his relationship with his wife, reestablish his social support system through his sporting friends and colleagues, and although he remained unemployed, his sense of purposelessness had, to a great extent, vanished. In short as he found new roles and renewed his relationships with a different set of rules, he no longer viewed himself as an invalid.

Mrs. D. Victim of Her Past

This thirty-eight-year-old woman was referred to the pain clinic by her neurologist who stated that "this pleasant health-care professional has been having severe headaches for a long time. They are mostly migrainous in nature but with a very prominent muscle contraction component. She has had very poor success in medication due to her lack of tolerance of side effects. She would like to explore your approach to this problem, and I would certainly appreciate your opinion."

Mrs. D. was married, with two young children. Her headaches dated back to her childhood, and she could not really remember a time in her life when she was without pain. Exploration of her family situation revealed that she was the younger of two siblings. Her father was a hard-working man and her mother a very domineering and controlling woman. She had no recall of ever receiving any affection from either parent during her growing-up years, although she remembered that her father, when he had time, was more inclined to take an interest in her schoolwork and in her general well-being.

Mother was extremely critical, and Mrs. D. spent a good deal of time thinking of ways whereby she could please her. She recalled how on one occasion she came home from school with what amounted to excellent grades, but her mother's only remark was that she could be a little more helpful around the house. As she grew older Mrs. D. became increasingly withdrawn, had frequent bouts of headaches, and spent an inordinate amount of time in her room.

She apparently grew up to be a rather shy woman who had virtually no friends and whose life revolved around her work. Curiously, she continued to live at home. While still in her early twenties she was raped by a fellow worker, but she kept the matter to herself and withdrew even further into her own shell. After the rape, she only left home to go to work, and spent her entire free time lying on the couch doing absolutely nothing. Neither of her parents recognized this seemingly abnormal change in their daughter's behavior, and not until she came into therapy with this author did she disclose the fact of her rape. Following the incident of rape, she met a man and fell in love, and for the first time in her life she felt valued as a person. A few days before the wedding the man broke off the engagement without any explanation and simply dropped out of her life. She went through a period of intense depression, but somehow managed to keep working. A few years after that event she did meet a man whom she married.

Mrs. D. described her married life as acceptable, but was devoid of any feelings of love and companionship. Her husband rarely consulted her on any matters of importance, and on one occasion decided to move the family to a different location 800 miles from her hometown without ever saying a word to her about this very important decision. The picture was somewhat complicated by the presence of Mrs. D.'s mother-in-law. She interfered greatly in family affairs and Mrs. D., who felt quite helpless with this problem as her husband always sided with his mother.

Mrs. D. had grown up in a home without any love, had been subjected to violence and rejection, and was in a marriage which gave her little pleasure. Her only source of gratification was her two daughters, and she also derived some satisfaction from her job. She had decided earlier in her life that her purpose was primarily to serve others as silently as possible, and never voice her disagreement, regardless of how strongly she felt about a given matter. She internalized all her feelings, negative and positive, with one exception: She was very demonstrative of her positive feelings toward the children.

Mrs. D. was a resistant patient. She had serious doubts about embarking on any kind of psychotherapeutic venture, and wondered out loud how that might indeed improve her headaches. However, despite her doubts, she engaged in therapy, and slowly and gradually discovered that she had many unresolved problems, much unexpressed anger, and guilt and shame that she could not account for.

Social Work Intervention. The practice of psychotherapy is certainly not the exclusive domain of social work, and is one of several intervention methods that social work has in common with psychology and psychiatry. Nevertheless, historically the social workers have engaged in psychotherapeutic activities ranging from psychoanalytic to cognitive. Psychotherapy in this instance was based on short term approach which has been previously described by Roy (1982). In essence, Mrs. D.'s problems were conceptualized in terms of pain proneness which is a concept developed by Engel (1959). Mrs. D. clearly manifested several of the attributes of a pain-prone patient; namely, prominence of guilt and use of pain to expiate guilt, history of a somewhat harsh childhood which was devoid of affection and love, a clear inability to express anger and a tendency to internalize feelings, a clear history of suffering and defeat, and her pain serving a multitude of unconscious functions.

Mrs. D. was seen over a period of eighteen months. The major sources of her conflicts and low self-esteem emanated from a pervasive sense of guilt over her inability to please her mother, accentuated by feelings of unworthiness by her experience of a violent rape, and the subsequent desertion by her boyfriend. All her hostile feelings toward her parents, toward the perpetrator of her rape, toward the man who had abandoned her just prior to her wedding, toward her husband and her mother-in-law were internalized. As these angry feelings began to crystallize, she experienced an enhanced sense of guilt because expression of negative feelings or even allowing herself to have those feelings was quite unacceptable to her. She struggled very hard to keep those feelings submerged, but in the course of therapy they emerged slowly but clearly.

She understood that at the interpersonal level the central problem was her fear of rejection, which had very much influenced her relationship with her husband. She stated on one occasion that she would rather maintain that relationship at any cost than openly argue with him. Her husband could thus take her completely for granted and do as he wished. She was, in the true sense, a silent partner. As the treatment progressed, she developed a clear sense about the sources of her conflicts and lost some of her earlier inhibitions about expressing negative feelings. Her interpersonal relationship outside the immediate family improved quite significantly. She formed a very close friendship with another woman with whom she openly discussed her thoughts and feelings. On the home front her husband noticed quite a change in Mrs. D.'s outlook and attitude and Mrs. D. was pleasantly surprised by her husband's willingness to accept her opinions and points of view without much opposition. Mrs. D. who had been on antidepressant and antimigraine medication for several years and had kept a meticulous diary of her pain, began to notice a decrease in the frequency of her headaches. She emerged from this therapeutic venture with a sense of liberation which was manifest in her attempt to realign her marriage relationship to that of equal partnership. If that did not work, she informed the author, then she might even consider divorce in order to enable her to make a fresh start.

Miss C. Case of Retirement, Pain, and Depression

Miss C. aged sixty-eight years was referred to the pain clinic with an unremitting complaint of backache, that had started three years earlier and continued unabated. The pain was severe enough to confine her more or less to her own apartment, thus almost completely isolating her from the community. She stayed a good deal of time either lying on the sofa or actually in bed, and was taking very inadequate care of herself. She was thoroughly investigated by a neurologist, an orthopedic surgeon, and other medical specialists, and their combined findings were essentially negative. She was very dismayed by that fact, and even when she came to the pain clinic she was determined to find a medical cure for her problem.

She was born and raised in a metropolitan area of western Canada and her childhood was essentially uneventful. She finished high school and worked in various jobs until she decided to start her own business. She developed her own retail business and spent all her working life running that business. She never married because, she said, she never really had the time. She looked after her sick and elderly mother for very many years. It was clear from her account that she was a very active woman in the business community and took an active interest in the chamber of commerce, and so on. As she approached retirement age, sixty-five, she sold her business in order to have more free time, and also to devote more time to her increasingly disabled mother.

Her pain problem started six months after her retirement, and to make matters worse, a year later her mother died. From all accounts Miss C. decompensated rapidly, and as she put it, became "an invalid." At the time of her inception into the pain clinic, she was angry, sad, and very despondent about her future. Underneath it all she was also afraid that she might have an incurable disease. She acknowledged that her only social contact was a sister who lived nearby, but whom she saw very rarely. There is indeed a temporal relationship between the development of illness or morbidity and life events that tend to be undesirable, uncontrollable, and unpredictable.

The individual perception of events is also significant in determining whether an event or events are perceived as negative or positive. It would appear in the case of Miss C. that loss of her occupational role proved to be a much more significant loss than she had anticipated. The only other source of gratification had been her caring role in relation to her mother, which she had lost. This created a type of social vacuum in which she found herself living. Given that climate, it is perhaps not altogether surprising that she developed a debilitating pain. This woman had no previous history of any kind of health problem.

Although she denied any feelings of depression, there was significant evidence of vegetative symptoms such as early morning wakening, a massive loss of appetite and weight, anhedonia, and lack of energy and drive. Many chronic pain patients deny any feeling of sadness, and pain becomes a substitute for dysphoric mood. In older chronic pain patients, however, the vegetative symptoms can be an integral part of the pain problem itself.

The diagnosis of clinical depression has to be made with some caution. Dessonville and his colleagues (1985) have suggested that symptoms of self-deprecation are key to acute diagnosis for clinical depression. In the case of Miss C., there was indeed much evidence of self-deprecation, and despite the fact that she had led a highly successful life, she regarded herself as a failure.

Intervention. Following her assessment, she was placed on 75 mg of tricyclic antidepressant by the pain clinic physician, and the social work intervention consisted of enabling this woman to reintegrate into the community at large. She was seen on a weekly basis for a period of two months. During this time she began to engage in a number of volunteer activities, took in a student in the person of her nephew, and resumed the relationship with her sister. She had somehow forgotten that she and her sister were the best of friends until about three years ago, which coincided with the onset of her pain problem. She and her sister decided to take a holiday. In a matter of just a few weeks, Miss C. reported a significant reduction in her pain problem. She was beginning to function at a level which effectively counteracted her sense of loneliness and low self-esteem. In other words, there was much evidence of improvement in her general outlook as well as in her mood. She was maintaining her improvement at the six-month review, following which she was discharged from the pain clinic.

Formulation in this case was relatively simple. Retirement proved to be much more hazardous than she had anticipated, and when this was combined with the death of her mother, she lost the only two sources of enjoyment and gratification in her life. Pain and depression could indeed be a natural reaction to such negative life events. In the context of Miss C., the meanings and functions of pain assumed a degree of significance that could not be overlooked. Pain is communication and always has a message. In her case the central task of the social worker was to unravel the message (Roy, 1984), which was one of loss. This woman's premorbid history of functioning was excellent, and for all practical purposes she really required very nominal help to resume her active and fruitful pursuits. Social work intervention in this case was a time-honored one. The concept of "person–environment" fit was very relevant in the case of Miss C. That fit had come unglued in her case, and the task of social work was to help this woman to find new means for gratification. Given Miss C.'s excellent premorbid level of functioning, it was achieved with relative ease.

Summary. The three aforementioned cases described problems of different orders and magnitude. A middle-aged man with a past history of accidents, illnesses, and surgeries, decompensates and becomes an invalid, only to make a partial recovery. A young woman with a history of neglect and abuse uses pain as a form of expiation of guilt and learns to internalize all her negative feelings. A successful businesswoman whose dreams of retirement collapse, with the situation further compounded by the death of her mother, becomes a victim of pain and depression. Social work interventions in these three cases exemplify the scope and range of clinical practice of social work. There is, however, a unifying thread that runs through the three cases, namely, that social work's primary focus is on the residual abilities of an individual and not on psychopathology. It is through the mobilization of healthy aspects of the personality that social work achieves its principal goal of enabling its clients and patients to regain a sense of congruence between themselves and their environment.

Patient and the Family

Social work preoccupation with the family is time-honored indeed. Siporin (1980), in his review of social work involvement with family in the historical context, claimed that such involvement did not begin until the early nineteenth century. He observed that "until recently, social workers were recognized by the general public and other helping professionals as being expert in and having almost exclusive domain in marital and family practice" (p. 17). He further noted the longstanding tradition of psychiatrists and psychologists treating individuals. However, there has been a dramatic decline in recent years in social workers working primarily with the family groups and spouses. He contributed this decline in large measure to "regressive competition from other helping human service professions and the passive response to such competition by social workers (p. 19). On the other hand, contributions to the theory and practice of family therapy by such eminent social worker family therapists such as Virginia Satir, Peggy Papp, and Lynn Hoffman, is to say the least very considerable.

Since the topic of chronic pain and family has come under serious review in recent years, only a broad outline of the issues is presented here (Roy, 1985b; Payne and Norfleet, 1986). There is indeed mounting evidence that the presence of chronic pain in a family system has far-reaching consequences for family members. Apart from the fact that family members in general, and spouses in particular, play a rather complex role in the perpetuation and maintenance of pain behaviors, impact of chronic pain on the quality of marriage, on the health of the spouse, and on the sexual functioning is both pervasive and serious (Roy, 1987a). A variety of therapeutic approaches that include structural, strategic, behavioral, problem centered, and others have been utilized to treat chronic pain sufferers and their families (Roy, 1985c). However, to date clinical as well as research reports on the efficacy of family treatment for chronic pain remains essentially limited.

Roy (1987b) has recently reported the pervasive nature of marital dysfunction in a group of chronic headache sufferers and their spouses. He assessed twenty headache sufferers and their spouses utilizing the McMaster model of family functioning (MMFF) (Epstein, Bishop, and Levin, 1978); MMFF allows assessment of family functioning on six dimensions: (1) problem solving; (2) communication; (3) roles; (4) affective responsiveness; (5) affective involvement; (6) behavior control. Briefly, he found that all twenty families functioned at the unhealthy end of the problem solving and the communication dimensions. Couples gave evidence of healthy functioning in the area of instrumental roles, but all twenty couples had difficulties in the performance of their affective roles. There were thirteen couples who had difficulty in giving expression to a range of emotions which included both positive and negative. They tended to express their negative emotions, but seven couples were capable of expressing both positive and negative emotions. In the area of affective involvement, twelve couples gave evidence of lack of involvement, and lastly, in relation to behavior control, sixteen couples gave evidence of unhealthy patterns of behavior control which included rigid as well as chaotic patterns. Fifteen of these twenty couples agreed to enter into therapy, and they were treated utilizing problem-centered systems family therapy (PCSFT), the product of over twenty-five years of research by Epstein and Bishop (1980). The model is predicated on a number of assumptions of systems theory, and the assessment tool for the problem centered system family therapy is the MMFF. The essential nature of therapy is short term and behaviorally oriented, and fourteen out of the fifteen couples at the termination of treatment gave evidence of substantial improvement, which they were able to maintain at the six-month follow-up. To illustrate the stages of assessment and of PCSFT treatment a case is presented.

Mr. and Mrs. T

Mrs. T., age sixty-seven, was referred to the pain clinic with the dual problem of severe headache as well as back pain. The history of her headache dated back to her childhood, and as far as could be accurately ascertained, her back pain was of some twenty-five years' duration. What was remarkable about this particular referral was that she had never had any significant level of disability with either of her pain problems. As a matter of fact she had enjoyed superb health and had only minimal contact with the health care system.

Her headaches began to worsen two to three years prior to her referral to the pain clinic. She was referred by her family physician for further investigation. Mr. and Mrs. T. were seen together and the story was that Mrs. T. was by far the more active partner in this marriage and carried major responsibilities for the upbringing of their five children. She reported that Mr. T., a retired professional man, was somewhat peripheral to the entire family system. Mr. T. did not agree with this characterization. In his view his wife tended to be overbearing and very perfectionistic, and continued to have unrealistic expectations of him. Despite the obvious conflict in this long-standing marriage, they had managed to raise five children who were all professionals. Nevertheless, since Mr. T.'s retirement, the marital situation had worsened rather sharply.

The inescapable fact was that Mrs. T.'s headaches took a turn for the worse soon after Mr. T. retired. At this point a battle of wills started between these two individuals. Mr. T. was unkempt, untidy, and most objectionable of all from Mrs. T.'s point of view, he deliberately pretended not to hear her. Mr. T.'s retort was he always heard when she had something important to say, which was of course only very rarely. The battle lines were clearly drawn for these two individuals.

Application of the MMFF to assess this couple led to the following findings:

Problem Solving

Family problem solving refers to a family's ability to solve problems to a level that maintains effective family functioning. Effective problem solving consists of seven steps:

1. identification of the problem(s);
2. communicating with the appropriate people about the problem;
3. developing a set of possible alternative solutions;
4. deciding on one of the alternatives;
5. carrying out the action required with the alternative;
6. monitoring to make sure the action is carried out;
7. evaluating the effectiveness of the problem solving process.

Healthy families solve most problems without much ado. In the course of their long marriage and in raising a large family, Mr. and Mrs. T. must have solved many problems, but at this point, with the changed circumstances, they were confronted with finding new ways of relating to one another. Obviously, Mr. T.'s retirement and the departure of all the children from their home had put Mr. and Mrs. T. together in a way that they had never experienced before. At the initial phase of the investigation Mrs. T. responded with some anger and hostility and suggested that removal of her head pain would basically solve whatever problems they had. Mr. T., on the other hand, indicated that the resolution of the pain problem might not resolve some of their interpersonal difficulties. Mrs. T., albeit somewhat grudgingly, conceded that he might be right. Of late, they had disagreed about everything, and although they were not confronted with any major problems, there was a great deal of bickering about mundane matters. They had some recognition of the nature of their difficulty—that they could barely agree on their problems, let alone solve them.

Communication

Communication is defined as the exchange of information within a family. Two aspects of communication are identified: First, clear versus masked dimension examines the clarity of the message, and second the direct versus indirect dimension determines whether or not the messages are received by the appropriate party. Probably of all the areas of family functioning, Mr. and Mrs. T. demonstrated the most pervasive problems in relation to communication. A very complex pattern of communication emerged. Mrs. T. on her part, was both clear and direct in her communication. As an example she would tell Mr. T. quite directly that it was time for him to change his pants because he hadn't done so for the past three days. Mr. T. would simply ignore this remark as though it had never been said. Mr. T. himself, however, rarely engaged in clear and direct communication with his wife. Without directly criticizing his wife, he would say what a wonderful person his mother was and what a happy life his parents had. Statements like that infuriated Mrs. T., and at the same time enhanced her feeling of helplessness and isolation. When she complained of pain he became unusually attentive and caring.

Roles

Roles are defined as the repetitive pattern of behavior by which family members fulfill family functions. Five role-related functions are identified;

1. provision of resources;
2. nurturance and support;
3. adult sexual gratification;
4. personal development;
5. maintenance and management of family system.

Throughout their marriage, the T.s maintained traditional roles. He was the provider and she was the wife and mother. Over the years they had grown apart, but despite a satisfactory sexual relationship, intimacy was a critical issue for them. They had not prepared for retirement in any sense, and they were struggling in their own way to come to terms with the issue of finding meaningful ways of spending their time. Mr. T. had taken to golf. Mrs. T. had attempted to involve herself in volunteer activities. Curiously, these activities were designed to enable them to stay away from each other but, they had not given any thought to the matter of developing common interests. The management of the instrumental matters in this family was very efficient. This was a very traditional couple with equally traditional roles and as such family affairs were well managed. Mrs. T. expressed a certain amount of dissatisfaction with her responsibilities and felt that Mr. T., now that he had more time, could contribute more. It was also she who identified lack of nurturance and support within this relationship. Mr. T. did not challenge her accusations.

Affective Responsiveness

Affective responsiveness is defined as the ability to respond to a given stimulus with appropriate quality and quantity of feelings. Mr. and Mrs. T. were certainly functioning at the pathological end of the continuum so far as affective responsiveness was concerned. Mrs. T. was angry and hostile and expressed what has been described as "emergency emotions" according to MMFF. She felt increasingly incapable of demonstrating any feelings of warmth or tenderness or love, or what has been defined as "welfare emotions" by MMFF. Mr. T. on his part, remained detached and did not verbalize his feelings at all. As was noted earlier, the only time he expressed feelings of concern and gave any evidence of welfare emotions was when she was in severe pain. In short, this couple was very restricted in their range of emotions; negative and angry feelings on one side and silence on the other seemed to be the dominant feature of this aspect of family functioning.

Affective Involvement

Affective involvement is the extent to which the family shows interest in, and values, particular activities and interests of individual family members. Six types of involvements are identified:

1. lack of involvement;
2. involvement devoid of feelings;
3. narcissistic involvement;
4. empathic involvement;
5. overinvolvement;
6. symbiotic involvement.

Mr. T.'s involvement with his wife ranged from lack of involvement most of the time to overinvolvement when she had pain. She herself gave evidence of overinvolvement, but there was also some evidence of narcissistic involvement. An example of the latter would be when she insisted that Mr. T. dress in a certain kind of way in order for her not to feel belittled by her friends or guests. She was very invested in her appearance, in sharp contrast to Mr. T. All in all, the nature of the involvement between this couple presented a rather complex picture.

Behavior Controls

Behavior control is the pattern a family adopts for handling bahavior in three areas: (1) physically dangerous situations; (2) situations that involve the meeting and expressing of psychobiological needs and drives; (3) situations involving interpersonal socializing behavior both between family members and with people outside the family. There are four styles of behavior control: (1) rigid behavior control; (2) flexible behavior control; (3) laissez-faire behavior control; (4) chaotic behavior control. Mr. and Mrs. T. had collided on their modes of behavior control much of their lives. Mrs. T. indeed was somewhat rigid and obsessional in her ways and Mr. T. tended to be quite laissez-faire. Under those conditions, there was no meeting of the minds. They constantly accused each other of failing to understand the other.

On completion of this assessment phase, the couple were invited to consider the possibility of entering into marital therapy.

Contracting

In the process of the assessment, there appeared to be some recognition on the part of Mr. and Mrs. T. that they were confronted with major conflicts. It was explained to them that the therapy was usually of a short-term nature, required a high level of commitment from them because the success of the therapy was totally dependent on their willingness to alter the situation, and that there were certain very firm expectations. First, that they would attend the family therapy sessions on a regular basis; second, that they would follow through on tasks mutually agreed upon by the family and the therapist; third, that they would participate in the follow-up part of the program. Mr. and Mrs. T., after some deliberation, agreed to enter into treatment. Not all couples with chronic pain quite so readily see the need for family therapy, and resistance is a very common problem found in the practice of marital and family therapy with chronic pain patients.

Following a detailed discussion of their problems, a contract was agreed upon which consisted of the following short-term goals:

1. that Mrs. T. would stop "badgering" her husband about his appearance;
2. that should Mr. T. feel bothered or infantilized by her, instead of resorting to silence, he would point it out to her and urge her to back off;
3. that they would plan and take a holiday together;
4. that once a week they would go out together to a movie or dinner or both.
5. that Mr. T. should be less solicitous during the time when Mrs. T. had pain and find other more appropriate ways of giving her attention.

These tasks were agreed upon by all parties, and were designed to interdict the problems of distancing, eliminate the pain-reinforcing behavior on the part of the husband, enable them to address categorically some of the problems associated with postretirement adjustment, and disengage from very destructive patterns of communication in which they regularly engaged.

Treatment Stage

After their initial skepticism, Mr. and Mrs. T. demonstrated a remarkable level of investment in their treatment. They gave evidence of working very hard. Together they were seen on nine occasions, including the assessment phase, over a period of some ten weeks. They seemed to be able to achieve the tasks almost too easily. For example, when on one occasion, out of sheer habit, Mrs. T. asked Mr. T. to have a change of clothes, instead of shying away he retorted that he was grown up enough to know when he should change his clothes. Mrs. T., instead of becoming angry, apologized, and said that was indeed so. These very early successes in the treatment propelled them into a higher level of activity. Instead of going out once per week, they were searching for other kinds of activities they could do together. They became more solicitous of each other, and Mrs. T. reported during one treatment session that for the first time in a very long time Mr. T. had expressed his love for her. She had genuinely felt for many years that he had ceased to love her.

Mrs. T., who was initially suspicious of this therapeutic venture, reported that the frequency of her headache had subsided, and quite inexplicably, she had not even thought about her back pain. In any event, the headache ceased to interfere either with their day-to-day living or with their social activities.

Closure Stage

A final session was held to terminate treatment. At this time the couple had accomplished all the tasks and more. Arrangement was made for a follow-up visit. It was emphasized that the treatment phase had indeed ended, and the follow-up was for the purpose of a review.

Discussion

Mr. and Mrs. T.'s case was complex. The couple gave evidence of lifelong difficulties in their marriage complicated by life-stage issues and Mrs. T.'s pain problems.

The life-stage issues for this couple were indeed quite critical. Mrs. T. had raised a very large family, and her children did not leave home until a fairly late age. However, the children had provided her with much of the succor and love she needed. All her attempts to pull Mr. T. into the family orbit had basically failed. Nevertheless, the family functioned quite adequately to a point, but the system came under severe strain with Mr. T.'s retirement. He was literally forced back into the family orbit, albeit a very small family by this time. Mrs. T.'s pain served two critical functions: (1) to protest against her husband's intrusion, and (2) as a means of receiving support from her husband. At a hypothetical level it can be argued that without intervention Mrs. T.'s pain would have assumed a very central role in their relationship.

Summary

Mrs. T., who presented at the pain clinic with a complaint of heightened back and head pain, was also confronted with ongoing marital conflicts which had worsened steadily since her husband's retirement. The couple engaged in short-term, problem-centered systems family therapy. They successfully completed the treatment, which not only had some beneficial effect on their relationship but seemingly Mrs. T. experienced a reduction in her pain to the point where she was discharged from the pain clinic.

It should be acknowledged that the problem centered systems family therapy is predicated on some of the same principles as the task centered approach described earlier. They are both rooted in systems theory, and emphasize clear definition of problems, certainly demand the family member's participation in defining issues and setting practical goals, and firmly place the onus for success of treatment on the family members. Like the problem centered systems therapy, the task centered approach is also short term.

The Patient and the World at Large

A chronic pain patient is frequently reduced to the status of an invalid, and experiences an inordinate amount of powerlessness in relation to his environment in general and to the bureaucratic systems that he has to contend with in particular. Arrival of a patient at the pain clinic is the termination of a long journey. In the process he has had many contacts with medical specialties, often been given contradictory messages, sometimes even undergone unnecessary surgeries, and generally found himself on a medical treadmill. He is in conflict with the medical system. He may very well be involved in litigation. Many patients commence their pain career with work-related injury. Their experience of the legal system leaves them bewildered and exasperated. Lawyers, in order to make a prima facie case, must have medical corroboration that the current pain problem is in some direct way associated with the accident, and that information is not always forthcoming. Thus, the patient is pushed and pulled between the medical and legal systems. The trial dates are set and postponed with almost clockwork regularity.

Many patients are in the unfortunate position of not being able to work, and there are many who are engaged in what is tantamount to warfare with the W.C.B., and in some instances with their ex-employers. W.C.B.s are designed to serve the interests of the employers without any input from the workers, so it is hardly surprising that many patients view the W.C.B. with a great deal of trepidation and distrust. The source of the distrust is the perception that the function of the W.C.B. is to attempt to minimize the degree of disability as much as possible and thereby deny the patients their legitimate financial dues. Conflict between pain clinic personnel and the W.C.B. is not unknown. The pain clinic may be convinced that the present physical and psychological state of a patient can indeed be explained on the basis of the work-related injury; the W.C.B.'s own physicians are often at variance with that opinion. One serious problem is the reluctance of the W.C.B. to accept that there are serious psychological consequences of trauma which potentially are just as debilitating as any physical trauma. Many patients live in constant fear of losing W.C.B. benefits. The struggle with employers for many of these patients is also palpable. Following any kind of work-related injury, many patients feel that they could still function in a lighter job. Such jobs are not easy to come by, and at times employers are less than eager to find alternative employment for injured workers. As these patients experience financial hardship and begin to hear a chorus of demands from banks, mortage companies, and other creditors, it is hardly surprising that they are gripped by a complete sense of powerlessness and alienation.

It is not within the power of a single individual to successfully fulfill all his or her needs; hence the need for social institutions. In relation to the chronic pain patient, the failure of institutions that are specifically designed to help this individual tend to be quite striking, at least from the patient's position of disadvantage and relative powerlessness. Not all institutions fail all patients at all times. At the same time each individual patient's catalog of complaints about mishandling or mismanagement by one or other of the bureaucracies can only be ignored at the clinician's own peril. Mr. L., whose case was discussed earlier in this chapter, lived in constant fear of losing his W.C.B. benefits. In spite of many representations made on his behalf by the clinic staff including social work, the medical staff of the W.C.B. remained unimpressed that his problem was chronic and that there was no hope whatsoever that he would ever be able to return to his job of truck driving. While on the one hand the message from the clinic to this particular patient was to make a new beginning, the pressure from the W.C.B. was in exactly the opposite direction. The relationship between the W.C.B. and the patient thus became completely adversarial. The sad truth is that the patient often finds himself in a struggle with almost all institutions that are in theory designed to provide help.

Mrs. F.'s struggle with her own lawyer and the legal system was no less impressive than Mr. L.'s perceived threat of losing W.C.B. benefits. Mrs. F., a woman in her late twenties was involved in an auto crash in which she sustained a back injury. Numerous medical investigations failed to elicit any discernible pathophysiology in her back, but she did decompensate rather dramatically, and for all practical purposes became an invalid. She lost her job, retreated from all physical and social activities, and became severely depressed. Her depression failed to respond to a variety of treatment. By this time she was ingesting an extraordinary amount of narcotic analgesics and spending much of the time in bed. She was married to a rather cool and distant character who provided her with very limited emotional support. This patient was in a state of almost complete dissonance with the external world. When she was initially seen by this author, her total preoccupation was to receive compensation for the accident.

She had hired and fired some three lawyers because of their inability to pursue her case with any degree of vigor. Her current lawyer was sympathetic and attempted to resolve the matter outside the court system, an approach that failed. Dates for court hearings were established and postponed on more than three occasions. Finally a court hearing was held and the process of cross-examination totally devastated the patient. Every fact of her past was explored, and her already compromised self-esteem was subjected to intense humiliation. This one court hearing succeeded in undoing six months of the pain clinic's work with this woman. Six years after the accident, her case still remained unsettled. Social and emotional consequences of that were clearly observable in this patient. Apart from being almost totally demoralized and having lost faith in the legal system, she demonstrated a singular inability to give any thought to her future. All attempts to get her involved in any kind of educational program, many of which she initiated, were nonstarters. Discussion of this case with her lawyer revealed the central nature of the problem, namely, that in the absence of any clear physical injury, her case was predicated on mental suffering and anguish, which from his point of view was not very satisfactory. He was still sanguine about procuring some compensation for the patient and was basically holding out for a more satisfactory settlement.

It is precisely a case of this nature that places the patient in a double bind situation. If the patient begins to give any evidence of improvement and progress, the case for the "opposition" is strengthened; at the same time, inability to arrive at a satisfactory resolution of the litigation may contribute to the maintenance of the patient's invalid status. It would be easy to dismiss this patient's dilemma by invoking the concept of secondary gain. This invocation will necessarily minimize or even trivialize the actual suffering of the patient. The notion that settlement of financial matters can result in miraculous recovery of chronic pain patients is at best suspect. Sheer poverty of data in support of the proposition is striking.

While Mr. L. and Mrs. F. lived in mortal fear respectively of losing their means of livelihood and not receiving justice, Mr. W., aged forty-seven, had little doubt that his pain problem was substantially complicated and worsened by the attitude of his employer. His medical history was equally remarkable. He received a work-related injury in a fire-fighting situation. He was seen by nineteen specialists, had four surgeries, and when he arrived at the pain clinic was on twelve different drugs. This man had no history of illness before the accident and had an excellent work record. He received regular promotions and, in his own mind, he was destined to reach the top.

Following the accident the employer denied any culpability, and to make matters worse, from the patient's point of view, severed all connections with him during his period of hospitalization and surgery. Mr. W. succinctly stated that "Twenty-five years of loyal service meant nothing." As he failed to make any significant recovery and his pain condition deteriorated even further, he was advised by his superior to seek psychiatric consultation. In the meantime he was assigned to a desk job which to his mind was not only humiliating, but was designed to create enough dissatisfaction in the patient that he would terminate employment. Mr. W.'s relationship with his employer was no less adversarial than Mr. L.'s with the W.C.B.

Interventions

These three individuals exemplify a few of the struggles that many chronic pain patients encounter in dealing with the world at large. These negative experiences tend to leave them aggrieved, alienated, and frequently severely depressed. Social work involvement with these sorts of problems can be multifaceted. A common theme that binds these three patients is their sense of powerlessness in combating powerful institutions, and conceptually, empowerment of these patients has to be the unmitigating objective under these conditions. Social workers have traditionally engaged in using multiple approaches to bring about some measure of balance of power between the individual and the institution. Political action, advocacy, networking, and formation of self-help groups are some of the proven means of action. It is critical that in utilizing any strategies designed to rectify the power imbalance between the individual and the institutions, the patient has to have an understanding about power dynamics. As Pinderhughes (1973), has observed: "The treatment goal for all times may be conceptualized as empowerment—the ability and capacity to cope constructively with the forces that undermine and hinder coping, the achievement of some reasonable control over their destiny" (p. 335). He further noted that "influencing the external social system to be less destructive may require power, pressure, negotiation or working jointly with extra-familial systems to link up with the existing support system or build new ones" (p. 336). The client urgently needs to lose his or her sense of isolation. An affiliation with an existing group, or creation of a new group to address power-related conflict, is critical. An example of such a development is the Injured Workers' Union or Chronic Pain Associations in various parts of Canada. They have had some influence, albeit quite norminal, in the practice and procedures of the W.C.B.

Many pain clinics, including the one that the author is associated with, run weekly groups conducted by ex-patients in which ongoing difficulties are discussed and strategies are devised to deal with structural and legislative problems. In addition, they serve as a support group for new patients. These groups are essentially self-help in nature. While in the early stages of the formation they may require some professional input, yet in a relatively short period of time they become self-governing, and are led by men and women endowed with considerable leadership qualities. Mr. L. joined such a group and experienced an immediate sense of relief from his recognition that several members of the group were experiencing similar difficulties with the W.C.B. Over a period of time his participation with the self-help group resulted in a much more realistic attitude toward the W.C.B. He partially lost his fear of losing his eligibility for compensation. Persistent representation was made on his behalf by the pain clinic to the rehabilitation and medical personnel to ensure continuation of his benefits. When he received some assurance that his benefit would not be arbitrarily discontinued, much of his anxiety vanished.

Advocacy is a time-honored method of achieving change. Ruth Willetts (1980) defines advocacy as "the act of pleading for, defending, supporting or espousing a cause, and such acts take on a special meaning when the persons for whom one advocates appear to be incapable of interceding on their own behalf." Almost all health care professionals at one time or another intercede on behalf of their patients. Considerable knowledge is required to comprehend the complexity of a modern social welfare state and the legislation that governs rules and regulations for individual entitlement (Albert, 1983). Patients need to be made aware of their rights. This important task is complicated by the unusual type of problems that many of the pain patients encounter. Generally speaking, lawyers are designated as advocates, but they can be expensive, and frequently the nature of the problem does not call for legal advice. Not infrequently patients' difficulties can be resolved by non-lawyers by initiating discussion among all parties. Problems that can lend themselves to resolution by discussion are far too many to enumerate, but some of the patients discussed above had problems that were resolved in that manner.

The case of Mr. W. is illustrative in this respect. It was brought to his attention after several phone conversations with his superior that there was a course of appeal open to him. More importantly, if he could make a convincing case that he was capable of assuming more responsibility, he would indeed receive a sympathetic hearing. An interesting discovery during the process of discussion with employers was made by this author. Mr. W.'s employer had a very ill-defined notion of chronic pain and had convinced himself that the patient was a psychiatric case, and, in short, was malingering. Information about chronic pain modified his view of Mr. W. sufficiently that the patient was reassigned to a somewhat more responsible position. The appeal process was avoided.

The process involved in this kind of advocacy can be protracted, and the complexities cannot be underestimated. The bureaucratic wheel turns ever so slowly and Mr. W. was fortunate that his situation was at least partially resolved in six months. In the case of Mrs. B. who was hesitant to explore the possibilities of a new career in case that would jeopardize her chances of winning her case, the task of the social worker was relatively simple. Discussion of this problem with her lawyer established that it would be a positive move on the part of the patient to start a career, but was unlikely to have any negative influence on the case. She is currently enrolled in a program for fashion designers.

Discussion

It is rather curious that Mr. W. was unable to negotiate with his employer for what he considered a more deserving position and Mrs. B., who had a lot of trust in her lawyer, could not bring herself to ask an important question. Their reluctance to do so is truly related to their sense of powerlessness. They viewed their relationship with the world at large as adversarial, sometimes correctly and sometimes not. The three cases presented here were carefully selected and essentially demonstrated a certain level of success of social work intervention. On the other hand, almost every practitioner in the field of chronic pain is aware of patients who have had horror stories to tell about their experiences with various institutions. Indeed, in one province in Canada, disgruntlement with the W.C.B. reached such a pitch that much pressure was brought to bear on the government, and an independent review of the Board's practices was conducted.

At the root of conflict between the individual and the external systems is the perception that authorities and institutions have only one goal, namely, to give the patient as little assistance as possible, and in that process, subject him to further humiliation by questioning the validity of his condition. Chronic pain remains somewhat of an elusive condition for many helping professions. Lawyers demonstrate wide variability in their understanding of this problem as well. Educating the public and the professionals that the patients have to interact with has to be a priority for chronic pain experts.

In a curious way in all the three aforementioned cases, education in the way of providing information to the relevant parties resulted in the amelioration of the problems. The social worker's principal role with the W.C.B., the lawyer, and employer was to furnish and receive information which essentially removed ongoing conflicts between the feuding parties, and beyond that enabled the patients to relinquish their somewhat paranoid stance. It is quite remarkable that when patients experienced success, however minimal, and had a sense of mastery over their environment, frequently their success in one area spilled over into other areas of their lives. As an example, one patient who was in a longstanding feud with the W.C.B. not only resolved his difficulties with that organization, but went on to organize the injured workers in his city. Besides, as he gained more confidence in the external world, it began to have some salutory effect on his intrafamilial relationships. He regained his self-esteem and gave evidence of functioning as a relatively healthy individual despite his ongoing pain problem.

Regaining self-esteem for the patients through a process of empowerment by a variety of means described above, is unquestionably a critical social work activity. Unfortunately, this particular aspect of social work strategy is not as actively pursued, or not given such high preference, as working with individual or family in a conventional therapeutic mode. This is, in part, due to the fact that an activity such as advocacy, which has political overtones, may be viewed negatively by an employer, and in some instances, social workers are discouraged from engaging in such activities. On the other side of the coin, many social workers themselves give priority to "clinical" work over being an activist. This type of dischotomy is essentially fruitless, and from the patient's point of view, altogether less satisfactory. Political activism in the way of advocacy is no more than the worker pleading the client's case with a degree of objectivity and relevant information, which the client could not possibly conduct himself. For social work to be fully effective with chronic pain patients, it is imperative that the strategies described in this section be used to address the problems that inevitably arise between the individual patient and the institutions.

References

Albert, R. (1983), Social work advocacy in the regulatory process. *Soc. Casework*, 64:473–481.

Dessonville, C.L. (1985), The patterns of depressive symptomatology in geriatric normals, depressives, and chronic pain patients. *Pain* (supplementary 2) S210.

Engel, G. (1959), Psychogenic pain and the pain-prone patient. *Amer. J. Med.*, 26:809–819.

Epstein, N., & Bishop, D., Problem-central systems therapy of the family. In: *Handbook of Family 'Therapy*, eds. A. Gurman & D. Kinskern. (1980). New York: Brunner/Mazel.

———Bishop, S., & Levin, S. (1978), The McMaster model of family functioning. *J. Marr. Fam. Counsel.*, 4:19–31.

Gallagher, E., & Wrobel, S. (1982), The sick-role and chronic pain. In: *Chronic Pain: Psychosocial Factors in Rehabilitation*, eds. R. Roy & E. Tunks. Baltimore: Williams & Wilkins.

Germain, C.B. (1980), Social context of clinical social work. *Soc. Work*, 25:483–488.

Holzman, A.D. & Turk, D.C. (1986), Chronic pain: A multiple setting comparison of patients' characteristics. *J. Behav. Med.*, 8/4:411–422.

Payne, B., & Norfleet, M. (1986), Chronic pain and the family. *Pain*, 26:1–22.

Pilowsky, I. (1969). Abnormal illness behavior. *Brit. J. Med. Psychol.*, 42:347–351.

———Murrell, T., & Gordon, A. (1976), The development of a screening method of abnormal illness behavior. *J. Psychosom. Res.*, 23:203–207.

———Spence, M. (1976), Illness behavior syndromes associated with intractable pain. *Pain*, 2:61–71.

Pinderhughes, E.B. (1973), Empowerment for our clients and ourselves. *Soc. Casework*, 64:331–338.

Reid, W., & Epstein, L. eds. (1978), *The Task-Centred System*. New York: Columbia University Press. pp. 12–19.

Romano, J.M., & Turner, J. (1985), Chronic pain and depression: Does the evidence support a relationship. *Psycholog. Bull.*, 97:18–34.

Roy, R. (1981), Chronic pain and social work. *Health & Soc. Work*, 6:54–62.

———(1982). Pain-prone patient: A revisit. *Psychother. Psychosom.*, 37:202–213.

———(1984), The phenomena of "I have a headache." Functions of pain in marriage. *Internat. J. Fam. Ther.*, 6:165–176.

———(1985a), Childhood abuse and Engel's pain-prone disorder: 25 years after. *Psychother. Psychosom.*, 43:126–135.

———ed. (1985b), *Family and Chronic Pain*. New York: Human Sciences Press.

———(1985c), Family therapy and chronic pain. State of the art. In: *The Family and Chronic Pain*, ed. R. Roy. New York: Human Sciences Press.

———(1987), Family dynamics of headache sufferers. A clinical report. *J. Pain Manag. Prac.*, 1:174–179.

———(1987a), Role of social work in the management of chronic pain. In: *Handbook of Chronic Pain*, eds. G. Burrows. Amsterdam: Elsevier.

———(1987b), Impact of chronic pain on family: Systems perspective. presented at the 5th World Congress on Pain, Hamburg, W. Germany, August 5.

———Thomas, M., & Matas, M. (1984), Chronic pain and depression: A review. *Comprehen. Psychiat.*, 25:96–105.

Siporin, M. (1980), Marriage and family therapy in social work. *Soc. Casework*, 61:11–21.

Sternbach, R.A. (1974), *Pain Patients: Traits and Treatment*. New York: Academic Press.

———Murphy R., Akeson, W.F., Wolf, S. (1973), Chronic low-back pain: The "low-back loser." *Postgrad. Med.*, 53:135–138.

Willetts, R. (1980), Advocacy and the mentally ill. *Soc. Work*, 25:372–379.

25

Chronic Pain and the Geriatric Patient

LOUIS L. JAY, R.PH. AND
THOMAS W. MILLER, PH.D.

INTRODUCTION

There are several, well-documented medical concerns facing the geriatric patient in our society (Arnoff & Evans, 1982; Bowsher, 1983). Medically, there are more multiple chronic conditions and a greater incidence of iatrogenic illness among the elderly. Most significant is the presence of pain associated with the aging process. This chapter addresses the diagnosis, multiplicity of pain-related disorders associated with the elderly population, and treatment strategies to address geriatric pain, and provides the reader with a clear perspective of chronic pain in the geriatric patient.

The impact of chronic pain on the geriatric population often affects their functional capabilities in multiple ways. Patients with chronic pain frequently display marked disability pervading all aspects of their lives, and are often unable to engage in meaningful life experiences. Clinical and research findings suggest that chronic pain patients often develop a syndrome characterized by marked functional impairment, chemical dependence, emotional distress, and marital and family disruption, in addition to the subjective experience of intractable pain (Wall, 1984).

For the geriatric patient with chronic pain, the scope and complexity is such that chronic pain patients often fail to improve with pain relief interventions, and their repeated efforts to find a successful intervention lead to overutilization of health care (Kuhn, 1984). Multidisciplinary chronic pain programs using multicomponent assessment and intervention packages have emerged but with mixed results. Although there is considerable diversity among these programs in the extent to which particular goals are targeted and treatment strategies emphasized, most seek to provide improvement in level of functioning and reduction in overall impairment.

Clinical researchers working in these programs have suggested that a number of cognitive factors, including cognitive distortion and irrational beliefs, are associated with patients' level of impairment, and these have increasingly begun to be targeted as part of treatment. Attitudes, beliefs, and expectations have been implicated in patients' responses to treatment, and have received attention as potential areas for intervention and predictors of outcome (Buckoms, 1985). Notwithstanding this perspective, chronic pain is distressing to all, but it affects the geriatric population through multiple diagnoses.

Chronic pain refers to pain that persists for a period of time longer than six months. It is usually associated with, and caused by, an injury, a disease, an organic, systematic, functional, psychosocial trauma, or psychosomatic disorder, and is transmitted through the central nervous system.

Diagnosis of Pain in the Elderly

A two-axis model for quantification and classification of chronic pain was based on the Emory "Pain Estimate" Model (EPEM) (Bowsher, 1983). This system operationally defines chronic pain through the analysis of three quantifiable sets of information: medical findings, behavioral data, and the relationship between medical–behavioral correlates. These correlates exist in four different classes of chronic pain patients. Assessment of the medical findings includes the evaluation of pathological and physiological–functional assessments, which are depicted on a 0 to 10 horizontal scale, while measurements of pain behavior are graphically depicted on a 0 to 10 vertical scale, crossing the horizontal scale at midpoint. Medical scores are based on a physician's assessment of all available medical data, and behavioral scores are based on information generated by the patients through paper-and-pencil testing (Schooff, Buck, and West, 1984).

Four classes describe significantly different groups of chronic pain patients:

1. Class I patients score above 5 on the behavioral vertical scale and low on the medical scale. These patients display conditioned behavior in excess of demonstrable medical findings. These patients best fit the description of patients with "psychogenic pain disorders" described in the *Diagnostic and Statistical Manual of Mental Disorders,* (DSM-III-R) (American Psychiatric Association, 1987).
2. Class II patients score low in both sets of variables. These patients are functional despite sometimes dramatized pain complaints with ill-defined anatomical patterns. Many headache patients fall into this case of chronic pain.
3. Class III pain patients score high on both the pathological and behavioral scales. They are disabled both by documented pathological conditions and by conditioned factors similar to those in Class I patients.
4. Class IV patients score high on the medical scale and low on the behavior scale. These patients are functional despite the presence of a well-documented pathological lesion. Class IV patients might be referred to as under-reactors to pain and, in general, display effective coping skills and adjustments to their pain situation.

Class I patients display primarily learned behavior, which is characterized by the following sets of symptoms referred to as the 5-D syndrome of chronic pain: *D*ramatization of complaints; *D*isuse—the consequences of inactivity on various body systems; *D*rug misuse; *D*ependency; and *D*isability.

Class II patients show normal levels of activity during daily living. Many of the patients in Class II are incapable of physically pacing themselves. Pain complaints are often responses to periods of sustained activity without appropriate rest, resulting in discomfort and decreased activity. Simple counseling can help these patients accept their limitations while training in relaxation and proper behavioral management skills may allow adjustment in life-style.

Class III patients display learned behavior secondary to a documented pathological condition. These patients may display many of the symptoms of Class I patients. When the pathological disorder cannot be corrected and/or when the condition is stabilized, these patients may be good candidates for programs of appropriate rehabilitation.

Class IV patients demonstrate competent coping in the presence of pathological conditions. Management of their illness should be careful and restrained so as not to interfere any more than is necessary with their ability to cope. Overtreatment of Class IV patients may convert this functional person into a Class III patient through iatrogenic complications.

A five-axis classification system recommended by the International Association for the Study of Pain was recently proposed for clinical use with chronic pain patients including geriatric pain patients (Pilowsky and Bassett, 1982). The axes include: (1) region of pain; (2) system of pain; (3) temporal characteristics of pain; (4) patient's statement of intensity and time lapsed since onset of pain; and (5) etiology of pain.

Etiology and Occurrence of Geriatric Pain

1. Chronic Tension Headache

Chronic tension headaches are the most common of all headaches for the geriatric patient. They are often induced by stress, tension, emotional problems and muscular contractions—usually in the occipital muscles in the sides and back of the head. (Sternbach, 1974). They cause pain by producing muscle spasms and pressing upon pain sensitive tissues.

It has been clinically established that Type A individuals, people who are generally overly ambitious, anxious, perfectionistic, worried, resentful, angry, easily frightened and frustrated, and more rigid in their attitudes and ideas, are prime candidates for chronic headaches.

2. Migraine Headache

Migraine is a recurring vascular headache, with geriatric patients being at increased risk due to vascular degeneration. It is characterized by a marked increase of symptoms such as severe pain, photophobia (sensitivity to light), and autonomic (involuntary) disturbances during the acute phase which may last for hours or days.

This disorder occurs more frequently in women than in men and a predisposition to migraine may be inherited. Statistics indicate that it affects 5 to 10 percent of the geriatric population.

The exact mechanism responsible for the disorder is not known. The head pain is related to dilation of extracranial (surface) blood vessels, which may be the results of chemical changes that cause spasms of intracranial (from within) vessels.

Migraine may be triggered by allergic reactions, excess carbohydrates, nitrates found in many processed foods such as hot dogs, or tyramine found in alcoholic beverages such as aged wines and other fermented foods, in pickles, cheeses, yogurt, caviar, pickled herring, and cured meats. Other triggering agents are bright lights, loud noises, slow or stalled traffic, drastic changes in the weather, disruption of sleep patterns, hormonal changes or treatment such as oral contraceptives, or various drug agents including vasodialators.

An impending attack usually manifests itself by visual disturbances such as flashing lights or wavy lines, by strange taste or odor, numbness, tingling, dizziness, ringing or buzzing in the ears, or a feeling that part of the body is distorted in size or shape. The acute phase may be accompanied by vomiting, chills, excessive urination, facial edema, irritability, and extreme fatigue.

3. Cluster Headache

Cluster headache (a variant of migraine) is characterized by a sudden onset of throbbing, excruciating unilateral pain. The pain is of short duration and subsides abruptly, but may recur several times daily and attacks occur most frequently during sleep. It is associated with symptoms of dilated carotid arteries (in the neck), fluid accumulation under the eyes, tearing or lacrimation, nasal congestion, and runny nose. The sharp pain involves the orbital area, frequently radiating to the temple, nose, upper jaw, and neck.

Geriatric patients with cluster headaches are afflicted by one of the most excruciatingly painful conditions.

4. Rheumatoid Arthritis

Rheumatoid arthritis is one of a group of arthritic disease states whose definitive cause is unknown but prominent in geriatric patients with arthritic conditions. It is an incurable (but manageable) chronic, progressive, degenerative disease that is associated with pain and swelling, and leads to deformity and crippling of the patient's joints, typically the small hand joints, feet, wrists, elbows, and ankles. Although any joint can be affected, it generally starts in the fingers. Rheumatoid arthritis usually begins with inflammation of the synovial membrane lining of the joint space. Chronic progression of this condition produces bone and cartilage calcification which compromises joint stability and causes dislocation to occur—which in turn produces joint deformities. There are several predisposing and contributing factors in the development of rheumatoid arthritis. One major factor may be interference with a person's autoimmune system, which adds to the aggravation and severity of the existing pain, inflammation, and deformities of the disease.

5. Osteoarthritis

Osteoarthritis, or degenerative joint disease (DJD), affects nearly 7 percent of the population and generally results from wear and tear in the mechanical parts of a joint. This disease commonly affects weight-bearing joints such as the hips, knees, and ankles, but also the hands. Osteoarthritis appears to be related to overuse and abuse of the joints, to certain types of occupational stress, possibly to injuries, to heredity, and to being overweight.

6. Osteoporosis

Osteoporosis generally affects one in four women over age sixty. This disease commonly causes fractures in the wrist, spine, and hips. Decreased levels of the female hormone estrogen and of the mineral calcium may play a role in causing bones to weaken and fracture. Exercise also appears to affect bone strength. Researchers recommend that women increase calcium in their diets and exercise regularly. Estrogen may be given to some women after menopause.

7. Low Back Pain

Most low back pain is related to degenerative joint disease of the lower part of the backbone between the hipbones and the ribs (lumbosacral area). It results from shear-strain in the lumbosacral junction caused by man's upright position.

Various studies and statistical data indicates that back pain afflicts about 80 percent of the U.S. population, at one time or another, during a lifetime. However, for individuals in whom pain originates in the lower back or lumbar region, the incidence increases with age. It usually becomes a significant problem in the third decade of life and reaches its highest peak in and after the sixth decade in industrial societies.

8. Angina Pectoris

Several types of angina pectoris have been identified from their clinical characteristics:

a. Stable angina is often referred to as classic or effort-induced angina. In this type of angina, discomfort is precipitated by physical activity or emotional stress, and is usually relieved by rest. Each episode of symptoms lasts about three to five minutes and is characterized by chest pain or discomfort, with radiation to the neck, jaw, back, shoulders, or arms. Nausea, sweating, palpitations, or shortness of breath may be present. It results from an increase in myocardial oxygen demand beyond that which can pass through narrowed coronary arteries.

b. Unstable angina describes chest pain occurring with increased intensity and frequency associated with decreasing levels of work and a decrease in responsiveness to treatment. Unstable angina may signal the forerunner of acute myocardial infarction and requires urgent diagnosis and treatment. The mechanism contributing to unstable angina is an increased myocardial oxygen demand in the presence of severe coronary artery constriction, clotting, or spasm.

c. Variant angina, or Prinzmetal's angina, is characterized by recurrent chest pain at rest and an electrocardiogram showing ST-segment elevation during pain. The pain associated with variant angina differs from that of stable angina in that it may be of longer duration, usually not precipitated by exertion, and it may occur only at certain times of the day. Decreased blood flow in this type of angina results from coronary artery spasm.

9. Dental Related Pain

Some of the most painful dental problems are caused by a toothache, an abscess of the tooth or gums, extraction, TMJ (temporamandibular joint) disorders, trigeminal neuralgia, and oral cancer among others. Periapical abscess is characterized as an acute or chronic suppurative process of the periapical region. It is secondary to an infection of the dental pulp usually due to decay. However, it may occur after trauma to the teeth or from periapical localization of organisms surrounding the root of the tooth.

10. TMJ Dysfunction

This problem is also known as myofacial pain dysfunction (MPD) syndrome. This abnormal condition is characterized by facial pain and mandibular (jaw) dysfunction, apparently caused by a defective or dislocated temporomandibular (temple/jaw) joint. Some common indications of this syndrome are the clicking of the joint when the jaws move, limitation of jaw movement, subluxation (a partial dislocation), and temporomandibular dislocation. The aging process may increase the risk of geriatric patients experiencing temporomandibular jaw dysfunction.

11. Trigeminal Neuralgia

This neuralgic condition is characterized by sudden bursts of excruciating pain of short duration radiating along the course of the fifth cranial nerve. The attack is often precipitated by touching a trigger point or by activity such as chewing or brushing the teeth. It is characterized by recurrent sudden attacks of sharp, stabbing pains in the distribution of one or more branches of the nerve. It generally occurs in people over forty, and the incidence is higher in the female geriatric population. Although each episode is brief, lasting one to two minutes, successive longer episodes may incapacitate the individual. The frequency of attacks varies from many times daily to several times a month or year.

12. Oral Cancer

Chronic irritation of the oral cavity often seen in geriatric patients such as that caused by chewing and/or smoking tobacco, by sharp jagged teeth, projecting fillings, or badly fitting dentures often may lead to the development of oral cancer, especially in the geriatric population. Excessive drinking of alcohol with or without tobacco use also appears to play a role in the development of oral cancer. Certain noncancerous mouth conditions that tend to become malignant include leukoplakia (precancerous condition) of the mouth, some tumors, and a tissue-wasting disease called Plummer-Vinson syndrome.

Treatment Strategies in Geriatric Pain

Medical/Surgical

In the treatment of all pain, whether acute or chronic, appropriate surgical and medical procedures should be applied only if the source of pain is known to be organic and such treatment is likely to improve it. Selected patients with ongoing nociceptive input may require nerve blockage or neurosurgical measures. In most chronic pain conditions which started with organic damage, there is considerable psychological overlay, and if the original pain-producing organic condition is stable and nonprogressive, a rehabilitation approach to restore coping skills and manage life with a minimum of discomfort may be attempted first with a good chance of successful outcome. When traditional medical intervention is necessary due to a life- or function-threatening condition, such intervention should be matched with structured pain rehabilitation (Roy and Tunks, 1982; Brena, 1984; Brena, Crue, and Stieg, 1984).

Pharmacological Management of Chronic Pain

Analgesia medications can be considered the first line of approach in all pain treatment. Aspirin, acetaminophen, ibuprofen, and other nonsteroidal anti-inflammatories can serve as a basis for most pain relief programs. When these fail to offer adequate relief, use of narcotic analgesia can be considered, but these are generally recommended only in acute cases in which rapid recovery is expected or when the condition is felt to be terminal.

When a narcotic analgesic is to be used over a long period of time, choice of medication should be made with extreme care. Propoxyphene napsylate has been successfully used as an opioid substitute and has both agonistic and antagonistic properties. Codeine is commonly utilized for extended periods. When a maintenance does of analgesic is used, the potential for abuse and tolerance must be considered. It is necessary to obtain informed consent from the patient, and use of medication must be closely supervised. A regular physical exam should be performed to minimize the possibility that physical problems have been hidden by the use of medication. Narcotics may thus

TABLE 25.1

CATEGORIZED ANALGESTIC MEDICATIONS PRESCRIBED FOR PAIN MANAGEMENT

Drug Agent	Usual Adult Daily Dose (mg)	Administration Route	Frequency PRN
Simple Analgesics			
Aspirin (ASA)*	325–650	P.O., Rectal	q 4h
Acetaminophen	325–650	P.O., Rectal	q 4h
Ibuprofen	200–600	P.O	q.i.d.
Sodium Salicylate	325–650	P.O., Rectal	q 4–8h
Non-narcotic			
Butorphanol (Stadol)	0.5–2; 1–4	I.V.; I.M.	q 4h
Nalbuphine HCl (Nubain)	10	S.C., I.M., I.V.	q 4h
Narcotic Analgesics			
Codeine Sulfate	15–60	P.O.	q 4h
Codeine Phosphate	15–60	P.O., S.C., I.M.	q 4h
Dolophine HCl (Methadone)	5–10	P.O., I.M., I.V.	t.i.d.
Hydromorphone HCl (Dilaudid)	2–4	P.O., S.C., I.M., I.V., Rectal	q 4–6h
Meperidine HCl (Demerol)	50–150	P.O., S.C., I.M., I.V.	q 3–4h
Morphine Sulfate**	5–15; 30–60	S.C., I.M., I.V., P.O.	q 4h
Oxycodone HCl (Percodan)	4–5	P.O., Rectal	q 6h
Pentazocine HCl (Talwin)	50–100; 30	P.O., I.M., I.V., S.C.	q 3–4h
Propoxyphene HCl (Darvon)	65	P.O.	q 4h
Propoxyphene Napsylate (Darvon-N)	65	P.O.	q 4h

*Larger dosage as appropriate to patient's condition. Some of the above agents are also available in other brand names.
**Clinical American and European studies indicate that controlled-release morphine given twice daily can manage moderate to severe pain in 90% of patients and that there are few side effects with this regime.

be used temporarily in conditions with ongoing nociceptive input, but they definitely are contraindicated and sedative hypnotics are vigorously discouraged in chronic nonmalignant pain patients, where such peripheral input is no longer thought to exist. Table 25.1 summarizes analgesics frequently prescribed for chronic pain management with geriatric patients, and Table 25.2 provides nonsteroidal medications prescribed in treating geriatric patients.

TABLE 25.2

CATEGORIZED NONSTEROIDAL GERIATRIC MEDICATIONS PRESCRIBED FOR PAIN MANAGEMENT

Drug Agent	Usual Adult Dose (mg P.O.)	Frequency	Maximum Adult Daily Dose
NonSteroidal			
Choline Magnesium Salicylate (Trilisate)	500–750	b.i.d. or t.i.d	2000–3000
Diflunisal (Dolobid)	500	q 12h	1000–1500
Fenoprofen (Nalfon)	200	q 4–6h	3200
Ibuprofen (Motrin)	400	q 4–6h	2400
Indomethacin (Indocin)	25	b.i.d. or t.i.d.	200
Meclofenamate (Meclomen)	200–400	Daily	400
Mefenamic Acid (Ponstel)	500, then 250	q 4h	1000
Naproxin (Naprosyn)	250	b.i.d.	750
Naproxin, Sodium (Anaprox)	500, then 275	q 6–8h	1375
Phenylbutazone (Butazolidin)	100	t.i.d. or q.i.d.	400–600
Piroxicam (Feldine)	20	Once Daily	20
Sulindac	150	b.i.d.	400

Some of the above agents are also available in other brand names.

NONPHARMACOLOGICAL APPROACHES TO GERIATRIC CHRONIC PAIN

Psychological factors and attitudes affect the pain experience in a very complex way. It is therefore not surprising that psychotherapy, both on an individual and a group basis, plays a large role in the treatment of chronic pain. Its value has been recognized for some time. Psychotherapeutic approaches allow patients to assess the role of pain in their lives, develop alternative coping mechanisms, deal with secondary gain, grieve for the loss of pain as a coping mechanism and life style, and learn ways of accepting a degree of disability without heavy reliance on medication.

Behavioral psychology (Grezsiak, 1982) uses operant learning as an explanation of the process of chronic pain development. Operant pain is pain expression shaped by reinforcement. Prolonged respondent pain can lead to operant pain. This may come about because of the effect of pain on its observer and the observer's altered behavior to accommodate the pain. These accommodations can be rewarding to the pain sufferer and increase the possibility of pain behavior. When pain behavior receives direct positive reinforcement it is likely to persist. Alerting contingencies so that health behavior is rewarded while pain behavior is not, is likely to have favorable results. Cognitive approaches (Cameron, 1982) train patients in strategies to enhance self-control. They include relaxation, imagery, cognitive relabeling, and reinterpretation of pain related to experiences, day-to-day problem-solving, assertiveness training and systematic desensitization. One cognitive treatment rationale is that disturbing moods and behaviors associated with the pain result from certain thought processes. Many cognitive approaches are designed to substitute rational coping skills and self-statements for catastrophic thoughts. Others reduce the psychological reaction to pain by training the patient to mentally create and focus on pleasant physical sensations.

Chronic headaches of vascular and tension types have

responded to cognitive treatment approaches, and cognitive approaches can be effective in treating groups as well as individuals (Melzack, 1980). Cognitive approaches can be applied to the sensory–discriminatory, affective–motivational, and cognitive–evaluative components of treatment approaches based on Melzack and Wall's Gate-Control Theory. The sensory–discriminatory aspect can be modified by training a patient to alter sensory input through relaxation and biofeedback. The cognitive–evaluation component and affective–motivational components can be modified by strategies designed to counteract thoughts of helplessness and reinforce thoughts of self-control. Behavioral techniques, including biofeedback, autogenic training, and deep muscle relaxation may be very beneficial. Biofeedback has been shown to be effective in controlling pain of tension headache and is also considered very useful in other pain syndromes by increasing relaxation. Biofeedback used in conjunction with hypnosis has been reported beneficial in 58 percent of the cases (Fields, 1981). It has been suggested that hypnosis operates through a mechanism of central nervous system analgesia not reversible with nalaxone.

Transcutaneous electrical nerve stimulation (TENS) operates by selective stimulation of large diameter, myelinated axons. It can provide dramatic relief, especially when used postoperatively and in cases of chronic pain associated with peripheral nerve damage. It is most effective when stimulation is applied proximal to the site of injury. Dorsal column stimulation with implanted electrophysiological devices is also effective in pain associated with nerve damage, but effectiveness has been noted to diminish in many patients with chronic pain. Infection, CSF leakage, and pain and cord trauma at the site of implantation have limited the clinical usefulness of dorsal column-stimulating devices.

The clinical use of cognitive behavioral approaches in treating conditions associated with the geriatric population has gained considerable recognition (Applebaum, Blanchard, Hickling, and Alfonso, 1988; Poppen, Hanson and Sav-Mei, 1988). Cognitive strategies, biofeedback, and behavioral medicine interventions have favorable applicability to the geriatric population (Carstensen, 1988). Various physiological processes are influenced by biofeedback procedures, including chronic pain, anxiety, general tension, and insomnia, which are often addressed through electroencephalographic behavioral medicine strategies. Cognitive-behavioral and behavioral medicine approaches to stroke rehabilitation and individuals who have partial impairment in physical or mental functioning have also gained considerable attention in the field of behavioral gerontology (Carstensen, 1988).

FAMILY THERAPY

Family members of geriatric patients should be involved in the treatment process when possible since they are providers of support, and may also have to adjust the family system to reaccept a more functional individual into it. Sometimes when it seems that a particularly strong need for homeostasis of the family system keeps the patient locked into the sick role, formal family therapy is necessary. It has been noted (Mohamed, Weisz, and Waring, 1978) that there seems to be a peculiar way of handling fantasy, affect, and cognition in families of chronic pain patients, most visibly affecting the "significant other." In such families, it may be impossible for patients to regain a higher functional status without encouraging major changes in family functioning.

Rolland's (1987) model of a chronic illness identifies critical phases of chronicity that influence the choice of intervention provided at any given time. These phases include crisis, chronicity, and terminal stages. Transition periods may occur between stages when families must reevaluate their functioning in view of a new change in the illness. Successful transition depends on the manner in which the family has completed the tasks of the previous phase.

The crisis phase of Rolland's model is that period when the patient and family are attempting to cope with the initial diagnosis and the accompanying symptoms. For the chronic pain patient, the crisis phase may be that moment when the label "chronic pain" is applied for the first time. After a prolonged period of discomfort, the patient may be told that the condition appears to be chronic. At this time, former hopes for a quick and simple solution to the problem may be erased.

The importance of including family members or significant others in treating chronic pain in geriatric patients is recognized as significantly important. This can often present problems for the geriatric person who may not live in close proximity to children or who may be confined to a nursing home. Models of conjunct treatment involving significant others with similar diagnoses have gained considerable attention and support and have been recognized for inclusion in the treatment process (Romano, Syrjala, Levy, 1988; Brockopp and Brockopp, 1988). There is consistent evidence in the literature that the family's interaction with the chronic pain patient significantly influences the context of the processing and adapting to the chronic pain condition. Family members or significant others can play a significant role in rewarding or inhibiting the geriatric pain patient's management of their chronic pain condition in conjunction with pharmacotherapy, individual cognitive models, and specific behavioral techniques. The chronic pain patient with the support of significant others including family members can move toward adaptation and the fullest of functioning within the parameters of the chronic pain patient.

The terminal phase is characterized by concerns related to separation, death, loss, and grief. For the chronic pain patient, the terminal phase applies to those individuals whose pain is related to the diagnosis of a life-threatening illness.

Rolland's model provides a framework against which the information gathered in relation to the family's development life cycle can be plotted. Judgments regarding the intensity of the difficulties facing both patient and family can usually be made on the basis of the objective data obtained and the clinical profile presented.

Family-related interventions, (Flor, Turk, Rudy, 1987) include intensive family therapy for those families in which serious pathology is found and a series of sessions for those families whose problems are related to the patient's condition. For those families whose suffering in relation to the patient's condition has depleted their energies, support can be offered.

Problem-solving skills can be taught to families who have difficulty modifying their former roles or behaviors in order to meet obligations and self-expectations. A comprehensive assessment of the family and patient should provide direction for the treatment team as to the kind of involvement that is most appropriate.

SUMMARY

The relationship that we have come to know between aging and chronic pain is indeed a complex one. The oldest and most general theory of aging compares the human body to a machine. Although the simplicity of this theory has appeal, a growing knowledge and understanding of the complexities of the human body warrant a more comprehensive theory. Aging and chronic pain need not be synonymous. While it is inevitable that an individual's physical functioning will gradually weaken with age, it is not inevitable that the individual will develop one or more of the summarized conditions of chronic pain. Chronic pain associated with the following conditions is more likely to appear in geriatric patients: osteoarthritis and rheumatoid arthritis, osteoporosis and the spectrum of degenerative bone, and joint and muscle disorders that accompany the aging process. A new era of creative scientific investigation in the fields of biomedicine, pharmacology, and the neurosciences holds great promise in understanding new mediums for the management, control, and, one may hope, the eventual alleviation of pain. More promising mediums to address the control of chronic pain, both pharmacological and nonpharmacological, await our geriatric patients who seek relief from this component of aging.

REFERENCES

American Psychiatric Association (1987), *Diagnostic and Statistical Manual of Mental Disorders,* DSM-III-R. Washington, DC: American Psychiatric Press.

Applebaum, K. A., Blanchard, E. B., Hickling, E. J., & Alfonso, M. (1988), Behavioral treatment of a veteran population with moderate to to severe rheumatoid arthritis. *Behav. Therapy,* 19/2:489–502.

Aronoff, G. M., & Evans, W. O. (1982), Evaluation and treatment of chronic pain at the Boston Pain Center. *J. Clin. Psychiat.,* 43(Sec.2):4–7.

Bowsher, D. (1983), Pain mechanisms in man. *Resident & Staff Physician,* 29:26–34.

Brena, S. F. (1984), Chronic pain states: A model for classification. *Psychiatric Ann.,* 14:778–782

———Crue, B. L., & Stieg, R. L. (1984), Comments on the classification of chronic pain: Its clinical significance. *Bull. Clin. Neurosci.,* 49:67–81.

Brockopp, G., & Brockopp, D. (1988), Family Issues in Treating the Chronic Pain Patient. Department of Psychiatry, University of Kentucky. Unpublished paper.

Buckoms, A. J. (1985), Recent developments in the classification of pain. *Psychosomat.,* 26:637–645.

Cameron, R. (1982), Behavior and cognitive therapies. In: *Chronic Pain: Psychosocial Factors in Rehabilitation,* eds. R. Roy & E. Tunks. Baltimore: Williams & Wilkins, pp. 79–103.

Carstensen, L. L. (1988), The emerging field of behavioral gerontology. *Behav. Therapy,* 19:259–281.

Fields, H. L. (1981), Pain II: New approaches to management. *Ann. Neurol.,* 9:101–127.

Flor, H., Turk, D., & Rudy, T. (1987), Pain and families. 11. Assessment and treatment. *Pain,* 30:20–45.

Grezsiak, R. C. (1982), Cognitive and behavioral approaches to management of chronic pain. *NY State J. Med.,* 82:30–38.

Kuhn, W. (1984), Chronic pain. *S. Med. J.,* 77:1103–1106.

Melzack, R. (1980), Psychologic aspects of pain. In: *Pain,* ed. J. Bonica. New York: Raven Press, pp. 143–154.

Mohamed, S. N., Weisz, G. M., & Waring, E. M. (1978), The relationship of chronic pain to depression, marital adjustment, and family dynamics. *Pain,* 5:285–292.

Pilowsky, I., & Bassett, D. (1982), Individual dynamic psychotherapy for chronic pain. In: *Chronic Pain: Psychosocial Factors in Rehabilitation,* eds. R. Roy & E. Tunks. Baltimore: Williams & Wilkins, pp. 107–125.

Poppen, R., Hanson, H. B., & Sav-Mei, V. I. (1988), Generalization of EMG biofeedback training. *Biofeedback & Self Regulation,* 13/3:235–244.

Rolland, J. (1987), Chronic illness and the life cycle: A conceptual framework. *Fam. Proc.,* 26:203–221.

Romano, J. M., Syrjala, K. L. & Levy, L. (1988), Overt pain behaviors: Relationship of patient functioning and treatment outcome. *Behav. Therapy,* 19/1:191–202.

Roy, R., & Tunks, E., eds. (1982), *Chronic Pain: Psychosocial Factors in Rehabilitation.* Baltimore: Williams & Wilkins.

Schooff, D. L., Buck, J., & West, W. (1984), Diagnostic issues in chronic pain. *J. Amer. Geriat. Soc.,* 32:489–494.

Sternbach, R. (1974), *Pain Patients: Traits and Treatment.* New York: Academic Press.

Wall, P. D. (1984), Introduction. In: *Textbook of Pain,* eds. P. D. Wall & R. Melzack. New York: Churchill Livingstone, pp. 1–16, 1985.

26

Concluding Thoughts on Chronic Pain

THOMAS W. MILLER, PH.D.

The attention of many clinicians and researchers is turning toward new directions in the diagnosis and treatment of chronic pain. These new directions, I trust, were obvious throughout the chapters in this volume, which have focused on theory, measurement, diagnosis, and treatment of chronic pain. Efforts to cover a diversity of topics and populations have also clearly been the focus of this compendium of clinical practice and research. An effort to focus on a cross-sectional perspective that takes into consideration the chronic pain patient, the family, the health care professional, and the social system within which these individuals function has highlighted the goals and objectives of this two-volume work.

The purpose of this final chapter is to bring into focus some of the major issues and trends in our growing understanding of the diagnosis and treatment of chronic pain in this decade:

1. While chronic pain is an intriguing phenomenon defying easy explanations and resisting generally accepted modes of treatment, we continue to be at an early stage in our understanding of both the mechanisms of the transmission of pain and the management and alleviation of pain.

2. The pathways and centers involved in pain transmission, evaluation, and modulation are not established with certainty, just as the chemical interactions involved in the pain process are not yet completely understood.
3. The medical community has, in the past two decades, begun to turn to professionals in clinical psychology, neuropsychology, nursing, social work, and rehabilitation counseling to address both the diagnostic and therapeutic aspects of chronic pain patients.
4. The use of a multidisciplinary team approach to consultation, diagnosis, and treatment of chronic pain conditions appears to be the most viable and beneficial medium in the management and alleviation of chronic pain.

The cost of treating either acute or chronic pain is approximately $90 billion annually in the United States. Of the 50 million accidental injuries that occur in the United States, nearly one-third are associated with acute moderate to severe pain. Annually, about 400,000 accidental injuries lead to partial or permanent disability. Approximately 65 million individuals in the United States suffer from chronic pain, and of these, 50 million are partially or totally disabled. In most patients with back disorders, arthritis, headaches, cancer, and other chronic painful conditions, it is not primarily the underlying pathology but the pain that prevents the patient from carrying out a productive life. On the basis of these data it appear that well over 700 million work days are lost from chronic pain, which, together with health care costs, total nearly $60 billion annually.

Pain may be described in terms of the individual's phenomenological subjective experience ("pain experience" or "pain perception") or in terms of the total organismic response—including but not limited to subjective awareness ("pain response"). A potentially more precise construct, "pain sensation," refers to the objective sensory detection of painful stimuli. This construct, however, is highly refractory to measurement and is probably inappropriate given current notions of pain as a psychophysiological construct. The more suitable term, *nociception*, refers to the body's neurophysical response to tissue damage. Pain may also be operationalized as the individual's verbal or nonverbal acknowledgment of pain experience along with his or her description of its intensity, quality, and temporal characteristics ("pain report"). Alternatively, pain may be operationalized as the entire repertoire of observable behaviors occurring in association with presumably painful stimuli, including but not limited to pain report ("pain expression").

More recently, physiologists have explained the condition of pain as being influenced by a function of sensory input that varies both as to the quality and the intensity of the sensory stimulus. Dallenbach and Melzack suggest that the amount of pain experienced is directly related to the amount of tissue damage incurred. In the sensory model of pain, the impact of tissue damage is transmitted from the damaged nerve endings or pain receptors through the peripheral A-delta and C-nerve fibers to the anterolateral spinothalmic tract, which ultimately conducts the nerve impulse to the thalamus and other higher brain centers and results in the sensory experience of pain.

A constellation of difficulties tends to develop in the chronic pain patient over time. Excessive physical disabilities related to disturbances in sleep and appetite are common and are often exacerbated by excessive medication. The ongoing struggle with pain frequently results in depression, somatic preoccupation, hypochondriasis, obsessive concerns with the possibility of fatal illness, and a tendency to formulate most life events and problems in the context of pain. Feelings of hopelessness, helplessness, and despair are common. Multiple visits to various physicians and clinics are common. With each new treatment, the patient experiences a resurgence of hope, which is followed by disappointment and eventually increasing resentment and bitterness toward the treating physician. Pain becomes a central focus and dominates life. External attachments and interests tend to be lost, resulting in withdrawal from family members and from customary social activities. Overuse of medication is a common complicating factor in that intoxication produced by high dosages of analgesics produces new elaboration of the problem in terms of addiction and toxicity.

Beyond patient and clinician, chronic pain affects others, especially family and other social systems. An energetic, productive individual may become a social and economic liability. Family and workmates have to make up for the loss of working capacity, which tends to weaken support for the pained individual and leads to anger toward him or her. Pain can become the central issue in a patient's life. It may begin to function as a major coping mechanism, allowing the patient to avoid stressful issues because of his pain condition. This leads to further incapacitation, which aggravates the problem, and a morbid fascination on the part of patients with their own decline.

Multidisciplinary pain clinics have emerged nationally. They offer individuals suffering from a variety of pain problems voluntary participation in research programs designed to improve the diagnosis, assessment, measurement, and treatment of all forms of acute and chronic pain. The knowledge generated by these clinical pain specialists benefits pain patients everywhere, as the results of their research studies are made available to all health professionals worldwide.

Increasingly, the medical community has begun to turn to professionals in psychology, nursing, social work, and rehabilitation counseling to address both the diagnostic and therapeutic aspects of chronic pain patients. The multidisciplinary team approach includes consultation, participating in team management, and collaboration in research studies involving chronic pain. There is considerable evidence to suggest that such an approach is most beneficial to the patient and to the medical professionals who have begun to realize that a systems approach to the treatment of chronic pain might well be the most effective method of treatment. It has been the purpose of this section to provide an overview of both the disciplines and concepts beneficial to the diagnosis and treatment of chronic pain. It has been well recognized that chronic pain patients often adopt a dependent and restricted life style characterized by overreliance on family members, bed rest, and habit-forming pain medications. A multidisciplinary model of diagnosis and treatment allows an alternative whose time has come in the treatment of chronic pain.

This two-volume series on chronic pain has attempted to bring together some of the most well-respected authors, clinicians, and researchers in the area of chronic pain to address from a multidisciplinary perspective this new and burgeoning area of clinical practice and research. As a measure of growth in our understanding of chronic pain, we realize the frequency with which concepts progress from being uncommon to being universally adopted. It is our intention that this compendium of information addressing the condition we have come to know as chronic pain be more than just another textbook, but rather, an organizer and heuristic medium that addresses the most relevant of concepts, principles, goals, and objectives in a growing body of information that will increase clinical sensitivity, develop new research directions, and enhance and enrich our present state of knowledge in treating the chronic pain patient.

Name Index

Subject Index